Never Bet Against Occam:
Mast Cell Activation Disease and the
Modern Epidemics of
Chronic Illness and Medical Complexity

Lawrence B. Afrin, M.D.

© 2016

Library of Congress Cataloging-in-Publication Data

Afrin, M.D., Lawrence, 2016-
     Never Bet Against Occam: Mast Cell Activation Disease and the Modern Epidemics of Chronic Illness and Medical Complexity / Lawrence B. Afrin, M.D. — 1st ed.
     p.cm.
Include bibliographical references and indexes

ISBN: 978-0-9973196-1-3 (Softcover)
ISBN: 978-0-9973196-0-6 (Hardcover)
ISBN: 978-0-9973196-3-7 (Digital)

Library of Congress Catalogue Number (LCCN): 2016934971

The author has worked to ensure that all information in this book is accurate as of the time of publication and consistent with standards of good practice in the general management community. As research and practice advance, however, standards may change. It is recommended that readers evaluate the applicability of any recommendations in light of particular situations and changing standards.

The web addresses referenced in this text were current as of February 2016, unless otherwise noted.

Managing Editor: Kendra Neilsen Myles; **Copyeditor:** Carol Schaengold; **Graphic Designer:** Kristi Posival; **Original Cover Designer and Artist (commissioned emblem painting on cover):** Kristi Posival (www.kristiposival.com); **Printer (Paperback):** Create Space; **Printer (Hardcover):** Ingram Spark

Printed in the United States of America.

Sisters Media books are available at special discounts for bulk purchase. Special editions or book excerpts can also be created to specification. For details, contact the Sisters Media, LLC.

Sisters Media, LLC
7717 Maryknoll Ct.
Bethesda, MD. 20817
240-687-7791
E-mail: info@sistersmedia.com
www.sistersmedia.com

For more information, please contact:
Mast Cell Research
Website: www.mastcellresearch.com
E-mail: info@mastcellresearch.com

Follow us!
Facebook: https://www.facebook.com/masttcellresarch/
Twitter: @MastCellHelp

Table of Contents

Foreword

They say, "Write what you know." Thus, the one book I likely will ever write.

I have no doubt there are many health care providers and scientists who will regard this book as premature, that there's not enough known scientifically yet about mast cell activation disease to warrant a book for the popular press like this.

I feel they're both right and wrong.

Let me be the first to acknowledge that what we have yet to learn about this subject dwarfs what we have learned already, and some might say we should know more before a book like this is written.

At the same time, I feel the time is ripe for a book like this because, in my opinion, the knowledge we already have is sufficient to help legions more than are presently being helped, if only this knowledge, heretofore confined largely to an obscure corner of medical academia, were spread more widely.

Label me however you wish. Whatever you suspect my motives to be, let me just state here for the record, simply and unequivocally, that, to the best of my awareness, all I ever wanted to do was help my patients (and would-be patients). That's all.

Let me also make clear that I hold all of my colleagues in the highest regard. At present, the challenges in diagnosing this disease are extraordinary (as I'll discuss), and no health care provider for years to come should be denigrated for not recognizing it or even not believing it exists. I truly believe the vast majority of my colleagues honestly do make the best effort they can at the time for every patient they see, but providing medical care in the early 21st century, in the U.S. or elsewhere, is an incredibly difficult job. As they say, "Walk a mile in my shoes…" I think it will be a long time yet before the public can reasonably expect the majority of the medical profession to know this disease, but as the reader will come to see, this reality is not anyone's fault.

I also apologize in advance to you, dear reader, for my long sentences and frequent parenthetic comments. Hard to change a writing style I've used for decades.

Finally, let me advise that I will be referring hereafter to health care providers as doctors and nurses. I recognize there are many other types of providers whose understanding of this disease will benefit many patients, but nobody yet has come up with a less cold-blooded term than "providers" or "clinicians," or a smaller mouthful than "practitioners," so I beg your understanding that my use of "doctors" and "nurses" is simply for the sake of simplicity and warmth and does not imply any thoughts of exclusivity. Also, of course, I have changed the personal information of the patients described herein as needed to protect their identities, but the rest of their cases are faithful descriptions of their presentations and the paths they are taking.

Acknowledgements

First and most important, I could not have learned what is reflected in this book without the unswerving support of my wife, Jill, and mother, Lois. More than once, when the easier path was to head in a different direction, their support helped me stay the course. And I certainly would be remiss in not also thanking my father, Michael. Though he passed long before my career took this new path, I firmly believe my ability to stand my ground in pursuing this path was because I had watched him, too, so consistently stand grounds he knew to be right, no matter the (sometimes great) personal cost. I also appreciate the mature-beyond-their-years manner in which both of my children, Jessica and Michael, have dealt with the challenges my pursuit of this work has brought my family.

I also want to thank my colleagues — especially my longstanding mentor, Dr. Robert Stuart, and another stalwart supporter, Dr. Neal Christiansen – who were willing to accept new realities when data and results defied expectations. I'd also like to thank my earliest mentor, Dr. Ron Schiff, my first supervising attending physician upon my starting the clinical training years in medical school. More than once in that first month on the hematology/oncology inpatient service in my junior year, I watched in awe as Dr. Schiff refused to give up on desperately ill patients, blending his almost obsessively thorough reviews of patients' cases with scourings of old and new medical literature and his own "out-of-the-box" creativity to devise innovative approaches that, more often than not, made the key difference for his patients' well-being and even their very survival. That's the type of doctor I wanted to become, and it is my hope that if Dr. Schiff sees this, he will know that at least one of his students took his lessons to heart.

I would like to thank, too, the eminent Dr. Gerhard Molderings not only for reaching out to this inexperienced pup immediately after I published my first case report in this area and subsequently spending uncountable amounts of his inestimably valuable time dialoguing with me and serving as a sounding board as I (painfully slowly, I'm sure) further developed my understanding of this area, but also for dedicating so much of his career to pursuits in this lonely area of biomedical science. The insights he has provided me and many other workers in this area are already resonating in the improved lives of thousands of patients, a number I am sure will continue exponentially growing.

Though I was terribly remiss in only coming to thank Dr. Horst Ibelgaufts six years after I first stumbled across his on-line cytokine encyclopedia which, in an instant, helped me gain crucial understanding how "one disease" could present so multisystemically and diversely, I would like to try to amend that oversight here and urge those who find my work helpful to also find a way to support Dr. Ibelgaufts (http://www.copewithcytokines.org), who for so many years (and continuing to this day) has toiled in obscure isolation on his labor of love which I am sure must have greatly benefited many researchers besides me who unfortunately have not yet chosen to express their support.

And I would be utterly remiss again if I did not thank here the many who assisted me in ultimately finding the best place at which to "blossom" in my pursuit of this work, including all those colleagues noted above plus Drs. Theoharis Theoharides, Dan Masys, Robert Means, Kalpna Gupta, and Dan Weisdorf – all gentlemen (and a lady!) and all true scholars and scientists open to new ideas.

Finally, I would like to thank the hundreds of patients with mast cell disease who allowed me the privilege of working with them these past few years to understand and try to improve their illness, for without their trust, there would not be this book and my prior screeds which I hope are beginning to bring understanding and hope to many others.

Preface: About the Cover

The charm shown on the cover and in more detail below was commissioned by a New Zealand patient as a gift for me soon after she was able to work with her local doctor and establish (with a little bit of help from me) a diagnosis of mast cell activation syndrome, in turn leading to some simple therapy which quickly helped her feel substantially better after six decades of mysterious unwellness. In the patient's own words:

This New Zealand jade pendant was designed and carved by Maori master carver and artist, Mr. Lewis Tamihana Gardiner. Mr. Gardiner is regarded as one of the most respected and innovative Maori jade artists of his generation. He is both a teacher and an artist, creating art that combines traditional practices with contemporary application. His work is born from deep within Maori tradition, but with an expression that is 21st century.

I commissioned the pendant to symbolise the inter-relationship, and timeless nature, of personal "connection" – Gratitude, Generosity, Knowledge and Aroha [in this sense, to mean empathy and compassion] – within a world that each of us is as close to, or distant from, one another as we choose to imagine.

New Zealand jade has a symbolism of its own – the source remains a mystery. The found deposits are, therefore, in themselves "gifts." New Zealand jade is therefore given to another person with the deepest sense of "gift."

The overall design is based on a rounded mast cell – with an outer membrane and cytoplasm and the inner nucleus. The cytoplasm has symbolic granules sandblasted into the surface.

One of the granules is sandblasted into a star shape. This represents an undiagnosed patient's call for help – her "wish upon a star" – that a physician on the other side of the world would read her emailed message and understand. The star symbol also represents the gratitude the patient felt when she received an understanding and compassionate, "one in a million star" response.

The inner nucleus is filled with the design of the Koropepe. Within the Maori world, the Koropepe represents the Foundation of Life – the cell.

Mr. Gardiner chose New Zealand kawakawa [flower] jade for its mottled appearance to enhance the overall design.

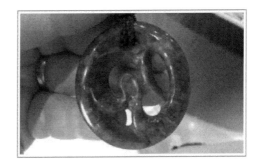

The pendant is shown here with Mr. Gardiner's permission.

Chapter 1: My First Case of MCAS: A Journey of a Thousand Miles

…as they say, begins with the first step, and so I will start this book by presenting you the first step – actually, a months-long effort – I took on my journey toward being able to recognize and understand mast cell activation syndrome (MCAS). This is the story of "Shelly," my first patient (or, as we say in this business, my "index patient") in whom I came to recognize this newly-recognized-but-not-truly-new disease which didn't even have a clear name at the time but now is called MCAS.

The First Visit

She was tired. When I walked into the exam room on the first day I met "Patient #1" in March 2008, her marked fatigue was obvious, almost palpable. She had other problems, too. Plenty of them. But "tired" was her "chief complaint," to use that implicitly whiny professional term. She had walked in to the clinic, and the exam room, under her own power, with no assistive devices, but hers was not the kind of tiredness one gets from exertion. And it certainly wasn't the kind of tiredness one gets from insufficient sleep. No, this was the kind of tiredness that the word "malaise" was meant for. A total lack of energy, and for no apparent reason. At merely 58 years old, her life had been ruined by this draining fatigue. Previously a high-energy, athletic, intelligent, highly productive, successful independent small businesswoman, she had been reduced over several years by this progressive fatigue to a shell of her former self. She couldn't even traverse the one flight of steps in her home, much less continue the daily jogs she had enjoyed for decades. Utterly exhausted, she eventually had to shutter her business. And the treatment she was getting for the one disease with which she had been definitively diagnosed only seemed to be making her worse.

As "Shelly" first explained her story to me, she had been fine until just a few years earlier. (As I would learn in the months ahead with her, this was a self-deceit I later came to see in many others, too, who had long been suffering the disease we eventually diagnosed.) She had been totally healthy, she assured me. Went running almost every day, tended to her small business, had a good life. But then, roughly a decade earlier, she had begun noticing the fatigue. Quite minimal at first. Business was good, so it had to be due to working too hard, right? For the first few years she managed to keep deluding herself, simply suffering the fatigue, but as time went on, the fatigue slowly but inexorably worsened, until it became obvious that her daily activities were not the cause. The fatigue waxed and waned from one day to the next, often from one hour to the next, but even at her best at that point, the fatigue was debilitating. She wasn't enjoying her jogs any longer, and the tiredness was beginning to affect her ability to keep up with her business. Something clearly was wrong, but the cause was just as clearly escaping her awareness.

Doctor visits previously had never been particularly significant affairs for her. Routine check-ups with the internist and gynecologist, for the most part. Menopause had come and gone fairly uneventfully years earlier, so there was no reason to suspect the fatigue was a hormonal issue. It was time to put her internist to the first true test he had ever had with her.

Her internist understandably wasn't impressed. At that time (2005), she was still (somehow) keeping up with all of her "activities of daily living," and though she said she was fatigued, she certainly didn't look it. Her physical examination, too, was equally unremarkable. Really, to all but those who knew her the best, she *looked* fine (other than perhaps a bit of fatigue to her usually stoic countenance), with no hints of anemia, thyroid disease, or cancer. But she certainly wasn't a chronic complainer, so this fatigue was real and was going to require a laboratory evaluation.

The internist got lucky. Routine blood tests indeed revealed what appeared to be the answer – but it certainly wasn't an answer he had been expecting. Although anemia (a low concentration of hemoglobin, the protein in red blood cells that carts oxygen from lungs to tissues and carbon dioxide from tissues to lungs) wouldn't have been any surprise at all in a fatigued patient, her hemoglobin was elevated, about 54%. Normal for a woman is roughly 36-42%. So she was "polycythemic," to be sure, but it wasn't to a life-threatening degree. Hospitalization wasn't required, but further evaluation by a hematologist was definitely in order to pin this down as the case of "polycythemia vera" it surely had to be.

"P. vera" is a type of blood cell cancer, specifically one of the "chronic myeloproliferative neoplasms," or MPNs, that's rooted in a bone marrow stem cell gone genetically awry. Like the acute leukemias, in which stem cell mutations lead rapidly to life-threatening overgrowth (and underneath) of blood cells, the MPNs also are rooted in stem cell mutations eventually leading to a life-threatening accumulation of blood cells. The natural history of an acute leukemia, though, is that the time from initial detection of the disease to death from the disease is usually weeks to a few months, whereas with the MPNs, the natural history from initial detection to death due to disease is usually several years, if ever. There are several types of MPNs. The most common one is chronic myeloid leukemia (CML) in which overproduction of white blood cells is the dominant feature. In essential thrombocytosis (ET), overproduction of platelets is the dominant feature. And in p.

vera (PV), overproduction of red blood cells, with an accompanying increase in hemoglobin concentration, is the dominant feature. Fatigue is a common symptom of cancer, including blood cell cancers such as acute leukemias and MPNs, thought to be a consequence of not only the diversion of energy to excess cancer cell production but also the inappropriate generation (by both cancer cells and normal cells) of many fatigue-causing chemical signals such as tumor necrosis factor (TNF).

Doctors learn early in training the more common of the relatively few causes of elevated hemoglobin levels. What we're taught is pretty simple: the marrow is genetically programmed to make red blood cells when it has the necessary raw materials and is exposed to the hormone erythropoietin ("epo") that's made by the kidneys. Given the right amount of epo, the marrow makes the right amount of red blood cells. Too little epo, too few red blood cells. Deficiency of epo is thought to be the principal reason why kidney failure patients are anemic.

Put more epo into the system, though, and one gets more red blood cells, which in naturally low-oxygen situations is a good thing. The kidneys sense the amount of oxygen in the blood, and when the oxygen content in the blood is low, the kidneys respond by producing and releasing more epo, thus triggering the marrow to make more red blood cells to ensure that sufficient oxygen still gets picked up in the lungs for circulation to the tissues. High-altitude living, heavy smoking, and obesity-related obstructive sleep apnea are the most common causes of low oxygen in the blood leading to increased kidney production of epo and increased red blood cell and hemoglobin production in the marrow. Less common causes of low oxygen in the blood include carbon monoxide poisoning and rare mutated forms of hemoglobin that simply cannot pick up as much oxygen from the lungs as normal hemoglobin does.

But Shelly was a decidedly non-obese coastal resident who had never smoked, nor was she regularly exposed to smoke. Her home was a modern one in a temperate climate, so there was no kerosene heater that might cause chronic carbon monoxide poisoning. And mutated hemoglobin is a problem present since conception, so it'll be diagnosed in childhood or young adulthood, not at age 58. So why did she have increases in red blood cells and hemoglobin?

Although she initially insisted she had been fine until the fatigue had come on about a decade earlier, a more detailed history quickly yielded more clues. She mentioned suffering sudden bouts of itching, for no apparent reason, all about different parts of her body, for many years. She had had a short period of a slow heart rate about 30 years earlier, but no cause was determined and it soon resolved on its own.

She said that a decade ago she had begun noticing a decreased tolerance for motion in vehicles, especially ships and planes. Five years later she had begun falling during her daily jogs, a problem that worsened as time went on. Two years after the falls began, she started suffering fatigue and dizziness and newly had to hold onto the bannister to safely traverse a staircase. The fatigue led her to her internist, who found the polycythemia and referred her to a local hematologist.

Her hematologist noted the polycythemia and immediately wondered whether polycythemia vera was present. Her hemoglobin in November 2004 had been mildly elevated at 15.5 g/dl on a routine check. When she had gone to her internist with fatigue in September 2005, her hemoglobin was minimally higher at 15.9. The rest of her routine blood counts (the so-called "complete blood count," or CBC) were normal. The hematologist ordered a red cell mass study (that's not a misspelling; it's "mass," not "mast"), a common test at the time for verifying whether the hemoglobin concentration was increased due to more red blood cells in the blood (polycythemia vera) or due to decreased fluid (plasma) in the blood (dehydration). The test, performed in October 2005 in the nuclear medicine department of an academic medical center two hours away, curiously showed only minor increases, about 10% above the upper limits of normal, in both the red cell mass and the plasma volume.

The hemoglobin wasn't nearly high enough to account for her symptoms, and the red cell mass study results weren't as expected in PV (which should cause significantly elevated red cell mass and normal plasma volume). Diagnosing PV by the international diagnostic criteria for PV at the time would have required additional tests, too, but nevertheless the hematologist was satisfied from the mild abnormalities found thus far that this was PV, and he ordered the standard treatment at the time for newly diagnosed PV in someone of Shelly's age: therapeutic phlebotomy, or a series of sessions draining the excess blood out of her through an IV.

Each molecule of the hemoglobin protein contains an iron atom, and when a person loses enough blood (no matter how), he becomes deficient in iron. Since iron is needed to make hemoglobin, and hemoglobin is needed to make red blood cells, the goal of therapeutic phlebotomy in PV is to make the patient sufficiently deficient in iron so that the marrow is necessarily throttled in its otherwise unregulated, mutationally driven production of excessive hemoglobin and red blood cells. And therapeutic phlebotomy indeed soon achieved the goal of making Shelly iron-deficient. Her hemoglobin, too, dropped to around 11 (a reasonable goal for a woman of her age with PV).

The problem, however, was that she didn't feel any better. The phlebotomies just weren't helping her in any discernible fashion. In fact, her fatigue, malaise, and dizziness were only worsening, and in October 2007 she began noticing shortness of breath and a much faster heart rate and higher blood pressure than her usually excellent runner's vital signs. In November 2007 she was feeling sick enough that she abandoned her longstanding exercise routine of running 5 days a week (typically 3-4 miles at a time) plus working on an elliptical trainer 20-40 minutes daily and going through an upper body workout 3 times a week.

She was referred to a cardiologist in December 2007 for further evaluation of these new problems, and even though PV wouldn't typically be expected to cause these problems as long as the blood counts are controlled, he wrote in his report that he felt her PV was indeed the cause of her new symptoms. Later that month, in view of both her worsening symptoms and the fact that the hemoglobin had edged back up to around 13, the hematologist increased the amount of blood being withdrawn at each phlebotomy session, briefly dropping her hemoglobin as far as 8, a degree of anemia that actually did make her feel even worse. Phlebotomy was adjusted and her hemoglobin improved back to around 10 by January. She also had become weak enough that she could no longer traverse the stairs in her home. She engaged some friends that December to help her move her office from the second floor of her home to the first floor.

The minor improvement upon recovering her hemoglobin to 10 was short-lived. January 2008 was a rough month for Shelly. New problems acutely hit her including nearly constant severe nausea and shaking chills. She had no appetite. She ached all over and was diagnosed with the flu (though no testing to prove such was done), and then when she began coughing up sputum, she was diagnosed with bronchitis, too. She was prescribed a course of a commonly used antibiotic, levofloxacin, but she quickly developed a rash from it and discontinued it. Because of her nausea, her hematologist ordered a CT scan of her body (with IV contrast so that the best quality pictures could be obtained), but the scan revealed nothing abnormal and only seemed to cause her extreme nausea and severe diarrhea during the following 24 hours.

Along the course of her phlebotomies, since they weren't helping her to feel any better, she had occasionally asked for a referral for a second opinion, but her hematologist had repeatedly expressed confidence in the diagnosis based on the original testing and declined to provide a referral. Finally, though, with her health seemingly doing nothing but continuing to decline, she decided to obtain a second opinion on her own. Through a network of friends, she determined she wanted a second opinion at the academic medical center where her red cell mass study had been done, and she wound up with an appointment to see me in late March 2008.

The worsening in December-January had begun to settle back to the prior baseline as February rolled on, but then in mid-March the shaking chills began again and this time were newly accompanied by soaking sweats every night.

Those were all the facts of her history when I first met her as scheduled. Other than appearing tired and appropriately concerned about her condition, her examination was unremarkable. Sometimes in PV the spleen or liver is enlarged, but there was no sign of this in Shelly. Her hemoglobin was 10.3, and she was as iron-deficient as one would expect given her phlebotomy treatments. Also, her platelet count was moderately elevated at 722,000, a common consequence of iron deficiency but also a potential feature of PV and the other MPNs. Her epo level was mildly elevated, an appropriate response by her kidneys to her mild phlebotomy-induced anemia.

I was puzzled. Yes, she had presented in 2005 with an elevated hemoglobin and a mildly elevated red cell mass, but PV – especially phlebotomy-controlled PV – just doesn't behave the way her illness was behaving. Nowhere close.

So, there were two possibilities. Either she had a (pretty odd) form of PV and coincidentally had one or more other mysterious diseases causing her assorted symptoms, or she didn't have PV and instead had one (or more?) other mysterious diseases causing her assorted symptoms and the initially elevated hemoglobin and red cell mass.

I wondered to myself, which scenario was more likely? One disease? Two diseases? Three diseases? More? And if her increased hemoglobin and red cell mass were not due to PV, what else could cause such findings? Something had to be driving her bone marrow to do this, and in such cases the culprit is usually excess epo, but there was no way to tell whether that was the case because she had not had an epo level checked when she first presented in 2005. One thing for sure, though, her prior athleticism told me she hadn't been low on oxygen in 2005, and so her kidneys had no reason to make more epo at that time. (She also had a normal oxygen level in the blood when she first saw me.) So if she had had an excess epo level in 2005, it had to be coming, in an unregulated fashion, from some source other than the cells in the kidney which normally make epo in a fashion that's very tightly regulated by the amount of oxygen in the blood. What might that source be?

She had never been competitively athletic in any meaningful fashion, so she certainly hadn't been surreptitiously doping herself with pharmaceutical epo. There are a variety of low-grade cancer-like diseases that occasionally show up with an odd ability to make epo and cause polycythemia. Among such diseases, the more common sources of unregulated epo are kidney and liver tumors, but even though Shelly had two relatives who had had kidney cancer, the CT scan done in January 2008 showed no sign of tumors of the kidney or liver, or any other tumors, for that matter. It was possible the scan might have missed a tiny kidney or liver tumor, but it was unlikely that such a tumor producing elevated hemoglobin in 2005 wouldn't have grown enough to be visible on a scan in 2008.

So if this wasn't a kidney or liver tumor, what other low-grade cancer-like diseases needed to be considered? There were several, but not a lot: diseases like fibroids (proliferation of connective tissue cells), hemangiomas (proliferation of cells from blood vessel linings), pheochromocytomas (proliferation of certain adrenal gland-related cells), and mastocytosis (proliferation of the body's mast cells, sentinels that help guard against and respond to infection, among many other functions). Mastocytosis, though pretty rare, was an interesting notion, as it's capable of causing all of the symptoms she had reported, plus it's a pretty slow-growing tumor in most people who have it, so it could have caused all of her symptoms over all of the years she had had them. The big problem with that diagnosis, though, was that the classic presentation of mastocytosis is unprovoked episodes of flushing and anaphylaxis (i.e., a life-threatening allergic-type reaction), and she hadn't had any of that. Yes, she had reacted badly to the contrast dye given IV during the CT scan in January, but many people react to contrast dye with various forms of gastrointestinal upset and flushing, and among such a contrast-intolerant population there are going to be those who react more and those who react less.

What to do next? The first thing to be done, clearly, was to prove this was not PV (or, at least, not the usual type of PV). In 2005 a remarkable discovery had been made: 98% of all patients with PV have a particular genetic mutation (virtually always acquired at some point in life rather than inherited) called JAK2-V617F. Testing for this mutation became available in 2006, but Shelly's hematologist hadn't run this test yet.

It was definitely time for a JAK2 mutation analysis, and that was going to take a couple of weeks to get a result. I also thought it worthwhile checking initial screening blood and urine tests for a pheochromocytoma because of her new problems with her pulse and blood pressure, even though it would have been an odd pheochromocytoma since ordinarily that disease causes far higher blood pressures than Shelly was having, and pheochromocytoma certainly doesn't cause the low blood pressure that Shelly had reported also occasionally having. Finally, I wanted to do a basic check on the total levels of the IgA, IgG, and IgM classes of antibodies in Shelly's blood, to see if there was an antibody-related problem with her immune system that was contributing to her recent infections and her general malaise. Unfortunately, there was nothing else I could do for her in the meantime, nothing I could prescribe, because I didn't have a diagnosis yet. There wasn't even any infection I know of that caused illness like hers, so there wasn't any infection testing or consultation that I could see might make a difference. However, because it was clear (from her hemoglobin of 10 and her iron deficiency) that she wouldn't need more phlebotomy treatment for some time, I told her I thought it would be OK to hold off on any more such treatments while we set about figuring out what was really going on.

The Second Visit

Shelly next saw me in the third week of April. For the most part, her rafter of symptoms was unchanged. However, she noted yet another new problem had popped up in the interim, namely, on random nights she was feeling very "revved up" and "wired" and just could not go to sleep. She actually looked a little better compared to the first visit, and the physical exam was otherwise just as unremarkable as it had been in March.

The initial test results were both helpful and unhelpful. The JAK2 mutation analysis was negative; she absolutely did not have the JAK2-V617F mutation or any of the few other mutations occasionally detectable in PV with presently available routine testing, making it highly unlikely that she had PV. So, then, what did she have? The IgM and IgA antibody levels were normal, and the IgG antibody level was low to only an insignificant degree. The hemoglobin was stable around 10, and the rest of the blood counts remained normal. The urine screening tests for pheochromocytoma were normal, but the blood screening tests were puzzling. The more sensitive blood tests (metanephrines) were completely normal, but the less sensitive tests (the catecholamines dopamine, epinephrine, and norepinephrine) definitely contained some abnormalities. The norepinephrine level was 805 pg/ml (picograms of norepinephrine per milliliter of blood, normal 80-520), and the dopamine level was 31 pg/ml (normal 0-20). The epinephrine level wasn't abnormal, but it was close: 27 pg/ml (normal 10-200). The comment provided by the lab on interpreting these results was interesting: "Small increases in catecholamines (less than 2 times the upper reference limit) usually are the result of physiological (i.e., normal) stimuli, drugs, or improper specimen collection. Significant elevation of one or more catecholamines (2 or more times the upper reference limit) is associated with an increased probability of a neuroendocrine tumor [such as a pheochromocytoma]. Measurement of plasma or urine fractionated metanephrines provides better diagnostic sensitivity than measurement of catecholamines."

As I said, helpful – "you don't have what you thought you had" – and unhelpful – "I still don't know what you have." Why were the norepinephrine and dopamine levels elevated? There were no obvious physiological stimuli at the time of the specimen collection, and she was on no drugs that should have boosted these levels. If anything, the beta blocker begun by the cardiology consultant in December 2007 would have been expected to lower the catecholamine levels. Hmmm. Perhaps the catecholamine levels would have been higher if she hadn't been on the beta blocker. Possibly an improper specimen collection? True, she was seated rather than lying down ("supine," as we say in the profession) when she had the blood drawn, but it would be somewhat unusual to see a norepinephrine level 50% above the upper limit of normal just from that.

Nevertheless, with at least some semi-significant abnormalities found in the catecholamines, it was time to repeat this testing more rigorously. I asked her to stop her beta blocker (which hadn't seemed to have been much help to any of her symptoms anyway) and return in a week for repeat blood and urine testing plus an "old-style" test, the clonidine suppression test, that we used to do to look for a pheochromocytoma before more modern blood and urine tests for this condition became available. In the clonidine suppression test, we draw a blood sample for catecholamines, then administer a single dose of a drug called clonidine, which should suppress catecholamine production, and then three hours later we draw another blood sample for catecholamines. If the elevated baseline catecholamines are being produced in an unregulated fashion (i.e., by a pheochromocytoma), clonidine should not be able to suppress those levels into the normal range, but if the catecholamines indeed are suppressed by the drug into the normal range, then there is some other, regulated process which is responding to some stimulus to produce those elevated catecholamines.

I also felt it worthwhile to order a special type of scan – "MIBG" – in the nuclear medicine department. MIBG scans look for pheochromocytomas. They're expensive, but a lot of money had already been spent since 2005 in treating her, to little avail, and the fact was that her life had been ruined by whatever she had. If we could figure out for sure what she had, we might be able to treat it and regain for her at least some of the pleasure of life and productivity she had formerly enjoyed.

Given my wonderings about a pheochromocytoma (which, when present, is almost always located deep in the belly), plus her gastrointestinal troubles (nausea, diarrhea), I felt it also worthwhile to take a more standard imaging of her abdomen and pelvis. Of course, she had had a CT scan in January, but CT scanning has long had a reputation for failing to pick up small abnormalities in the abdomen. While more expensive than CT, MRI scans are thought to be at least somewhat better able to pick up small abnormalities, so I ordered an MRI of the abdomen and pelvis, too. Again, this was not the time for being a tightwad with the testing. This disease, whatever it was, had ruined her life.

I naively noted in her chart at the time, "As I told her today, I'm fairly optimistic we'll figure this out in fairly short order, as there just aren't that many possibilities in the differential diagnosis for secondary polycythemia [polycythemia not due to PV], and even fewer possible explanations for secondary polycythemia which also explain her other symptoms."

The Third and Fourth Visits

Shelly returned in mid-May solely to submit her second 24-hour urine collection, and then she returned again three days later to undergo the clonidine suppression test. I wasn't able to see her at that visit, but I later learned the test was done with her seated rather than the proper supine position, an unfortunate event but not surprising given that, as I said, it's an old test and the clinic staff were no longer familiar with it.

The Fifth Visit

Shelly returned next a week after the clonidine suppression test to review the results. She told me that the chronic fatigue was getting worse and that the very morning of the visit, while out for a walk before driving to our center, she had suddenly become lightheaded and fell, fortunately not sustaining any significant injury. But she found her blood pressure, upon returning to her house, to be not low but rather quite unusually high for her, at 160/98. Within an hour, shortly before starting the drive to our center, it had fallen to 122/72. She still felt a little bit lightheaded at the visit, but she declined my offer of hospitalization or alternative transportation and felt she could make it back home safely.

She also offered the additional tidbit that in 2006 she had begun noticing that every time she tried to lie out in the sun, the soles of her feet quickly became intensely tingly, itchy, and mottled in their appearance. Another sunbathing-related problem, too, had been present since long before 2006: acute development of a patchy red rash at various points about her abdomen. The rash didn't happen with every sunbathing, just some of the time – though it seemed to be happening more frequently as time went on. She said it was most definitely a different rash than a sunburn. These problems with the feet and with the abdominal rash came on only with sunbathing. Curious. More clues, but what did they mean?

She also provided more family history: it turned out there were three, not two, fairly close relatives who had had kidney tumors, and another fairly close relative had had a tumor of some type of the adrenal gland – the same organ where pheochromocytomas are thought to arise.

Her physical exam that day was notable only for the obvious worsening of her fatigue.

The results were in on all of the tests from the prior week. The 24-hour urine showed the catecholamines, metanephrines, and two other related metabolites with even longer names – allow me to just abbreviate them as VMA and HVA – to all be normal. The blood catecholamines obtained prior to the dosing with clonidine showed a similar pattern as before, but even more impressive in magnitude, at least with respect to norepinephrine, which now was measured at 1,271 pg/ml – 50% higher than what we had found previously and definitely more than twice the upper limit of normal. This was certainly a piece of evidence (if the lab's comment was to be believed) in favor of the notion that a neuroendocrine tumor was present, most likely a pheochromocytoma in this case, even though – again – the overall presentation here really wasn't all that consistent with how a pheochromocytoma ordinarily behaves.

In addition to the higher baseline norepinephrine, the dopamine was still elevated (30) around the same level we had seen previously, and the epinephrine, at 16, was even a bit lower than the "low-normal" level we had seen previously. So the overall pattern we had seen initially was certainly still holding up, but what did it mean?

As for the repeat blood catecholamines determined from the sample taken three hours after the clonidine dosing, they were all normal. Dopamine was "< 20," epinephrine was unchanged at 18, and norepinephrine, at 492, had been snuffed back to just under the upper limit of normal.

Egad. Things were even more confusing now. On the one hand, the normalization of the norepinephrine level after the clonidine dosing argued strongly against a pheochromocytoma. Also, the radiologist reported that the MIBG and MRI scans were completely normal. Not a hint of a pheochromocytoma – or any other abnormality, for that matter. It still remained possible that she had an extremely unusually behaving pheochromocytoma, but the odds of such – poor to begin with – were rapidly becoming ever more remote.

What, then, was causing the baseline norepinephrine level of nearly 1,300? Could it be some other type of neuroendocrine tumor than a pheochromocytoma? Highly doubtful, as all other such tumors that I knew of were expected to have clinical presentations considerably different than what Shelly's illness had presented for our consideration. Thinking ahead about this possibility, I had also checked another special blood test, a chromogranin A level, when she had come for the clonidine suppression test. Chromogranin A is expected to be elevated in a variety of neuroendocrine tumors, but the level in Shelly turned out to be totally normal.

Meanwhile, her hemoglobin on the fifth visit was still about the same as it had been (10.8, slowly but steadily edging up in the absence of therapeutic phlebotomy, as usually happens in PV – which she didn't have).

Things were really getting puzzling. This really was not coming together as a single disease. Was she in fact diagnosable? Or would she wind up with just a long list of "idiopathic" problems – polycythemia of unknown cause, fatigue of unknown cause, nausea of unknown cause, attacks of lightheadedness and high blood pressure of unknown cause?

As I said, the situation was getting more confusing, and I was getting less confident of figuring it out quickly, but I refused to believe it couldn't be figured out. I have always believed that, except for the very occasional new infectious disease, there are no "new" diseases. There are enough patients and physicians and medical journals in the world that every way the human body can go awry has been seen and has been reported in the medical literature. The cause of a described illness may not be understood, but fundamentally all illnesses have been described, and it is one of our tasks in modern medicine to learn the true causes of, and treatments for, all of the described illnesses.

And it still was far more likely that all of her many idiopathic problems, past and present, were due to a single root cause. It was severely stretching the bounds of credulity to imagine that Shelly was so special a person, so uniquely unlucky, as to have acquired, around the same time, multiple mysterious ailments all completely independent of one another.

No, this had to be one and only one problem, and it had to be a problem that had already been described in the literature. There may not be a name for it yet, there may not be any understanding yet of its cause or prognosis, and there may not be any treatment for it, but it had to have been described in the literature.

All in all, the only things I could take away from this visit were that she almost certainly didn't have a pheochromocytoma. Meanwhile, the new history of the rash was curious, and I thought about another set of rare disorders, the porphyrias. There are several forms of porphyria, but they all are rooted in defects in the enzymes needed at various steps in the process of manufacturing hemoglobin. Some forms of porphyria cause rash; some can cause elevations in red blood cells. Some cause unprovoked acute attacks of abdominal pain and/or acute neurologic abnormalities such as seizures or, perhaps, the odd feelings in her feet when sunbathing. Sun exposure sometimes is a trigger of porphyric attacks.

Sometimes diagnosing porphyria is as simple as identifying a particular color change in the urine under fluorescent light. I checked that, but I didn't see even the slightest hint of a color change. I decided to send off more sensitive blood and urine testing for the porphyrias and asked her to return in a few weeks to review the results. I really didn't have much suspicion of porphyria – there were too many odd aspects to her presentation that didn't fit any of the porphyrias – and with the ordering of the porphyria screening I really was more buying time for additional thinking than tracking down a good lead.

The Sixth Visit

It was mid-June now, nearly three months since she had first come to me for help. I'd proven she didn't have the PV she had been thought to have for the last three years, but otherwise I hadn't made much progress. I had long felt myself to be "the dumping ground" for mysterious cases in my division, and most such cases I had managed to figure out (or so I thought; to be further discussed later in this book). Shelly was really beginning to task me, though, and I was disheartened at the prospect of not being able to help this previously highly active and productive woman.

Shelly told me about a curious development since the fifth visit. She reminded me she had been experiencing, at unpredictable intervals over the last several months, episodes of rapid fluctuations in her blood pressure. With absolutely no provocation that she could identify, her systolic blood pressure would suddenly soar to 180 and then plummet to 104 in less than a half-hour.

Curiously, this problem seemed to intensify in the two weeks following the fifth visit – and then, suddenly, in the few days before the sixth visit, she started feeling better. Much better. At the sixth visit, in fact, she said she felt "well" and "normal" for the first time in longer than she could remember. She really had no complaints at that time.

However, she also recalled more rash-related history. She noted that around 2000 she had begun experiencing, at unpredictable intervals, sudden outbreaks of a somewhat punctate red rash ("like I've been exposed to poison ivy," she said), principally on her arms and trunk. Sometimes it seemed to be related to sun exposure (though different from the patchy smooth rash she had noted at the fifth visit), but sometimes not. This "poison ivy" rash had always puzzled her because she had never actually been exposed to poison ivy.

More curious family history emerged at this time, too. She noted that her sister had recently relocated to a new city a considerable distance from where she had used to live, and she had begun noticing sun-exposure-related "blotchy" red rashes, similar to what Shelly had described about herself at the prior visit.

The physical exam at the sixth visit again showed nothing remarkable except for my general impression that she did indeed appear the healthiest and most energetic I had yet seen.

The results from the porphyria tests were all normal. The hemoglobin continued its slow rise, now 11.0.

I now began wondering more about an odd form of mastocytosis. I took some time in the exam room, using the computer there, to review some medical journal articles about the types of rash seen in mastocytosis. I found an article about a type of rash in some cases of mastocytosis that I had never heard of before, telangiectasia macularis eruptiva perstans (TMEP). The article included color photographs of sample TMEP rashes. I asked Shelly to come around to the computer and look at what I had found. She immediately said that the rashes in the pictures in the article looked just like the sun-related patchy red rashes she had been seeing erupt at various points about her abdomen for many years. But, on exam, there wasn't any of it on her now.

Even though she still hadn't had any of the flushing or anaphylaxis I had been trained to expect to see in mastocytosis, it was time to start doing some testing for mastocytosis. Off to the lab she went for blood testing and urine testing for the two "mastocytosis markers" my training had told me to check when suspecting this disease: tryptase in the blood and N-methylhistamine in the urine. I also referred her to our dermatology department so that her story could be reviewed and so that her skin could be biopsied to look for the increased numbers of mast cells that would define mastocytosis.

Reading is Fundamental

While Shelly waited for her appointment with the dermatologist, her case continued to bother me. If this was mastocytosis, it was an awfully strange form of the disease. One of the key techniques I had learned early in my career for figuring out and managing strange cases was to "hit the literature" (i.e., search the available medical literature, which used to involve physically going to the medical library but now fortunately could be done much more thoroughly and efficiently on-line). I had learned by this point in my career that there was virtually nothing new under the sun in the range of diseases known to medicine. If there was a form of mastocytosis that could behave the way Shelly's disease was behaving, then it was highly likely it was already described in the medical literature. I just had to find it.

As recent decades have rolled on, the medical literature has swelled like a tsunami approaching the shore. Finding reports of unusual cases has become harder due to exponentially growing haystacks amidst which to hide the needles, but also somewhat easier thanks to modern software tools.

Textbooks are the time-honored ultimate authority in medicine. I read chapters on mastocytosis in hematology, oncology, and endocrinology textbooks, and I quickly learned the disease was far more a multi-headed Hydra than I had ever been taught, let alone what I had ever previously seen. Every system in the body could be – but didn't necessarily have to be – affected. And most of the symptoms were utterly non-specific, that is, could easily be caused by a host of other ailments. A presentation with unprovoked anaphylaxis, flushing, and rapid fluctuations of blood pressure was classic for mastocytosis. In most cases, the proliferation of mast cells seemed to be limited to the skin, and there were a couple of fairly classic rash patterns (urticaria pigmentosa [UP] and TMEP) that one might see in those cases, but otherwise mastocytosis was difficult to suspect from its highly variable presentations in the skin. The rare "systemic" form of mastocytosis, though – spread throughout the body in multiple (and potentially all) tissues, but most commonly the bone marrow – often presented few easily visible clues. Again, without the anaphylaxis, flushing, and blood pressure fluctuations, each of the symptoms could easily be potentially attributed to many other diseases, making it very difficult to put together "the big picture" and think about this rare disease (literally roughly one to three cases per million people in the population) as the unifying cause for a bewildering array of presenting symptoms and findings.

Shelly certainly had rapid fluctuations of blood pressure, but it wasn't really clear whether she had flushing – she had never described her symptoms to me in a way that I interpreted as "flushing" – and she certainly hadn't ever suffered any anaphylactic episodes, whether to known or unknown triggers, that she knew of. So if she had mastocytosis, it still wasn't looking like a "textbook-classic" case.

Textbooks, though, start becoming obsolete the moment they're released, and medical journals obviously are the premier reference source for the latest developments in any field. So after my textbook reading, I went on to read the most recent reviews I could find in assorted journals – and dawn began breaking in the form of three recently published articles. Just the year before, a group led by pre-eminent European mast cell researcher Peter Valent (based at the University of Vienna) described a small group of patients who had symptoms of abnormal mast cell activation and were investigated for mastocytosis. Although a small population of abnormal mast cells was found in the marrow in each of these patients, these populations weren't nearly large enough to qualify the patients as having systemic mastocytosis. The authors "tentatively" labeled this new diagnostic entity, "monoclonal mast cell activation syndrome" (MMCAS).

This paper was followed less than a year later by another report of a similar discovery by a team led by the pre-eminent mast cell researchers Cem Akin at Harvard and Dean Metcalfe at the U.S. National Institutes of Health (NIH), who often collaborate with Dr. Valent. Their report, too, described a small group of patients suffering anaphylaxis of unknown cause ("idiopathic anaphylaxis") whose marrows were found to harbor only small populations of abnormal mast cells which did not qualify them for being diagnosed with systemic mastocytosis.

Oddly, though, the particular mast cell abnormalities found in the patients described in these two reports were largely the same as those found in patients with systemic mastocytosis, thus raising a new question: if the patients in these two reports and patients with systemic mastocytosis had largely the same abnormalities, then what else was different between the two groups that produced far more mast cells than normal in those with systemic mastocytosis but only a few (if any) more mast cells than normal in those with MMCAS and idiopathic anaphylaxis?

The likely answer appeared in yet another paper that was published, around the same time (spring 2007) as the Harvard/NIH report, by a team led by pharmacologist and geneticist Gerhard Molderings at the University of Bonn. Dr. Molderings and his team had examined 17 patients with a form of systemic mast cell activation disorder in which GI symptoms were pronounced, but the testing they did on their patients was different in an important way from the testing done by the other two teams. This different testing focused on genetic mutations in the abnormal mast cells. For almost a decade by that point, it had been known that one key mutation (called D816V) was present in a key protein called KIT in abnormal mast cells in the great majority of patients with systemic mastocytosis. KIT is thought to be the dominant regulator of the mast cell's functions. In their 2007 reports, both the Vienna team and the Harvard/NIH team did the standard ("PCR," for polymerase chain reaction) testing looking specifically for the KIT-D816V mutation and found it in some (not all) of their patients, but they didn't do any other testing looking for any other mutations (in KIT or any other mast cell regulatory gene).

Dr. Molderings and his group, though, did far more extensive testing for mutations in KIT in mast cells they extracted from their patients' blood. The Bonn team determined the *full* sequence of KIT messenger RNA (mRNA). (When cells want to make a particular protein out of the genetic blueprint for that protein contained in the corresponding gene, they first translate the DNA sequence in the gene in question into a complementary string of nucleic acid molecules called mRNA, and then that mRNA string is transcribed (by the cell's protein making units called ribosomes) into the corresponding string of amino acids which is the desired protein.)

Lo and behold, when the Bonn team fully sequenced mast cell KIT mRNA in their patients with mast cell activation syndrome (looking for any and all mutations instead of just the D816V mutation sought by the Harvard/NIH team), they found roughly 35 different mutations – interestingly, *none* of them D816V – in the mast cell KIT mRNA sequences in their 17 patients. That's right: 100% of their patients not only had mutated KIT but in fact had multiple mutations in KIT, but it seemed that virtually every patient had a unique set, or pattern, of KIT mutations (just not the D816V mutation almost always found in mastocytosis). (The Bonn team later (2010) published another paper showing even more mutations across the larger group of patients they had found by that time, and again virtually every patient had a unique set of multiple mutations in KIT – including, in this report, D816V, though just in a single patient. Importantly, in this study they also sequenced KIT in a set of seemingly healthy control subjects, finding only a few mutations in a few of them. Perhaps the mutations found in the healthy controls were biologically insignificant, or perhaps these "healthy" controls would eventually develop MCAS symptoms, but regardless of that matter, the bottom line was that there was a clear difference between the few mutational findings in the healthy controls vs. the copious mutational findings in the MCAS patients.)

At this point things were starting to click together for me. It appeared that abnormal mast cell activation was associated not only with the KIT-D816V mutation classically associated with systemic mastocytosis (and might it be the case that actually there were usually a lot of mutations in systemic mastocytosis beyond KIT-D816V? later research would indeed find that to be the case) but also with a wide variety of other mutations which evidently aren't associated with the significant excess accumulation of mast cells seen in mastocytosis. It certainly wasn't clear yet whether the mutations were the actual *cause(s)* of the abnormal activation, but I nevertheless found the association intriguing and provocative.

An important puzzle, though, remained for me. Like most physicians, I had been taught that, under normal circumstances, mast cells – present in all tissues, albeit in scarce numbers and sparse distributions – produce and release small amounts of very potent biochemical signals, generically called mediators, which interacted with other cells and tissue to cause adjustments needed to maintain a state of health. The problems in mastocytosis, I was also taught, not only stemmed from there being too many mast cells but also that they were releasing their mediators inappropriately, causing other cells and tissues to make adjustments which were unnecessary, counterproductive, and causative of illness. However, like most physicians, I was taught that the list of mediators produced by mast cells is pretty short. In my textbook readings, the lists I saw contained roughly 10-20 different mediators. This was a dilemma for me. How could a disease capable of presenting with so many different symptoms be due to the inappropriate release of only a couple handfuls of different mediators? It just didn't make sense…

…until my searching for more information about mast cell mediators led me to discover the fabulous "COPE With Cytokines" online encyclopedia of information about "cytokines," some of the potent biochemical signals used by cells to influence the behavior of other cells. (The array of mediators produced by the mast cell includes cytokines as well as other molecular signals that belong to other molecular classes assigned names other than cytokines.) COPE, as I learned, is the remarkable result of the almost obsessive (meant kindly!) work over two decades by Dr. Horst Ibelgaufts, who trained as a molecular biologist in Germany and has come to teach the subject at a medical school in, of all places, the Philippines, where he has continued to work on COPE, surely a labor of love since it seems that, unfortunately, few of COPE's users contribute to support the site. (He deserves better; support him if you can. I suspect that, for the most part, a little bit of money goes a long way in the Philippines, but at the same time, certain resources that are critical to him, like Internet bandwidth, are probably a lot more expensive than in first-world countries.)

COPE's listings, as with most encyclopedias, are arranged alphabetically, so I clicked on M, and down amongst the long list of entries beginning with M, I found an entry for mast cells. A click on the link took me to a page that initially looked innocent enough – a few paragraphs of well-referenced, dense text generally describing mast cell function, below which was the beginning of the (similarly well-referenced) list of cytokines known to be produced by the mast cell.

I reviewed the introductory text and then started scrolling down through the list of mast cell cytokines – and scrolled, and scrolled, and scrolled, and kept scrolling, my eyes getting steadily wider. Clearly, the world of mast cell function I had previously been taught was but the tiniest portion of the true, and far more complex, world of mast cell function. Now I could see how it might be that different patterns of mast cell mutations (in KIT and perhaps other mast cell regulatory genes, too) could lead to different patterns of aberrant release of a large spectrum of mast cell mediators, in turn leading to not only a large spectrum of clinical presentations but also a large spectrum of responses to therapies targeted at mast cells and assorted mediators.

Out of curiosity, since each of the cytokines listed in that encyclopedia page was hyperlinked to another page in the encyclopedia chock full of information about that specific cytokine, I started clicking on each link, starting with the first, and continuing my reading to learn more details about the function of each cytokine.

You can imagine my surprise as I read the page of information about merely the second cytokine on the list, activin A (which I had never heard of before), learning that one of its activities is promoting red blood cell growth. One of the things about Shelly I could not understand is why she had become polycythemic (i.e., produced too many red blood cells) despite an unremarkable epo level. Here, now, merely at item #2 in a list of more than 200 entries, was a cytokine product of the mast cell that had potential for causing Shelly's polycythemia. There was no need to find a cause for her polycythemia that was distinct from causes of her other problems. Instead, it might take just one particular mutation, or set of mutations, in her mast cells to overproduce activin A (or any of the several other mediators made by the mast cell which also directly or indirectly promote red blood cell growth), among a spectrum of mediators, to simultaneously cause her polycythemia together with her other symptoms. (Interestingly, at the time of this writing there now is a pharmaceutical company that is trying to develop an activin-A-like product into an epo-like drug that will boost hemoglobin and red blood cells in anemic patients.)

On a hunch, I then searched the literature to see if norepinephrine, too, was a known mast cell product. Indeed, I soon found not only a paper demonstrating exactly that but also another paper describing how mast cells produce and release a hormone called renin which, through a chain of reactions, then leads to increased norepinephrine in the blood. Just as with activin A and polycythemia, there was a way to connect mast cell activity with increased norepinephrine. This didn't prove, of course, that it was inappropriate mast cell activity causing increased norepinephrine in Shelly herself, but at least I wasn't just imagining/hoping that there would be such a connection. Instead, such a connection was already known to exist in at least some patients. And while it remained possible that something other than inappropriate mast cell activity was causing Shelly's norepinephrine level to rise, the odds – Occam's Razor, about which I'll have much more to say later – said it was more likely that the elevated norepinephrine was due to the same root explanation causing her other problems than due to some other explanation.

A systemic mast cell activation syndrome – a "new" disease – was now really beginning to look like the cause of Shelly's "weird" illness with JAK2-normal polycythemia and other features, but the number of times in a doctor's career when he discovers a "new" disease in one of his patients is usually zero, so I knew I was still far from proving the case in her. More evidence had to be found.

The Seventh Visit

It was now the second week in July. On Shelly's seventh visit to my center, she saw not me but one of my colleagues in the dermatology department. She told the dermatologist the same story she had told me and also noted that these rashes were "extremely" itchy ("pruritic") when they came on. She felt she had some of these rashes scattered about her legs at the time of the visit, and the dermatologist obtained a biopsy and sent it to the pathologist with instructions to do the special processing needed to look for mast cells (since normal processing of skin biopsies by pathologists usually won't reveal mast cells even if they're present).

The Eighth Visit

Shelly returned next to see me a week later. She told me that after enjoying that brief period of feeling quite well, her symptoms had returned with a vengeance beginning a week before her visit to the dermatologist, finally simmering down somewhat the day after the visit to the dermatologist. She said the symptoms this time included "waves of nausea 24 x 7" which were not relieved with scopolamine (an anti-nausea drug commonly used for seasickness) or famotidine (a "histamine H_2 receptor blocker" used mostly to reduce stomach acid), episodes of assorted spots of intense itching on exposure to heat (whether sun or bathing), insomnia, fatigue, intermittent dizziness and lightheadedness, intermittent fast pulse ("tachycardia") upon minimal exertion, soaking sweats at night, decreased exercise endurance, diffuse swelling (more so in the legs than her arms), and a couple days of great difficulty initiating her urine stream. The day after the visit to the dermatologist, all of these symptoms suddenly vanished, but then, about four days later, she developed shortness of breath and tachycardia with minimal exertion, and on attempting to exercise that day, she found a blood pressure during exercise of 180/104 compared to her normal 140/76 with exercise. By that evening, though, she once again felt completely fine and had remained so since.

The physical exam at that visit showed only the slightest traces of the leg rash that had been biopsied. The biopsy wound seemed to me to be healing well, though Shelly felt it was taking much longer to heal than she had typically experienced with small wounds in the past.

Her hemoglobin that day had increased yet a bit further, to 11.6, almost normal, though frankly, with her wide extent of inflammatory symptoms, I would have expected her to be more anemic, as inflammation has long been recognized to cause anemia, and she certainly was markedly, chronically inflamed. The serum tryptase level was in the middle of the normal range (certainly not typical for systemic mastocytosis), and so was the urinary N-methylhistamine level – though I again noted in her chart at that time that she had been feeling well when the specimens were collected, and my reading on systemic mastocytosis at that visit had told me that these markers would be expected to rise and fall in accordance with how she was feeling. The pathologist reported the biopsy of her rash was showing "dense infiltrate urticaria" (exactly what one would get with a skin reaction to a noxious chemical or an insect bite), but there was no increase in mast cells. However, I saw that he had not used the tryptase and toluidine blue stains that I had requested. I spoke with him, and he said those stains were not readily available to him and that he had felt the stains he had used, Giemsa and chloroacetate esterase, would yield equivalent results. That was OK by me; there was no reason for him to not know his business.

I noted another bit of strangeness, too, in the labs that day. Her iron stores were not improving. It had been more than four months since her last phlebotomy, and although her hemoglobin was returning to normal, there was no sign whatsoever that her iron stores were improving. To be sure, I wouldn't have expected her to rapidly develop marked improvement in the iron deficiency she had shown at her first visit because she was using iron to make the increasing amount of hemoglobin shown in her blood – but there nevertheless should have been some improvement in iron stores, and yet there in fact had been none.

As there was nothing about her history to suggest an ongoing bleeding issue of any sort, in my chart entry that day I wondered whether intestinal mastocytosis might be interfering with her ability to absorb her dietary iron. I decided to check an oral iron absorption test that day. It's a simple test in which a baseline iron level in the blood is determined and then the patient drinks a certain quantity of liquid iron, after which the iron level in the blood is re-tested at certain intervals. If an increase in the blood iron level of at least a certain degree isn't seen within a certain amount of time, then the patient clearly is not properly absorbing iron, and the question then becomes "Why?"

I also pondered that day about checking a brain MRI for any signs of a pituitary gland issue that might explain her malaise, insomnia, nausea, and swelling. I decided, too, to check levels of markers for a class of cancers called germ cell tumors, which sometimes can cause odd symptoms despite having only very small sizes. I also began thinking about doing a bone marrow biopsy, a key test for diagnosing the "systemic" form of mastocytosis in which significantly increased numbers of mast cells are found in the marrow.

The Ninth Visit

Shelly returned for the ninth time a month later, in mid-August. She told me she had just gotten over another "spell" of her symptoms that had started about four days earlier and lasted about two days. Symptoms had included fidgetiness, nervousness, inability to sit still, exertional shortness of breath ("dyspnea") and tachycardia, nausea, indigestion, disrupted sleep (for example, she would sleep for three hours and then suddenly wake for a 3-4 hour period afflicted with pruritus, tachycardia, and indigestion), unsteady balance, and tachycardia and hypertension. She also noticed onset of a very pruritic rash near her belly button; she brought out-of-focus pictures suggesting a 2-3 cm wide lesion of a central clear blister surrounded by a red base. The day of the visit was one of her better days. She had smartly taken advantage of the just-passed spell to collect another 24-hour urine for N-methylhistamine and had submitted it to the lab. Thanks to some additional reading I had done by that point on mastocytosis markers, I asked the lab to also test the specimen for a prostaglandin D_2 level. However, I found out that even though Shelly had been very careful to keep the specimen chilled throughout collection and transport, the lab personnel had left the specimen on their desk, unchilled, for about three hours before beginning to check it in, so I wasn't sure I was going to get an accurate level of PGD_2, a notoriously short-lived, heat-sensitive metabolite.

On the physical exam, she looked a little bit tired but otherwise appeared healthy. There was no rash on her abdomen or elsewhere.

Thyroid function tests (ordered while wondering whether her spell had been some sort of very odd "thyroid storm") were normal. Blood testing for pituitary gland issues and germ cell tumors was negative. I was inching closer to ordering an MRI of the brain looking for any lesion that might cause a hormonal storm of some sort to explain her episodic malaise, insomnia, nausea, and swelling.

I performed a bone marrow biopsy at this visit. In fact, because I had just read an article showing that one-sixth of the marrow biopsies in mastocytosis cases fail to show the disease, I obtained two cored biopsies plus the usual "aspirate" sample sucked up into a syringe. As is the case with bone marrow aspirations and biopsies in most patients, she tolerated these procedures well.

Although her hemoglobin was still rising (11.9 on this visit) and the oral iron absorption test had been unequivocally normal, the iron stores on the ninth visit remained very low. It was time to ask the gastroenterologist to "scope her" (both "upper" and "lower," i.e., esophagogastroduodenoscopy (EGD) and colonoscopy), not only to see if any bleeding lesion could be found that might explain why her iron stores were not improving but also to see if there were the increased mast cells in the walls of the intestinal tract that I was increasingly suspecting had to be present to explain at least some of her symptoms.

I called the gastroenterologist I had in mind for performing this procedure and explained Shelly's history to him. I told him that because all of her imaging to date had been normal, I was doubtful he would find any specific lesions in the walls of her esophagus, stomach, or intestinal tract on upper or lower scoping. I told him that if he did find any lesions, he certainly should biopsy them, but regardless of whether specific lesions were seen and biopsied or not, I wanted him to obtain random biopsies of seemingly normal areas all throughout the upper and lower portions of the intestinal tract.

I then also called the pathologist who I knew would be receiving the specimens. I described Shelly's history to him, too, and asked that he perform not only the normal staining on all of the specimens but also the special staining ("CD117") best suited to identifying mast cells. Like the gastroenterologist, he agreed to my request.

The Tenth Visit

Five weeks later she returned to our center, not to see me but rather to see the gastroenterologist for the upper and lower scopings. She tolerated the procedures well. The gastroenterologist called me during the procedure. "I've looked all up and down through her, and it all looks completely normal. Are you really sure you want those biopsies?" Yes, I assured him, I was sure I wanted those biopsies. "OK, I'll go back in…"

Meanwhile, the hematopathologist had finished his analysis of the bone marrow aspirate and biopsies, reporting everything to be completely normal except for no signs of any iron stores in the marrow (where iron is typically stored). There definitely was no sign of mast cell disease in the marrow. A chromosome analysis (usually called a "karyotype" or "cytogenetics") was normal. Another test on the aspirate, "flow cytometry," looking for increased or abnormal mast cells, was negative, too.

The Eleventh Visit

On the first of October, a week after the scopings, Shelly returned to our center for the eleventh time. She said she had done well for the two weeks between her last visit to me and her scopings, but in the week following her scopings she had suffered an ongoing flare of her symptoms including one particular bad 17-hour-long bout with hypertension and tachycardia, insomnia despite marked fatigue and malaise, nausea without vomiting or diarrhea, and dyspnea on mild exertion but without wheezing. She had not suffered any pain and had not noticed any rash. She had again remembered my prior instructions to take advantage of such flares to collect and submit another chilled 24-hour urine specimen.

She provided the additional sad family history that her mother had just been diagnosed with acute leukemia.

The physical exam that day was unchanged from what I had last seen. She obviously was tired, but otherwise the exam was normal.

I reviewed the results from the blood tryptase and urinary N-methylhistamine and PGD_2 tests from the ninth visit. They were all normal, but it was possible such readings were lower than the true levels because my institution's lab (or perhaps the shipper who transported the samples to the distant lab subcontracted to actually ran some of these tests) had not kept the specimens properly continuously chilled.

The hemoglobin that day had edged up further again to 12.7, and finally there were signs in her lab tests that her iron stores were beginning to improve.

The pathologist coincidentally called me during Shelly's visit that day to report that my suspicions had been wrong. "These are most 'textbook normal' biopsies I have ever seen in my 30 years of doing GI pathology," he told me. I asked him whether he had done the special processing I had requested, although I already knew the answer since at that time it took our pathology department three weeks to do CD117 staining, and yet he had called me just one week after the procedure. To his credit, he acknowledged he had not sent any of the specimens to his staff to have the special processing done. "Why not?" I asked. "Because these are the most normal biopsies I have ever seen, so there's no point." We argued collegially for a while about the situation. He noted the biopsies were completely normal on standard processing. He also noted the CD117 staining was significantly more expensive than the standard processing. I objected to cost being an issue and noted that in addition to the treatment and evaluation to date having cost far more than what CD117 staining would cost, there was the far more important fact that a previously highly active and productive life had been ruined by this disease, so it was important to do all we could to identify a (hopefully treatable) diagnosis, and at the moment the disease that best fit her symptoms from a clinical perspective was mastocytosis.

In the end, he agreed to do the special processing. Meanwhile, he filed a report stating the regularly stained biopsies showed "benign" stomach, small intestine, and large intestine tissue.

The long assessment I wrote in her chart that day was as follows: "I remain pretty confident that this not only isn't p. vera but also isn't a pheo (at least not a classic pheo), which still leaves us to figure out what caused the presenting (and now coursing along a path toward eventually re-emergent) mild normocytic erythrocytosis (and assortment of other symptoms) in this otherwise very healthy, thin, non-apneic non-smoker. Much of the history continues to suggest a mastocytic or pheo-like disorder, but I can't find any clear evidence of either, merely a persistently elevated plasma norepinephrine. And why is she being so slow to improve her iron stores despite normal oral iron absorption? She's either consuming every bit of iron she takes in, or she's losing iron, but there's no obvious bleeding, let alone extensive diarrhea. Endoscopies and routine urinalyses are negative, so there's nothing more to be done to look for GI or urinary blood loss at this point (the endoscopist felt the upper and lower tracts appeared so normal that capsule endoscopy [to look at the middle portion of the intestinal tract that upper and lower scopings can't see] was not warranted). Previously I had been considering ordering an MRI of the brain to look for pituitary issues that might account for possible hormonal storms explaining her malaise, insomnia, nausea, and fluid retention, but at this point I think I'm going to hold off on that and instead send some additional blood and urine testing looking for other potential causes of flushing (carcinoid, medullary carcinoma of the thyroid, VIPoma) and ask for an Endocrinology consult to help me find the neuroendocrine disorder that must be going on here (which, like sometimes happens with a pheo, is also causing a secondary erythrocytosis). Note that I've also thought about a PET scan, as there's some preliminary data suggesting its utility in finding neuroendocrine tumors, but in addition to my doubts about whether a malignancy could be responsible for the very long duration of this illness, I doubt a PET would be able to anatomically or functionally see a mass so small as to escape detection on the MRI we've already done of the abdomen and pelvis (though there admittedly remains the possibility of a thoracic neuroendocrine tumor). Thus, I will defer on a PET, too – at least until I get Endocrinology's opinion. In addition to sending the 24-hour urine received today (and collected during one of her acute episodes) for a repeat N-methylhistamine and prostaglandin D_2, we're going to recheck it for metanephrines, catecholamines, and VMA/HVA, plus we're also going to check it for 5-HIAA [a marker for a type of neuroendocrine cancer called carcinoid]. Plus, we'll send more blood today for a serum serotonin, CEA [a marker for colon and certain other cancers], calcitonin [a marker for a neuroendocrine cancer called medullary carcinoma of the thyroid], VIP [a marker for a neuroendocrine tumor called a VIPoma], and repeat plasma norepinephrine, chromogranin A, epo, a vitamin B_{12} level, inflammatory markers, and a repeat set of general antibody levels. I'll see her back in another month, or perhaps a bit later if the Endocrinology consult gets scheduled within the next 6-7 weeks."

The next day I reviewed Shelly's entire case with one of our senior pathologists for the third time. As I wrote in her chart, "he, too, cannot think of anything other than a pheo which would explain the symptoms, the elevated norepi level, and the erythrocytosis – but he also agrees with me that if this is a pheo, it's got to be one of the [most] bizarre pheos ever.

The Twelfth Visit

A week later, Shelly returned to see one of our endocrinologists, who wrote that mastocytosis and pheochromocytoma seemed to have been ruled out. She ordered a rafter of labs assessing pituitary, thyroid, and adrenal function and gave the patient a glucose meter to check her glucose level during a symptomatic episode to look for low blood sugar, though she felt that was unlikely given that the last major episode had lasted 17 hours.

The Breakthrough

Three weeks to the day after Shelly's eleventh visit, the GI pathologist called me. Ordinarily very articulate, he was struggling for the words to describe what he was seeing. He told me, "I've never seen anything like this before. On the regular ['H&E'] stains, all of the biopsies are completely normal, but on the CD117 stains, the biopsies all appear flooded with mast cells."

Finally we're getting somewhere, I thought.

(Later the pathologist actually counted the mast cells and found areas of up to about 70 mast cells per high power field in the microscope. He told me that about 20 was thought to be the upper limit of normal, though as I learned later, there's a bit of controversy as to what that limit should be (some say as low as 15, others say as high as around 50 – but most I've questioned about this, including several prominent mast cell disease experts, say 20 is reasonable). He also went on to check stains with CD25, a marker for abnormal mast cells (and certain other types of cells), and found the slides similarly "flooded." They weren't "aggregated," or arranged in clusters, as is needed to satisfy the current diagnostic criteria for systemic mastocytosis, but they definitely were significantly increased in number.)

The Thirteenth Visit

A few days after the breakthrough, and a few days before Halloween, Shelly returned yet again. She reported continuing frequent episodes of assorted symptoms that she had mentioned previously. She noted that the itching was becoming more generalized. She was feeling a little bit weak that day.

On the physical exam, she did indeed look a bit more tired than I had last seen, but once again everything else was normal.

The labs that day showed the hemoglobin had edged up further to 13.7, again, technically "normal" but nevertheless considerably higher than I'd expect for someone acting so chronically and markedly inflamed. Other than proving her to have the menopause we already clinically knew she had, the labs ordered by the endocrinologist had all returned normal results. The labs I had ordered at the eleventh visit also were all normal (or virtually normal) except the norepi and dopamine levels were still elevated (978 and 31 pg/ml, respectively) similar to before. And, finally, we had gotten back an elevated PGD_2 level. It wasn't elevated much – just 304 ng (normal 100-280) for the 24 hour collection period – but it sure wasn't normal, all the more impressive given that this metabolite (whose extreme sensitivity to heat I certainly didn't fully appreciate at the time) had been 24 hours in the collection process followed by transportation to our lab before being sent by our lab to a reference lab roughly 2,000 miles away for actual processing (though as I later learned, that lab itself did not truly perform the test and instead just reshipped the specimen to another lab about another 2,500 miles distant to undergo the actual testing).

As I told Shelly that afternoon during her visit, "I think we've got it." But it was still a bit early to decide on treatment, because I knew that with mastocytosis it's important to determine whether the mast cells contain the KIT-D816V mutation that's found in about 90% of cases of systemic mastocytosis. It's important to figure this out for the simple reason that mastocytosis, when it doesn't bear that mutation, appears likely to respond to a very expensive drug called imatinib, but when the mutation is present (which, again, is the great majority of the time), there almost never is a response to imatinib.

As I wrote in her chart that day, "I reviewed the new pathology findings with the pathologist, who tells me that other than mastocytosis, the only conditions which might produce this staining are a gastrointestinal stromal tumor (GIST, for which there certainly is no clinical, radiologic, or pathologic evidence) and irritable bowel syndrome (which, simply, she doesn't have). A lymphoplasmacytic lymphoma of the Waldenstrom's type sometimes can produce the antibody abnormalities seen here, but that's certainly no explanation for the CD117$^+$CD25$^+$ overexpression in the intestinal tissue, not to mention there's been no other evidence of lymphoma and lymphoma wouldn't be expected to produce the particular constellation of symptoms seen here. The pathologist agrees with my interpretation that the immunostaining findings strongly suggest she has systemic mastocytosis, and as if that isn't rare enough, she appears to have a relatively uncommon form with malignant mastocytes residing predominantly in the intestinal tissue (and possibly the skin, based on her history, though we don't have biopsy proof of such yet) rather than the more common form of marrow, nodal, and/or splenic involvement. I've asked the pathologist to try to obtain the KIT-D816V mutation analysis on the CD117-overexpressing tissue [unlike the team in Bonn, I had no way of fully sequencing KIT (whether DNA or mRNA) in a routine clinical specimen, and D816V was the only KIT mutation I could test for], as positivity for this mutation would be the ultimate proof of mast cell disease. Meanwhile, now that we have more convincing evidence of a malignancy, I'm ordering a PET/CT to see if there's evidence of focal metabolic hyperactivity missed on (mostly MR) imaging to date that might indicate other foci of disease suitable for further biopsy if felt necessary and suitable for monitoring for response once treatment begins."

The Fourteenth Visit

This was a visit, on Halloween, specifically for the PET/CT scan. She seemed to tolerate it OK.

The Fifteenth Visit

Shelly returned for the fifteenth time in early December. She was no better, and her flares/spells/episodes had continued with full force. She had suffered another flare of her abdominal rash over the Thanksgiving holiday (what holiday-related exposure might have triggered it?), and since it was gone by the end of the holiday weekend, she couldn't come to our center to have it biopsied.

The physical exam showed more fatigue but again was otherwise unremarkable.

Her hemoglobin that day was down just a trifle to 12.9, but iron stores were continuing to improve. The total body PET/CT scan was completely normal. Regrettably, the pathologist had not yet sent the GI biopsies off to the reference lab where the KIT-D816V mutation analysis was to be performed.

We had a long talk that day in my clinic. What, exactly, was this disease? It didn't fit any of the forms of mastocytosis I had learned about in training or had read about over the last several months. And how should it be treated? Should we keep waiting for the mutation analysis? Given that her "mastocytosis" was presenting so differently from usual, wouldn't we expect the odds of finding the KIT-D816V mutation to be much lower than what's seen in systemic mastocytosis? And since we know that KIT-D816V-negative mastocytosis often responds well to imatinib, should we go ahead and try that stratospherically expensive drug? Or should we first try cheap drugs such as antihistamines or aspirin, even though they often help only a fraction of the symptoms? Or, given her nausea and the increased mast cells in the gastrointestinal (GI) tract, should we try moderately expensive cromolyn, which isn't well absorbed from the GI tract and may not help any of her symptoms beyond nausea?

All in all, given that the rare KIT-D816V-negative form of the rare disease of mastocytosis had a good track record of response to imatinib, and given that I estimated her mast cells were unlikely to bear the KIT-D816V mutation because of how different her disease was behaving compared to (ordinarily KIT-D816V-positive) systemic mastocytosis, I naively recommended that she should first try imatinib. I felt we likely would figure out quickly if it was helping, and it could easily be stopped if she didn't soon show significant improvement.

But how to dose it? Imatinib was a breakthrough once-daily oral drug originally developed for a type of leukemia called CML (chronic myeloid leukemia), and it does a spectacular job of controlling most cases of CML. Soon after it was introduced into the market, it was found to also be helpful in KIT-D816V-negative or -unknown aggressive systemic mastocytosis and received FDA approval to market the drug for that purpose. Recommended initial dosing for CML and mastocytosis was 400 mg daily, but many patients eventually proved to need mildly higher or lower doses for a wide variety of reasons, so the drug was manufactured not only in a 400 mg tablet but also in a 100 mg tablet.

We had no idea how her odd form of mastocytosis would react to imatinib (or any other drugs, for that matter), so for safety's sake I decided to start her at just 100 mg once a day. (I also had read about some cases of mastocytosis that responded well to very low doses of imatinib, just 100 mg per day.) I figured it would take her about a week to figure out whether she was tolerating it OK and whether it was helping significantly at that dose, so I told her that if she felt she was tolerating it OK after a week but hadn't yet noticed any improvement in how she felt, she should try increasing the once-daily dose to 200 mg.

I sent a message to the pathologist re-requesting the KIT-D816V mutation analysis, and I prescribed the imatinib with instructions for her to return in a month.

The Sixteenth Visit, or, Patience Pays Off

A few days after New Year's Day 2009, Shelly returned for her first check-up on imatinib. I entered the exam room, and it was immediately obvious she was hugely improved. She was radiating energy and beaming a smile at me. I asked her what had happened. She said, "I did just what you told me to do. I tried one pill a day for a week, and I didn't get any worse, but I didn't get any better, so then I started taking two of them every morning." She then described how she woke on the morning of the fifth day in that second week, after having taken the 200 mg dose for only four days by that point, and she was acutely aware – while still lying in bed, without even having stirred yet – that every single one of her symptoms was completely gone. She hadn't even gotten out of bed yet, but she knew all of her symptoms were gone. She then leaped out bed (compared to her previous daily ultra-fatigued, achy crawl/stumble out of bed about a couple hours after waking) and had been going full steam ever since. She felt "gloriously better, all full of energy, simply could not remember the last time I've felt anywhere close to this good." She also noted her blood pressure had improved, her exercise tolerance had improved, and she had had only a single episode of tachycardia since the higher dose of imatinib was begun. She had had no further recurrences of her solar-induced rash. She just was really, really happy that day. She also noted that all of her acquaintances, too, had commented to her about her obvious marked improvement.

On a physical exam, everything appeared normal. Her hemoglobin was stable at 12.7, and the rest of her routine blood cell counts and blood chemistries remained normal. The GI biopsies still had not been sent for the KIT-D816V mutation analysis.

"Don't mess with success" has always been a useful credo for me. I asked her to stay on the 200 mg dose and return in three months.

Meanwhile, I began wondering: if mast cell activation disease could present – likely as a consequence of some combination of mutations in assorted mast cell regulatory elements leading to some aberrant pattern of expression of some subset of the mast cells' huge repertoire of mediators – as so odd an entity as JAK2-unmutated polycythemia, what range of other odd presentations might be possible as a consequence of other combinations of mutations leading to other aberrant patterns of mediator expression? Food for thought, for sure...

The Seventeenth Visit, or, This Might Actually Stick

Shelly returned the second week of April 2009 and told me she did extremely well through January and February but had modest brief relapses ("spells") of weakness, tachycardia, and other "routine" symptoms for a couple of 2-3 day periods in March. Since then, though, she had been back to feeling fine. She additionally noted she had returned to essentially her full pre-illness exercise regimen, and she just as proudly noted that the past winter was the first winter in many during which she had not suffered a single upper respiratory infection. She thought she still was slow to heal, though, because she suffered a minor cut while gardening a few weeks earlier, and it took about three weeks for the cut to heal. She again noted she had had no further recurrences of her solar-induced rash. She remained just as happy that day as when I had seen her in January.

Her exam was again normal. Her hemoglobin had increased to 13.6, still well within the normal range for a woman. Iron stores were much better. I re-checked the catecholamine levels. The dopamine was normal (< 20), the epinephrine was a bit higher at 24, and the norepinephrine, while still elevated at 684, was by far the best (non-clonidine-suppressed) level she had yet shown. The GI biopsies still had not been sent for the KIT-D816V mutation analysis, and I gave up asking for it at that point since her excellent response to low-dose imatinib obviously rendered the mutation analysis a moot point from anything but an academic perspective.

We talked about tracking the number of spells she might continue to have and possibly increasing the dose if the relapses proved too numerous, but at that time we left the dose at 200 mg.

The Eighteenth Visit

Shelly returned for another three-month check-up in July 2009. She had done very well through the interval with absolutely none of her previously typical "spells" even in spite of marked stress from dealing with the death of her mother from acute leukemia and the death of her mother-in-law from a stroke. However, she had had a different type of four-day "spell" with intermittent diffuse cramping and edema about a week before the visit and in the aftermath of a short bout of a "GI virus" that she was pretty sure she had acquired from her visiting sister. She hadn't missed a dose of imatinib yet.

The exam was again normal and her hemoglobin had risen a bit further to 14.3.

I suspected a virally triggered modest flare of her mastocytosis was the explanation for her four-day "spell" and that once the virus was gone, the trigger was gone, so her mast cells settled back down to their usual baseline on imatinib. We kept her dose at 200 mg and extended her follow-up to six months.

The Nineteenth Visit

Shelly next returned in January 2010, reporting a "mild relapse" for a couple of weeks in December 2009. The only truly new issue was her observation of occasional small bruises developing about various aspects of her skin, never with any clear provocation.

Very interestingly, she also noted that she had begun putting her business back together and had gone off to a conference to engage in some networking, but she had forgotten to take her imatinib with her. Eighteen hours after the first missed dose, she acutely became substantially fatigued. She withdrew from the conference, returned home, immediately resumed her 200 mg daily dosing, and twelve hours later began feeling much better again and had maintained the improvement until the mild relapse in December 2009. At the time of this writing in December 2015, she has not missed a single additional dose to my knowledge.

Her exam was again unremarkable (she had no bruises at the time), except at this point I also tested her for dermatographism (redness and/or hives along the track of a light scratch; it's a rough indicator of more "twitchy" mast cell activation than normal), and indeed she showed the redness.

Her hemoglobin had settled back down a bit to 13.7; clearly, she was no longer trending toward polycythemia. Because of her report of minor spontaneous bruising, I checked a couple of basic screening tests on her blood clotting ("coagulation") system – a prothrombin time (PT) and a partial thromboplastin time (PTT) – and they were normal.

We agreed that in the event of future relapses, she would try temporarily increasing her daily imatinib dose to 300 mg but otherwise would keep the regular dose at 200 mg.

As of her last visit to me in September 2014, Shelly has continued to do very well on 200 mg a day of imatinib as her only treatment for what is now termed a mast cell activation syndrome (MCAS). She has learned that on the (rare) occasion of a flare, escalating her imatinib dose to 300 mg a day quickly (within a couple of days or so) settles the flare back down, at which point she can safely return to the 200 mg dose. More than once we have discussed trying to see whether she might do just as well on less expensive medication, but she understandably has not been interested in such medication trials. Her physical examination shows occasional minimal bruising but otherwise remains completely normal. Her hemoglobin seems to have stabilized around 14.5, right around the upper limit expected in a woman.

Short of outright cure (or equivalent improvement) with a cheaper drug, it is hard to imagine a more successful – or more spectacular – outcome. Hopefully you can appreciate that when I first saw Shelly's phenomenal response to imatinib, I was inspired – and intrigued. Given all that I had learned up to that point about what the mast cell *normally* does, I couldn't help but wonder how many different ways that different variants of inappropriate mast cell activation might clinically present. Was it possible I (and others?) had been missing this diagnosis from time to time? If so, surely it must have been merely an occasional miss. After all, mastocytosis was a rare disease, so this "atypical mastocytosis" must be at least as rare, if not even rarer, right?
Of course, at that point I couldn't possibly predict just how wrong that assumption was going to turn out to be.

Chapter 2: My Second Case: Double, Double Toil and Trouble

…fire burn, and cauldron bubble. I never did much care for Shakespeare's writings, but the second patient in whom I figured out a diagnosis of MCAS certainly was troubled and toiling because of a fire burning and a cauldron bubbling – and in such a strange place at that.

"Marlene" was hurting. Badly. The standard pain rating scale is 0 (no pain) to 10 (the worst pain you could ever imagine suffering), and she tearfully rated her pain at 11. Any doctor can tell you about innumerable patients seen with self-described pain ratings well beyond what the patient appears to be suffering, but there was no question her actual pain level was fairly close to what she was reporting.

The weird thing about it, though, was the location of this pain: it was her mouth that hurt, all the tissues lining her oral cavity (a bit less so the tongue), and the rest of her intestinal tract. And it wasn't a "normal" pain as if she had suffered a trauma to her oral tissues. No, this was a severe "burning" sensation. Her mouth was the worst of it, by far and without question, but she could also feel the burning to a lesser degree all down her throat and esophagus, down into her stomach and vaguely through the entire abdomen, and throughout the perineal area, too (anal and vaginal tracts).

As the 58-year old Marlene first explained her story to me in December 2005 – yes, 2½ years before I first met "Shelly" – she had been feeling well, with no chronic health problems except for high blood pressure and osteoporosis, which never really bothered her, and a one-pack-a-day smoking habit for the last 40 years, until about ten months earlier when, out of nowhere, she seemed to develop a diffuse itchiness (worst on the skin of her abdomen), and then a few days later the area became red and warm but not really tender. A trip to our center's emergency room led to an empiric diagnosis of an abdominal wall cellulitis (infection of the under-the-skin, or subcutaneous, tissues). She was admitted to our hospital, during which time she was given an intravenous antibiotic appropriate for fighting any of the bacteria that typically cause skin infections. She was discharged on a 14-day course of a similar oral antibiotic. She returned to our ER on the last day of the antibiotic because she had seen no improvement at all; in fact, she was now having chills and lower back pain. A CT scan of the belly showed some odd nodules about the adrenal glands but didn't really show a clear reason for her cellulitis. The ER physician though she was having an allergic reaction to the oral antibiotic and prescribed a one-week course of a different antibiotic. Over the course of that antibiotic, the patch of cellulitis (though not the itchiness) seemed to resolve, but then a week later it acutely recurred just how it had initially presented, centered around the umbilicus. She also reported a general malaise at that time. She was readmitted to the hospital with a diagnosis of an inadequately treated abdominal wall cellulitis and was started on yet an entirely different class of (intravenous) antibiotic, and by the next morning the redness and warmth and size of the affected area had dramatically decreased. She was sent home on a 9-day course of a similar oral antibiotic. She was also prescribed loratadine and hydroxyzine (both antihistamines) for her itching in the hospital, and for the first time the itching seemed to settle down a good bit, so these medications were continued on discharge.

Unfortunately, as soon as she finished the antibiotic, the cellulitis recurred. Marlene was restarted on the same antibiotic, but nearly two weeks later a similar rash appeared on her neck and she was briefly rehospitalized out of concern for spreading infection, but by the morning after admission the neck and abdominal rash had resolved. Evaluation for a battery of rheumatologic diseases was negative. An infectious disease consultant recommended stopping the antibiotic since the rash had resolved. A dermatology consultant found no rash to biopsy and recommended a biopsy if it recurred. She was advised to use hypoallergenic soaps and detergents and avoid fragrances and dyes.

About three weeks later Marlene began suffering seemingly unprovoked episodes of nausea followed by face and neck flushing and then shaking tremors and abdominal pain. These episodes were also associated with a burning sensation in her eyes, a metallic taste in her mouth, lightheadedness, and tightness in her chest along with shortness of breath and wheezing. Watery diarrhea, up to six times a day, also came on around this time. She was also beginning to notice a burning sensation diffusely about her abdomen. Two weeks later she was hospitalized for further evaluation of these ongoing problems. An abdominal MRI scan did not add anything to what the earlier CT scan had revealed. A red rash at the left hip was noticed, but a biopsy looking for mastocytosis showed only a pattern consistent with contact dermatitis and not any increase in mast cells. Testing for pheochromocytoma and another type of neuroendocrine tumor called carcinoid was negative. Another CT scan of the belly showed nothing new. She was discharged with minor improvement, to continue evaluation as an outpatient.

At an evaluation by an endocrinology consultant a week later, Marlene reported all of the previous symptoms had continued. She also noted she was feeling extremely weak and tired and that her flushing episodes were associated with tingling sensations about her upper trunk and palpitations. She also was noticing intermittent headaches and occasional brief episodes of blurred vision. She would feel anxious and frustrated when the symptoms flared up, and there was nightly insomnia in spite of her fatigue. She did not feel depressed. The consultant did additional testing for thyroid and adrenal diseases. Two weeks later she returned, unimproved. The results of the prior testing were all normal. The endocrinologist performed additional testing for thyroid diseases and repeated testing for a pheochromocytoma. These tests, too, yielded normal results. The endocrinologist repeated yet further testing for a pheochromocytoma.

Marlene next saw her primary doctor to be evaluated for jaw discomfort, but an X-ray of her jaw was normal. Her primary doctor started her on an antidepressant for anxiety, but she thought the drug only made her symptoms worse and she soon stopped it.

It was now July 2005. Marlene returned to the endocrinologist, who noted the latest testing for pheochromocytoma was negative. He ordered repeat testing for carcinoid disease and thyroid cancer. He also ordered a serum chromogranin A level.

Marlene returned two weeks later to find that her chromogranin A level was 8-fold elevated above the upper limit of normal. The endocrinologist repeated the test, and she returned two weeks later to find the repeat level was 13-fold elevated. She was referred to another center to have a special PET scan performed to try to find the tumor that presumably was the source of the elevated chromogranin and her symptoms. She was told it would be a long time to get set up to have this scan done.

Marlene then returned to the endocrinologist in mid-August reporting worsening symptoms. He ordered repeat urine testing for signs of carcinoid, pheochromocytoma, and mastocytosis. Previous testing of serum tryptase and urinary N-methylhistamine – traditional markers for mastocytosis – had repeatedly been normal, but this time a urinary test for a prostaglandin D_2 level – a trickier test to perform because of the special handling required for the specimen – was ordered. Despite this additional testing effort, she returned a week later to find that the results were all normal except for the 24-hour urinary prostaglandin D_2 being elevated at 445 ng (normal 100-280). The endocrinologist never commented on this result, so it's not clear whether he ever saw it. She also learned that her insurance company had denied coverage for the special PET scan. The endocrinologist ordered a special scan at our center for a pheochromocytoma as well as repeat blood testing for a type of thyroid cancer. She was referred to the dermatologist for an opinion.

In October 2005 Marlene was evaluated by another rheumatologist, who concluded, with a bit of additional testing that largely repeated prior testing, that she did not have any rheumatologic disease.

At this point, because of ongoing suspicions of a neuroendocrine cancer in view of the elevated chromogranin A levels, Marlene was referred to my division and was assigned to me because all of our other staff at that time were focused in areas other than neuroendocrine tumors and because I was always happy to see patients with any kind of hematology/oncology problem. I initially saw her in December 2005, and her symptoms were the same as they had been for many months by that point. Her burning mouth was by far her worst symptom, and though she had been referred for evaluation for cancer, which surely must be at an advanced stage to produce a chromogranin level as high as hers, she didn't *look* like she had advanced cancer of any sort. Nevertheless, surely nothing but a neuroendocrine tumor could produce such a high chromogranin level, so I sent blood tests looking for a few other rare types of neuroendocrine tumors. They all soon showed normal results, and meanwhile the chromogranin level was still about 10 times the upper limit of normal. Also, like the endocrinologist, I had missed the prostaglandin D_2 level because of the way in which such esoteric test results were filed in our electronic medical record system. (Of course, even if I had seen the level, I'm not sure I would have understood its significance at that time, though I'd like to (egotistically) think that seeing such a significant elevation would have driven me to figure out its significance.)

Marlene returned next to see me a month later, in early January 2006 – after a normal repeat CT scan of the belly and a normal standard PET scan – and underwent a bone marrow aspiration and biopsy looking for signs of mastocytosis. The chromogranin level was repeated, too. She returned in mid-January to find the marrow results were normal. I ordered another MRI of the abdomen to try again to find a tiny neuroendocrine tumor. I also ordered a special CT scan of the small intestinal tract for the same purpose, and I ordered an MRI of the brain to look for a pituitary tumor since by that point I had read a few case reports about rare pituitary tumors capable of secreting chromogranin. Additional special blood testing looking for parathyroid cancer and other rare neuroendocrine tumors and immunologic diseases was sent.

A week later she saw her primary doctor for bilateral ear ringing ("tinnitus") and burning. She was started on a two-week course of an antibiotic for a presumed ear infection. She returned to my clinic at the end of that course reporting no improvement in any of her prior symptoms, and she also noted new problems with aches and pains moving all about her body seemingly at random. All of the recent testing again showed no cause for her symptoms. I quizzed her extensively regarding her home environment but could not identify any such factors of concern. We discovered that in August 2004 she had had an upper denture plate made and initially suffered some reactions from it that were treated with antibiotics, but these problems eventually resolved, she was still using the plate, and it had a been a long time since she last noted any reaction upon inserting it.

I discussed the matter at that point with another rheumatologist at my center and five neuroendocrine cancer experts of national repute. None had any new ideas; all thought that the elevated chromogranin level virtually guaranteed the problem was a neuroendocrine cancer whose location eventually would be revealed through persistent repetition of testing.

Marlene next returned to my clinic at the end of February 2006, again unimproved. I repeated testing for some rare neuroendocrine tumors along with another urinary test for prostaglandin D_2. I also referred her to the gastroenterologist for upper and lower endoscopies to look for tiny neuroendocrine tumors in the GI tract which might not be detectable by any of the scans done to date, but I thought it unlikely such a tiny tumor would be able to cause her so many, and severe, symptoms.

In April 2006 Marlene noted a small ulcer on her vaginal labia. A gynecology consultant thought she had an immunologic disorder called Behçet's disease, but a biopsy of the ulcer revealed none of the expected inflammation (or any other notable findings, for that matter), and other general blood tests for inflammation had been repeated many times by that point and had always been normal, which would have been highly unusual for Behçet's disease. Nevertheless, I arranged for consultations with another rheumatologist and an ophthalmologist to look for other signs of Behçet's disease. In May 2006 both consultants found no sign of this disease.

Marlene required two ER visits in the next couple of weeks for episodic worsening of vaginal burning. A course of antibiotics was prescribed at each visit, but these treatments were unhelpful.

She returned next to see me at the end of May, again unimproved. I noticed at the time that her chromogranin level was showing odd fluctuations rather than the relatively steady course of escalation to be expected of an untreated, and thus progressing, neuroendocrine tumor. Hmmmm. Perhaps her disease was not the neuroendocrine tumor that it had been presumed to be for the prior nine months. But if it wasn't a neuroendocrine tumor, and if it wasn't any of the other, many diseases that had been ruled out, what on earth could it be? I noted, too, that the other special testing I had sent in February had all yielded normal results.

In June 2006 I gave Marlene an "octreotide challenge test," trying to see if an injection of this expensive medication for controlling carcinoid might reduce her chromogranin level, but her chromogranin level clearly did not change in response to the injection. Nevertheless, after consultation with colleagues, I decided to empirically prescribe her a short trial of octreotide.

She returned in August 2006, again unimproved. I wondered at that point about atypical presentations of rare forms of porphyria, but testing was negative. I asked her to undergo testing for a variety of vitamin deficiencies, metal toxicities, and other immunologic diseases, all of which yielded normal results. In my ongoing reading at that time, I newly learned of a disease called burning mouth syndrome, which certainly described her oral problem "to a T," but didn't seem to be able to account for any of her other problems.

Evaluations by a dermatologist and an otolaryngologist in September 2006 found no explanation for her many problems. The ENT doctor did not feel repeat biopsy of the lining of the mouth would be helpful.

Marlene returned again to see me a week later and now additionally reported intolerance to heat exposure; a hot shower would cause diffuse itching. She also reported her symptoms reliably worsened 2-3 hours after eating. She had had a waxing/waning coating on her tongue for several months by that point and was convinced she had a fungal infection even though many cultures had shown otherwise and even though no known fungal infection could come anywhere close to accounting for her full range of problems. She had had modest brief periods of improvement with courses of antifungal antibiotics previously, so I tried her on a different antifungal. She returned a couple weeks later reporting the same result. I asked for another evaluation by an infectious diseases specialist and also performed additional special testing for various rheumatologic diseases. All of this work proved unhelpful.

In October 2006, following a brief hospitalization for constipation, Marlene relocated to Baltimore. She spent the next year and a half there undergoing extensive evaluation at another major academic medical center, still with no diagnosis or effective therapy being identified. She did briefly return to our center in October 2007 for another upper endoscopy, but the gastroenterologist found nothing remarkable. He also took random biopsies throughout her upper GI tract given the perplexity of her case, but the pathologist (who had not performed the special staining needed to see mast cells since the gastroenterologist had not advised him of any clinical suspicion of the disease) reported these tissue samples to be normal.

Shortly after returning to our area in March 2008, Marlene required several ER visits for worsening symptoms and eventually was rehospitalized at our center in April 2008 for worsening symptoms. A repeat evaluation by a consulting rheumatologist again yielded no new ideas. I was asked to see her in the hospital (and thus became aware she had returned to our area). Although I was months away from figuring out what was going on with "Shelly" (the first patient, described in Chapter 1, in whom I diagnosed MCAS), I was already beginning to suspect "atypical mastocytosis." I also saw that although the October 2007 duodenal biopsy had been reported with a summary impression of "benign," in fact the pathologist had also observed a modest increase in that tissue sample of a type of white blood cell called an eosinophil. Eosinophils tend to flock to areas of allergic reactions. Why were increased eosinophils in her duodenum? Did this relate to her symptoms getting worse an hour or two after eating? I also noted that her bone marrow biopsy had shown a modest increase in eosinophils. If her problems were all "allergic reactions," why was the allergic trigger so inapparent, and why would she have such severe symptoms but only modest (instead of marked) increases in eosinophils in the duodenum and the bone marrow?

Marlene was hospitalized for yet another week at the end of April 2008 for recurrent worsening of her symptoms, especially mouth pain. I asked for additional special testing for rare eosinophil diseases; results were all negative. A repeat chromogranin level came back spectacularly elevated at about 100 times the upper limit of normal. I repeated scans looking for tumors; they showed nothing more than the few non-specific findings previously noted. Repeat serum tryptase and urinary prostaglandin D_2 levels were again normal. Additional biopsies of the lining of the mouth and the skin and the bone marrow were obtained to look for increased mast cells; they were negative. Repeated upper and lower endoscopies found mild inflammation in the duodenum and a few colonic polyps. Her pain improved somewhat with high doses of the anti-inflammatory steroid prednisone, and she was discharged.

On additional review of the literature, I stumbled across another rare syndrome – only 400 cases described in the literature since the initial report in the 1950s – of something called Cronkhite-Canada Syndrome (CCS), typically presenting with intestinal polyps (with a propensity for becoming cancers), diarrhea, and difficulty in the GI tract absorbing protein from the diet. Although I didn't appreciate the significance of this at the time, the medications empirically recommended for treatment of CCS were a mast cell stabilizer called cromolyn and (anti-inflammatory) steroids such as prednisone. I noted that various subtypes of CCS had been defined, and with her burning mouth and altered (metallic) sense of taste, it seemed she might possibly fit Type

II CCS even though her colonic polyps weren't anywhere as numerous as typically reported in CCS patients. Nevertheless, I asked Marlene to try cromolyn. She contacted me a day later to report she had almost immediately experienced significant relief of her mouth pain with the first dose. However, this benefit seemed to disappear after a few days.

She was rehospitalized for yet another severe exacerbation of symptoms (primarily her mouth discomfort) in late June 2008, staying for nearly another week. Her internists did not think she had CCS. Extensive evaluation included a repeat brain MRI scan, a special evaluation for pancreatitis called MRCP, and a "HIDA scan" looking at gallbladder function. All of these tests again showed no cause for her problems. The chromogranin level was repeated and was found to have plunged to the lowest level seen yet, barely above the upper limit of normal. She was started on a proton pump inhibitor and a histamine H_2 blocker and improved enough to be discharged.

Marlene was referred to pain management physicians, but by the end of 2008 those physicians had concluded they could not help her pain and they discharged her.

Another gastroenterology consultation in September 2008 yielded the opinion that she did not have CCS and her pain was not of any GI origin. She was referred back to ENT for repeat evaluation of her altered sensation of taste. The ENT physician thought her altered taste was due to dryness in her mouth, and he recommended she keep her mouth moist.

I saw Marlene again in October 2008. Some cognitive dysfunction, especially short-term memory loss, was becoming apparent. I repeated a wide range of special blood and urine testing and special scanning for neuroendocrine tumors; all of this was again normal.

In January 2009 – a couple days after observing Shelly's excellent response to imatinib – I completely reviewed Marlene's case yet again. This time I found the elevated prostaglandin D_2 level from August 2005 (and, of course, by that time I understood its significance). I asked for a repeat serum tryptase and chromogranin A, plasma free catecholamines, and urinary N-methylhistamine and prostaglandin D_2. I also asked the pathologist to go back to Marlene's old biopsies (especially the GI biopsies) and re-process them, this time doing the same "CD117" special staining that had been needed to find the increased mast cells in Shelly's GI biopsies. I saw her four days later, noting her catecholamines were showing the same pattern I had seen in Shelly. Also, the pathologist had called me that morning to report that the very first biopsy (duodenal biopsy from April 2008) he had re-examined with CD117 staining showed practically the same result he had seen upon re-examining Shelly's biopsies. Marlene had "only" 55 mast cells per high power field in her duodenal biopsy compared to Shelly's 70, but it was still a significantly elevated number. I decided to also check a plasma histamine level and wait for the rest of the pending test results.

Marlene returned 10 days later. Her plasma histamine level had come back mildly elevated. We learned the pathologist had found the same level of increased mast cells in her GI tract biopsies from 2006, too. (Testing for the KIT-D816V mutation, too, soon returned negative.) However, all of the skin biopsies remained negative on re-testing with CD117. I diagnosed her as having a systemic mast cell activation syndrome and started her on imatinib with the same approach to dosing I had used in Shelly.

Marlene returned a month later (February 2009) noting that her pain had improved from "12/10" to 2/10 within 2-3 days of starting imatinib but then had relapsed to 6/10. The repeat urinary N-methylhistamine and prostaglandin D_2 testing had come back normal. Not having any idea at that point whether different patients with this "mast cell activation syndrome" might do better with different doses of imatinib, and since we already knew that the safe starting dose of imatinib in aggressive systemic mastocytosis was 400 mg, I asked her to double her daily imatinib dose to 400 mg.

She returned in March 2009 reporting no improvement. We recalled the prior brief improvement with cromolyn. I wondered whether Cronkhite-Canada Syndrome might actually be a variant of mast cell activation syndrome, and I also wondered whether cromolyn might work better now with her being on imatinib, so we restarted her on this.

Marlene again returned in late March 2009 reporting mild improvement with pain 5/10 on average and even having a several-hour period each afternoon with almost no pain. I was not enthusiastic about trying traditional chemotherapy for traditional mastocytosis since she didn't appear to have traditional mastocytosis, and besides, traditional chemotherapy is usually fairly poorly effective against traditional mastocytosis. Instead, I added a trial of another drug, hydroxyurea, reported in some case reports to help mastocytosis.

She returned in April 2009 reporting her pain declined to 1/10 by the third day of hydroxyurea, but by the sixth day her pain began increasing again, peaking at 9/10, at which point she stopped hydroxyurea, then seeing her pain decrease back to the 5/10 baseline she had previously "enjoyed" on just imatinib and cromolyn. I asked her to re-try hydroxyurea, but all it did the second time was worsen her pain back to 9/10, so she stopped it and her pain returned to 5/10 on continued imatinib and cromolyn. (In retrospect, I wonder if her initial improvement and then worsening with hydroxyurea was due to response to the drug followed by reaction to its fillers and/or dyes, but that scenario is a story for a later chapter.)

In May 2009 I asked Marlene to try the immunosuppressant azathioprine and then, if unimproved two weeks later, try adding celecoxib. Four weeks later she reported these drugs hadn't helped at all and things were back to her old 9-10/10 baseline. She didn't even think imatinib or cromolyn were helping any longer. I asked her to stop imatinib, cromolyn, and azathioprine and to try doubling the H1 antihistamine diphenhydramine (from 25 to 50 mg) she had long been taking every six hours, doubling her celecoxib from once to twice daily, and adding a twice-daily dosing of the H2 antihistamine famotidine. At that time I also newly learned she had had an anaphylactic reaction to aspirin in her 20s and had been told to never use that drug again.

Marlene's husband reported two weeks later by phone that she was doing much better, with pain consistently down to 3-5/10 and much reduced use of the methadone pain medication that had been started by her pain management physicians the prior year, but she was sleeping 12-14 hours per day. I elected to make no changes.

She returned in June 2009 reporting pain was 0-1/10 and she was sleeping 10 hours a night. Her energy level was greatly improved.

Marlene certainly had her ups and downs in the years following her diagnosis, but each time she "flared," we were successful in finding other medications, reported in the literature as helpful in some patients with mast cell activation, that helped settle her flares back down. The inexpensive, short-acting benzodiazepine drug called lorazepam proved particularly helpful ("when the pain comes on, I take one little pill (0.25 mg), and the pain is gone in 5 minutes"), and the inexpensive old antihistamine antidepressant doxepin also was of some help. Other drugs, though, such as the leukotriene inhibitor montelukast, did not help at all. Her spells of inattention were finally diagnosed on EEG study in December 2009 as partial complex seizures, and though the anti-seizure drug levetiracetam didn't help, oxcarbazepine did. She had to come off celecoxib in October 2010 due to emerging problems with kidney function, but once the kidneys improved, we had her try simple aspirin, starting very cautiously at a very low dose she had to obtain from a compounding pharmacist, and she found she tolerated it without any problems and did progressively better as the dose was increased. Her kidneys (and stomach) appeared to hold up fine with the aspirin. Unfortunately, repeated efforts to taper her off her methadone reliably, rapidly led to relapse of her burning mouth pain.

A presenile dementia (possibly Alzheimer's disease) was clearly coming to take hold of Marlene as 2014 came along, and I lost track of her upon closing my practice at the Medical University of South Carolina, a couple months before I moved to the University of Minnesota that summer. Unfortunately (or perhaps fortunately, depending on one's perspective), her husband messaged me in July 2014 that she had passed. I sent condolences but felt it improper to request details, and thus I can't say what happened to her in the end.

The very brave Marlene taught me so much about the up-and-down, twist-and-turn course, and many potential oddities, of mast cell disease. She also taught me – perhaps more than any other patient of any type that I've ever encountered (and I certainly have seen a lot of awfully sick patients in my career) – about the huge human potential for strength and survival in times of severe suffering. (I've said many a time that her pain (before achieving diagnosis and effective therapy) always appeared to be so bad that I can't imagine how she didn't commit suicide in those first four years of the severe burning in her mouth, but clearly she had a strength that I doubt I would have had.) I will always miss her.

I'll end this chapter with a final note that the above-recounted odyssey is actually a significant simplification of her story. It is hard to imagine a disease more complex than mast cell activation disease, whether the rare subtype of mastocytosis or the seemingly far more common mast cell activation syndrome.

Chapter 3: My Third Case: Three Strikes and Yer...Onto Something?

Just two weeks after I had first met Shelly, serendipity struck again.

At age 61, "Betty" was referred to me for a fifth opinion regarding her anemia, and in April 2008 I saw her for an initial evaluation (coincidentally, just two weeks after I had first met Shelly). It was an unusual referral simply for the fact that she was coming from outside of South Carolina, and even though she was only "one state over," I don't think I had ever before been asked to provide an opinion for an out-of-state patient.

Betty's back had been hurting, and she had been terribly tired, for a few years now – and the frequent transfusions she had been getting for her severe anemia didn't seem to be helping much.

She and her husband weren't too clear on the past details of her illness – they thought she had been sick from her anemia for only a year and a half – but the full set of records her referring physician had thoughtfully provided were very helpful in showing her problems with the anemia dated back to '04.

A convenience store manager for nearly a couple decades until retiring due to her illness in '07, Betty had already acquired a rafter of problems by the time her presenting fatigue set in in '04. One of the physicians she had consulted in '07 had noted chronic problems of emphysema (from heavy exposure to customers' smoke, she said, as she herself had never smoked), gastroesophageal reflux (i.e., heartburn), depression, anxiety, chronic diarrhea of unclear cause, and chronic neck pain from cervical disc disease. She had been suffering night sweats since a hysterectomy 30 years earlier and also had been suffering migraine headaches for many years along with obstructive sleep apnea that had gone untreated when she was found to be intolerant of the "continuous positive airway pressure" (CPAP) device often used to treat this. She also had survived an early stage breast cancer found a decade earlier, treated with surgery and radiation treatment but not chemotherapy or any hormonal therapy. Other information in the chart also showed that for several years she had been having diffusely migratory aching that had been diagnosed in '02 as fibromyalgia and rheumatoid arthritis, but assorted treatments hadn't helped much. And as if all of that wasn't enough, she had suffered multiple blood clots ("pulmonary emboli," or "PEs" (plural of "pulmonary embolus")) in her lungs and the deep veins of her legs ("deep venous thromboses," or "DVTs") over the last decade. No cause had ever been identified.

The fatigue that had worsened so much in the fall of '04 had soon led to discovery of pretty severe anemia for which Betty was immediately referred to an oncologist in her community. A cause for her anemia was not immediately apparent. She was tried on epo shots and transfusions, but, quite oddly, these potent treatments didn't seem to improve her anemia much at all. She was then referred to a hematologist in her community, who performed a bone marrow biopsy and found that the elements of her marrow, which make red blood cells, were virtually absent. This, then, appeared to be a case of the pretty rare "benign" (as opposed to malignant, but nevertheless serious) hematologic disorder called pure red cell aplasia (PRCA), in which the marrow just gives up making red blood cells. Usually the cause of this is infection with a virus called parvovirus B-19, but a check for that was negative. Sometimes an uncommon cancer of the thymus gland in the chest called a thymoma causes it (though we've not yet figured out how), but a CT scan of her chest didn't show any thymoma to be present. For that matter, CT scans of her abdomen and pelvis didn't show anything else abnormal, either. She was tried on the usual treatments for pure red cell aplasia, first a stiff dose of the steroid prednisone and then the chemotherapy (and immune-system-suppressing) drug cyclophosphamide, but neither helped. She continued to require transfusion of two units of blood every 3-4 weeks just to maintain her hemoglobin level around 7-8, roughly half of normal. Her hematologist recognized that with all of these transfusions, she was at serious risk for developing iron overload, a problem that can "rot out" most of the organs in the body over time, so he tried to treat her with "chelation therapy" (medications which leech iron out of the places in the body where it's stored, to then be dumped out of the body through the urine), but an oral chelator, deferasirox, caused nausea in her, and an older chelator, deferoxamine, injected under the skin caused marked bruising. IV deferoxamine treatments weren't tried, for reasons not clear from the records provided me.

Betty was next referred in April 2005 to a hematologist at a major academic medical center in her state, but no new findings came of that evaluation. Transfusions continued until her local hematologist decided nearly three years later to get another opinion. To this day I don't know why he decided to send her to my institution, and I'm virtually certain she was assigned to my clinic by the luck of the draw, as I certainly had no more experience with PRCA than the average hematologist, which is to say, virtually none. As I said, it's a rare disease.

When Betty first came to my clinic in April 2008, she told me about all of the symptoms noted above (she even mentioned occasional episodes of blurred vision, too) – and she looked the part, too: pale, tired, achy, mild back pain behaviors, but other than those constitutional findings and diffusely dry skin, I found nothing remarkable on her physical exam.

Unsurprisingly, she was on many medications: oxycodone (long and short acting forms), montelukast, tizanidine, potassium, pramipexole, fluconazole, zolpidem, furosemide, venlafaxine, paroxetine, primidone, and albuterol. Curiously, on her allergy list, she noted the narcotics morphine and meperidine caused hives, while the non-steroidal anti-inflammatory drug (NSAID) called naproxen caused her an upset stomach.

Egad. What to make of all of this? The hematologic data made a convincing case for parvovirus and thymoma-negative PRCA which, as usual for that entity, hadn't responded well to treatment, but there simply was no way that PRCA could have caused all of her rheumatologic issues that had come on at roughly the same time as the PRCA, let alone any of her blood clots. But maybe I was looking at it backwards. Maybe there was a rheumatologic disease which had "spun off" her PRCA, but if so, which rheumatologic disease? She really didn't seem classic for any of them. Maybe her PRCA was some weird autoimmune disease. Lymphomas, especially T-cell lymphomas, sometimes spin off autoimmune diseases, and cancers of virtually any sort can cause clotting. Could this be a "really weird" lymphoma? T-cell lymphomas, in particular, have a reputation for causing odd "paraneoplastic" phenomena. Or maybe it really was a parvovirus infection and the initial testing was just falsely negative.

I decided to check Betty's blood for a wide range of rheumatologic and clotting conditions, plus a re-check for parvovirus and a few other viruses, and a check for B- and T-cell lymphomas. I also repeated her chest and abdominal CT scan, but no thymoma or other concerning abnormality was seen other than the expected iron overload in her liver. I also looked at her peripheral blood smear, with the only finding of note being the clear presence of a significantly minority subpopulation of neutrophils (a type of white blood cell) called a "pseudo-Pelger-Hüet form" which usually is a hint of a pre-leukemic blood malignancy called myelodysplastic syndrome (MDS) – except she clearly did not have MDS. I also obtained her original, diagnostic bone marrow biopsy and had it reviewed by our long-time chief hematopathologist, a master in that specialty if there ever were one. (Interestingly, he had trained in internal medicine but quickly became enamored of hematopathology and soon turned his career in that direction, a perfect case in point that sometimes passion and commitment and experience are sufficient to achieve success in an area without necessarily undergoing formal training.) The diagnostic marrow indeed showed a virtual absence of red blood cells, pretty classic for PRCA, and no signs of the "giant pronormoblasts" – altered

red cell precursors – which suggest parvovirus infection. There was another small curiosity, too, though – small clusters of another type of white blood cell called an eosinophil – that hadn't been commented on by her previous doctors. Increased numbers of eosinophils can be seen in many conditions, including rheumatologic and T-cell diseases – and in allergic situations.

Two weeks later I entered an addendum in Betty's chart, noting all the tests had been negative except for a subtle suggestion of a T-cell malignancy (the "T-cell-receptor gene-rearrangement" (TCRGR) test in the blood was positive) and a couple of significantly elevated markers of inflammation. Specifically, her erythrocyte sedimentation rate (ESR) was off the scale, and her anti-nuclear antibody (ANA) titer, too, was pretty high at 1:1280 (normal is roughly 1:40 or less). Also, her epo level was extremely high – exactly as would be expected in a severely anemic person – so it was very clear that there was some force acting very strongly in her marrow to completely counter the high epo level's very strong pro-red-blood-cell-growth (i.e., pro-erythropoietic) force. Given that her marrow exams and scans had not shown a lymphoma, I wasn't too sure about the TCRGR finding – the test has a roughly 20% false-positive rate – but it clearly was time for her to see the rheumatologist. I also made arrangements with her local hematologist to start her on IV treatments of deferoxamine, which would help leech the excess iron in her body (that she had gotten from all the transfusions) out through the urine. As I previously noted, he had already tried her on an oral chelator for doing this, and he had also tried her on subcutaneous deferoxamine, but she hadn't tolerated either of those approaches. Iron overload (hemosiderosis) from transfusions clearly hadn't been the cause of all of the symptoms she already was having back when her severe anemia was first found, but there definitely was some overlap between the symptoms she was presently having and the symptoms one can have from hemosiderosis, so significantly reducing her iron overload would be a big step toward sorting out how much of her present trouble was due to hemosiderosis vs. something else.

The rheumatology consultant saw Betty several weeks later and did a careful evaluation but could only conclude "I cannot classify her as having a specific connective tissue disease. She does not meet classification criteria for lupus, rheumatoid arthritis, or other connective tissue disease at this time." Not surprising, but frustrating nonetheless.

It was time to take another look in her bone marrow. There obviously was an epic struggle going on there between pro-erythropoietic and anti-erythropoietic forces, and perhaps now, a few years after the anemia first became apparent, we would be able to see an obvious root cause.

I did the procedure in August '08. To the inexperienced, bone marrow biopsies look brutal but actually are usually well tolerated without any need for pre-procedure sedation or peri-procedure pain medication, and indeed Betty tolerated it quite well. I saw her back the following month to review the results with her. At the time of the procedure there was no question the pathologist was going to find little red blood cell production under the microscope because the biopsy core, instead of being the usual rich red color, was virtually all white.

As it turned out, though, the results made an already ridiculously complicated situation even more complicated. To start with, as I had expected, there was essentially no red blood production found under the microscope. Small clusters of eosinophils, still of uncertain significance, were again seen. There certainly was no lymphoma (B- or T- or NK-cell) anywhere in the biopsy (under the microscope, or by a more sensitive test called flow cytometry), and there were no cells that didn't fundamentally belong in the marrow. And a chromosome analysis only showed the normal pattern of 46 chromosomes with the two X chromosomes every normal human female should have.

But, very curiously, there were two other, completely unexpected findings. One was that a little bit of "hemophagocytosis" was found. This term refers to an unusual situation in which a type of white blood cell called a macrophage literally incorrectly comes to regard red blood cells as the enemy. The macrophage then engulfs perfectly normal red blood cells, taking them into the macrophage's own cytoplasm, and proceeds to break them down, or eat ("phagocytize") them. In a rare, aggressive, usually acute and terribly sickening and often fatal disease called hemophagocytic lymphohistiocytosis (HLH), hemophagocytosis is prominent. It's a disease that features severe anemia and diffuse aching, just like Betty had, but HLH usually has many other features that Betty wasn't showing, not the least of which was that her illness had been going on at that point for a few years. If Betty had HLH, it would have had to be a pretty weird and rare form of that rare disease, one for the record books.

And the other unexpected finding? "Increased mast cells." Not anywhere near enough, to be sure, to raise concerns for, let alone officially qualify for, systemic mastocytosis. But increased nonetheless.

On the one hand, we're taught in our medical training that increased mast cells show up all the time as a normal *re*action – a so-called "secondary" phenomenon – to a wide variety of inflammatory and cancerous situations. But Shelly's case, and all the reading I was doing by that point, made me wonder if it might just be possible for these increased mast cells to be a "primary" phenomenon – i.e., the root of the trouble – in Betty, even if they weren't so increased as to constitute a case of systemic mastocytosis.

As I wrote in her chart at the time, "I continue to think what's going on here is a spectrum of autoimmune disease due to a subclinical clonal T-cell disorder which also is suppressing erythropoiesis by disrupting the normal cytokine network needed for this component of hematopoiesis." But I also noted, "Though I find it hard to believe that a woman with one rare disease already (PRCA) now also has [one or more other rare diseases] such as mastocytosis and/or HLH, I'll send today a serum tryptase, urinary N-methylhistamine and urinary prostaglandin D_2, serum ferritin and triglycerides and a soluble interleukin-2 receptor." (The first three look for mastocytosis and mast cell activation; the latter three typically show very high levels in HLH.)

I also decided to try Betty on a cautious dose of a commonly used immunosuppressive medication called cyclosporine to see if it would help combat the "weird T-cell-based autoimmune process" I was increasingly suspecting to be the root of her trouble.

Money and travel were getting increasingly difficult for Betty. She and her husband next returned two months later, in early November '08. Betty reported that she had had too much gastrointestinal upset at the planned dose of cyclosporine but was tolerating it OK at half that dose. Her transfusion interval seemed to have been slightly improved from feeling like she needed blood every three weeks to feeling that way every four weeks, but even if that was a real improvement from the cyclosporine, it was a pretty modest improvement (certainly none of her many other symptoms had improved at all), and it was clear she wouldn't be able to tolerate any higher a cyclosporine dose.

Meanwhile, the additional special labs were all normal except for a minimally elevated urinary prostaglandin D2 and a double-the-upper-limit-of-normal soluble IL-2 receptor (sIL2r). The ferritin was elevated in her usual range (about 7,000 ng/ml), and though this is quite high relative to normal (roughly 20-300 ng/ml), it was far below the extremely high levels often seen in HLH.

So, except for the sIL2r, this was all more evidence that this wasn't HLH, but there was little evidence of mast cell disease. I decided to switch Betty's treatment to another immunosuppressant, azathioprine, again starting with cautious dosing.

She next returned after another two-month interval, now early January '09 – and the day before I saw Shelly's response to imatinib. Nothing had improved, and in fact her local hematologist's partner had stopped her azathioprine two weeks earlier for just that reason.

In fact, she was now noting fairly steady achiness in many of the areas about the body containing concentrations of lymph nodes such as the armpits and the hollows above the clavicles. There weren't actually any enlarged lymph nodes that I could feel on her examination, but she sure hurt in those areas when I palpated about, trying to find the enlarged nodes I thought I'd be able to find there in view of her pain.

My diagnostic assessment was unchanged, and I spoke with her local hematologist at length and we decided to have him try her on another immunosuppressant, cyclophosphamide.

Betty returned in early February '09. She seemed to have tolerated the first couple of doses of cyclophosphamide OK (it was being given IV every three weeks), but it hadn't appeared to help her in any way. She not only was unimproved in any way but in fact reported further worsening of the new pain in the lymph node-bearing areas. Whereas in January she had felt the pain in some of these areas, now she was feeling it in all of these areas – but there still wasn't a single enlarged node I could feel in any of these (obviously tender) areas on my exam of her.

I was getting more concerned for an "occult" (hidden) T-cell lymphoma. I decided to repeat a number of the previous tests including the bone marrow biopsy and also check a type of scan she hadn't had before, a positron emission tomography (PET) scan, that was showing increasing usefulness for finding lymphomas and other cancers. In fact, I repeated the bone marrow biopsy that day.

Nine days later, with the PET scan still pending for the following week, I noted in her chart the results of all the other testing that had been done. The ANA titer, pretty high to begin with at 1:1280, had doubled to 1:2560. The TCRGR was still positive. The sIL2r level was now off the scale. Surely a lymphoma! However, there still were none of the classic signs of lymphoma (enlarged lymph nodes on physical exam or scans). And to confound the situation even further, the repeat marrow was unchanged from the prior marrow except that now, in addition to seeing the same spotty increases in eosinophils as before, there also was a subtle increase in another type of white blood cell called a basophil which, like the eosinophil, tends to increase in allergic situations – and allergic situations are a lot more suggestive of mast cell disease than lymphoma of any type.

I wrote in her chart at the time, "Now the question arises, is her autoimmunity (the ANA, and perhaps other autoantibodies not yet apparent) born out of T-cell lymphoma or out of mast cell disease? The subtle basophilia is rapidly turning to my attention to the possibility of mast cell disease, even though the marrows to date haven't shown mastocytosis per the WHO diagnostic criteria." I decided to check additional markers in the blood and urine for certain types of T-cell lymphomas and for mast cell disease when she returned for the PET scan.

She got the PET scan and the other labs, and then returned a month later. She was tolerating IV chelation fine, but nothing had changed with any of her symptoms. Her exam was unchanged: markedly fatigued, diffusely achy and pained. The PET/CT scan was normal – but the 24-hour urinary prostaglandin D_2 was "sky-high" (especially for somebody without mastocytosis) at 1,849 pg/ml, more than six times the upper limit of normal.

Surely with a PGD_2 level that high, this had to be systemic mastocytosis, and perhaps it was just a "sampling error" (i.e., luck of the draw) that my biopsy needle hadn't hit a patch of what is known to be a patchy disease. Given that imatinib rarely works for systemic mastocytosis with the KIT-D816V mutation, I felt it important to find out whether that mutation was present before making a treatment decision, so I asked the lab to process the February marrow specimen for that mutation, and I asked Betty to hang in there another month while we waited for results.

Unfortunately, when she returned a month later (April '09), it turned out the lab had lost track of the test request and hadn't even begun to process the test. I also noted that, as I had seen in Shelly, Betty's plasma norepinephrine level was twice the upper limit of normal, and, as I had seen in Marlene, the chromogranin A level in the blood was elevated. This was looking more and more like it was overlapping with what I had found in Shelly and Marlene: inappropriate mast cell activation, clearly with some features common to all these cases (for example, fatigue and aching and elevated prostaglandin D_2) and some features different amongst the cases (too many red blood cells in one, a burning sensation from stem to stern in the GI tract in another, and way too few red blood cells in another). There were just too many signs by that point in Betty that she had "more or less" the same thing as Shelly and Marlene, both of whom had improved to varying degrees on imatinib, so I started Betty on imatinib, too.

She returned six weeks later reporting no improvement – in her symptoms. However, stunningly, she hadn't needed a transfusion in two months, and her hemoglobin was up to 8.8 g/dl. I asked her to step up her imatinib by one notch, from 200 mg once a day to 300 mg once a day. Because aching was still her chief complaint, I also decided to have her try adding aspirin, which has long been known to help some patients with mast cell disease – and cause reactions and even anaphylaxis in others. Betty, though, had tried aspirin on occasion in the past and knew she didn't have a problem tolerating it, so I asked her to start with two adult-strength aspirin tablets twice a day. I also started her on a proton pump inhibitor, omeprazole, to try to reduce the chance of the aspirin causing an ulcer. I also wrote in her chart, "I will hold for now on adding histamine blocking since her plasma histamine and urinary N-methylhistamine testing has been normal."

Betty returned a month later. Her aching was unimproved, but nevertheless she felt distinctly better overall. Intriguing – but was it due to the increased imatinib dose, or to the aspirin, or both? Also, her hemoglobin, which had peaked at 10.6 g/dl determined two weeks earlier at her local hematologist's office, had fallen to 10.4 g/dl by the following week and was down even further to 9.7 g/dl by the day of this early July visit with me. I wondered whether the higher imatinib dose was now suppressing red blood cell production, so I asked her step the imatinib back down to 200 mg once a day. And since the aspirin had been aimed at the aching but hadn't helped it one bit, I decided to stop it. What to try next? I thought about oral cromolyn, but her insurance company wouldn't cover it and she certainly couldn't afford it (about $1,000 per month) on her own. I wondered whether my prior reasoning for holding histamine blockers was valid. What difference would it make, other than in histamine-mediated symptoms, if her particular variant of mast cell activation syndrome released elevated levels of histamine or not? Instead, what I should have been thinking about was that mast cells, normal or not, have cell-surface histamine receptors which, when engaged by the histamine the mast cell itself releases, stimulate further mast cell activation. And the drugs to block those histamine receptors – the classic antihistamines – are cheap. So I asked her to try adding into her regimen a full histamine receptor blockade with the "H_1" antihistamine loratadine (10 mg twice daily) and the "H_2" antihistamine famotidine (40 mg twice daily).

Betty followed up with me again six weeks later, in mid-August '09. She felt generally somewhat worse, and the diffuse aching was still unchanged. Her hemoglobin, though – I remember literally doing a double-take and my jaw dropping open – had jumped from 9.7 to 12.8! Totally normal! Holy moley!

Great progress, to be sure, but look at the trouble I had created for myself: by making so many changes so quickly, how could I know which drugs were responsible for which portions of the improvement? Was imatinib at 200 mg a day all she needed? Were the antihistamines (or perhaps even just one antihistamine or the other) all she needed? Or did she need a combination of imatinib and one or both antihistamines? And since her malaise had returned, did she need aspirin, too? What to do?

Clearly it was time to begin making changes more cautiously. I asked her to decrease imatinib to 100 mg once a day and keep everything else the same.

Six weeks later (late September), symptomatically she was unchanged. Her hemoglobin had gotten as high as 13.3 back home, but on the day she saw me it was virtually the same – 12.9 – as the last time I had seen her.

It was really beginning to look like the antihistamines were doing the "heavy lifting" here. Since imatinib was not available in 50 mg pills, I asked her to decrease her imatinib to a 100 mg dose every other day, plus I added montelukast to try to help with her itching (and perhaps other symptoms) since by that point I had seen the drug help itching in some other MCAS patients I had diagnosed and treated by then.

Another five weeks went by. Her local hematologist called me. Betty's hemoglobin was now *too high* at 15.8 g/dl (i.e., now she was polycythemic), and nothing else was better. Even though she had kept up with the chelation treatment pretty faithfully, her ferritin level was not improving – though it was impossible to tell how much of that high ferritin was due to iron overload and how much was due to inflammation. We batted back and forth for quite a while whether to now perform therapeutic phlebotomy (as Shelly had initially undergone for her misdiagnosed polycythemia vera), but in the end decided to change nothing and watch her just a while longer.

She saw me again a week later for her "mast cell disease of some sort" (as I had taken to writing her diagnosis at the beginning of each of my progress notes on her). Now mid-November '09, her hemoglobin here was 13.3, and she told me multiple symptoms (night sweats, stomach discomfort, and others) had worsened since the imatinib was decreased to a 100 mg dose every other day.

As I wrote in her chart that day, "Very complex situation, 'pure red cell aplasia' effectively resolved thanks to some combination of imatinib and antihistamines, but her resurgence of symptoms soon after the decrease in imatinib dose suggests the imatinib really will be important on an ongoing basis in this patient for controlling at least some of her symptoms. I've thus asked her to go back up to 100 mg/d on the imatinib, and if after two weeks she feels she is completely unimproved, she will increase further to 200 mg/d. Meanwhile, we'll continue antihistamines as above. Montelukast doesn't appear, by her history, to have helped with anything, so we'll ditch it. It's clear now that her hemoglobin has rebounded beyond what I would expect in someone who so obviously continues to have a severe systemic inflammatory state, so what's going on here? Two possibilities, as I see it: either (1) her disease has *always* been elaborating both anti-

and pro-erythropoietic mediators, and in the past the anti-erythropoietic factor(s) dominated (leading to the 'pure red cell aplasia') but now her medications are controlling those factors but not the pro-erythropoietic factors; or (2) it might be pure coincidence that her pure red cell aplasia has become borderline polycythemia at the same time we have initiated imatinib and antihistamines, i.e., perhaps her disease (which we may or may not be controlling to any degree with her medications) is evolving such that it is no longer elaborating anti-erythropoietic factors and now instead is elaborating erythropoeitic factors. (Certainly in the literature there is a well-established, if rare, association of polycythemia with mast cell disease.) A third possibility, less likely, is that polycythemia is emerging due to a JAK2-mutation-based chronic myeloproliferative disease having emerged out of her underlying mast cell disorder. Any way you look at this, increasing her medications (imatinib) targeted at the underlying aberrant cell is the treatment of choice for right now (at least until we can get the epo level and JAK2 mutation analysis we're requesting today). Thus, we'll see what the increased imatinib can do for her."

Betty returned on December 30, 2009 reporting that shortly after resuming imatinib on a daily basis (at just 100 mg), she noticed a significant improvement in her fatigue, sweats, and stomach discomfort. She also was very pleased with the significant improvement in her platelet count since increasing the imatinib (I hadn't mentioned it before, but her platelet count had been slowly but steadily declining through most of 2009); in fact, it had doubled from November to December, from 83,000 to 150,000. (How many cases of idiopathic thrombocytopenia labeled by default as "chronic ITP" (immune thrombocytopenic purpura) might be unrecognized MCAS?) Her latest hemoglobin, checked locally two days before seeing me, was 14. She repeatedly thanked me for the assistance I've provided her. Unfortunately, however, chronic shortness of breath (dyspnea) remained a significant problem, requiring her to use Advair 3-4 times daily. She also noted a significant element of orthopnea to this problem (breathlessness when reclining) and was regularly using 3 or more pillows under her head to gain enough comfort to permit sleep. She said an echocardiogram done locally about six months ago was reported to her as normal. I didn't have results on the epo and JAK2 testing I had requested in November because, as it turned out, she had never gone to the lab for some reason.

What to do? "Very complex situation, 'pure red cell aplasia' effectively resolved thanks to some combination of imatinib and antihistamines, and the recent attempt to wean her off imatinib has clearly shown she needs imatinib as part of her regimen for controlling her mast cell disease. I think her persistent asthmatic-type symptoms (and her ocular symptoms) are signs of continued aberrant mast cell overactivity. I've asked her to first try increasing her loratadine to 10 mg twice daily (this is certainly the cheaper and less toxic approach; note I had originally prescribed it twice daily, but it turned out today she actually had only been taking it once daily), but if after two weeks she feels her symptoms are not significantly improved, she is to increase her imatinib to 200 mg/d. She will return here in a month to see how she's doing and to review the results of the epo and JAK2 analyses. (I made sure she went to the lab today to have these tests drawn.) Due to the orthopneic aspect of her dyspnea, we will recheck an echocardiogram today. She is to continue her chelation regimen."

The echocardiogram was unrevealing; certainly, heart failure (of any cause) was not causing her shortness of breath.

Betty returned a month later, at the end of January 2010. She had increased her imatinib to 200 mg/d, but it hadn't helped her feel any better. In fact, her breathing was worse and her local pulmonologist had started her on continuous oxygen therapy a week earlier, and then, the day before visiting me, she contracted the gastrointestinal virus that had already run through the rest of her family. The last hemoglobin, checked locally one week earlier, was down to a still very normal 13 g/dl, the JAK2 mutation analysis from late December was negative (that is, this almost certainly wasn't polycythemia vera) – and, very interestingly, her epo level from late December, when her hemoglobin was a completely normal 14, was three times the upper limit of normal.

What to do? As usual, I copied and pasted and edited my prior assessment (documentation requirements keep growing and growing, so thank goodness copy-and-paste is available in our electronic medical record systems, though it of course incurs an obligation to edit what you paste to make sure it agrees with the findings in the present visit rather than the prior visit): "Very complex situation, 'pure red cell aplasia' effectively resolved thanks to some combination of imatinib and antihistamines, and the recent attempt to wean her off imatinib has clearly shown she needs imatinib as part of her regimen for controlling her mast cell disease. I think her persistent asthmatic-type symptoms (and her ocular symptoms) are signs of continued aberrant mast cell overactivity, but increased H1 blocking and imatinib haven't helped, and she previously tried montelukast to no benefit. I find myself wondering whether nebulized cromolyn would be helpful." I decided to discuss it with her local hematologist first, and when we had this conversation later in the week, he said he would prescribe it.

Betty returned two months later, at the end of March '10. All of her symptoms were worse, and although we hadn't changed any medications in late January, her hemoglobin had declined to 11.5 by

March 1 and then crashed to 8.5 by March 22. Her local hematologist restarted transfusions.

The next two years was a series of unrelenting disappointments, as Betty tried numerous maneuvers with her medications, including trials of many other medications (dasatinib, doxepin, pentosan, hydroxyurea, ketotifen, and others). She also dealt with new problems including hypothyroidism, megaloblastic anemia from excessive folate consumption from the time with polycythemia, and new scarring (fibrosis) in her marrow, creating some concern for a hematologic malignancy called myelofibrosis, except that the disease usually causes the spleen to massively enlarge, yet she had no enlargement at all. Along the way, too, there was a deep vein thrombosis, and warfarin anticoagulation had to be added to her regimen. Finally, in April 2012, when she mentioned to me that her insurance had changed that year, I recalled that I had wanted to try oral cromolyn near the beginning of all of this but couldn't due to insurance problems. Her new insurer, though, would cover it.

She returned in August 2012, and though nothing else had improved, she hadn't needed a transfusion in two months and her hemoglobin had risen from 7.3 in April to 11.2. She was pleased with that, but seeing as how she was still otherwise quite symptomatic, we discussed having her try yet other medications. In the end, though, we decided to make no changes. I asked her to return in another four months, but I haven't seen her since and I've received no follow-up from her local hematologist.

And, as with Marlene, I'll end Betty's story at this point with a final note that the above-recounted odyssey is actually a significant simplification of her story.

Chapter 4: OMG, It's Everywhere, and I've Been Missing It All Along, Or, So Who Is This Occam Guy, and Why and How Is His Razor Making Bets That I Shouldn't Take?

It was May of 2009. I had diagnosed MCAS in Shelly, Marlene, Betty…and several others, to wit:

> The 24-year old woman with JAK2-positive essential thrombocytosis, Budd-Chiari syndrome (clotting in the liver's portal vein), a "lupus-like syndrome," hypothyroidism, chronic headaches, fatigue, and many other chronic, waxing/waning symptoms. 24-hour urinary prostaglandin D_2 661 ng/ml and plasma free catecholamines just like Shelly had. Tryptase normal.

> Multiple "poor-phenotype" sickle cell anemia patients (male and female) with findings that could not possibly be attributed to sickle cell anemia including various autoantibodies (but without the diseases usually associated with those autoantibodies), chronic modest monocytosis, and intermittent modest eosinophilia and even occasional modest basophilia.

> A 45-year old woman whose relatively new autoimmune hemolytic anemia, controlled on azathioprine, couldn't possibly explain her undefined connective tissue syndrome ("fibromyalgia vs. ANA/dsDNA-negative lupus vs. relapsing polychondritis"), severe obstructive sleep apnea, vitamin D deficiency, episodic flares of type III (idiopathic) angioedema and multisystem inflammation. 24-hour urinary prostaglandin D_2 803 ng/ml. Normal bone marrow.

> A 34-year old schoolteacher with unrelenting fatigue, always feeling cold, chronic mild eye irritation, waxing/waning general abdominal discomfort, frequent acute onslaught of hives, and premature menopause. 24-hour urinary prostaglandin D_2 377 ng/ml.

> A 52-year old professor with beta-thalassemia major, transfusional hemosiderosis, osteoporosis, hypoparathyroidism, hypothyroidism, type 2 diabetes mellitus, gastroesophageal reflux disease, cardiomyopathy, history of deep venous thrombosis, hepatitis C, osteoarthritis, kidney stones, pseudoxanthoma elasticum, modest eosinophilia, slight basophilia. Chronic fatigue and malaise way out of proportion to her degree of anemia (quite mild, actually, thanks to the intensive transfusion schedule she insisted on out of thinking that her fatigue was due to her anemia, yet the transfusions never really seemed to help her feel better), chronic itching, diffuse aching, insomnia. Elevated random urinary prostaglandin D_2. Normal bone marrow.

A 74-year old woman with longstanding stable Stage I chronic lymphocytic leukemia and a rafter of other symptoms not easily attributable to CLL including fatigue, depression, aching, fevers, chills, sweats, anorexia, nausea, constipation, and modest abnormalities in laboratory coagulation tests. Elevated plasma histamine, increased mast cells in stomach and colon biopsies.

A 75-year old man with cutaneous lupus, lifelong environmental allergies, skin cancers, fatigue, multiple anti-phospholipid antibodies, well controlled diabetes mellitus type 2, peripheral neuropathy, longstanding difficult-to-control hypertension, chronic kidney disease, gout, mini-strokes, and an IgE level of 3,300 without other signs of hyperIgE (Job) syndrome. Mildly elevated tryptase, elevated histamine, and a "Shelly" pattern to his plasma free catecholamines.

A 50-year old hospital worker with iron-deficiency anemia of uncertain cause, severe colonic diverticulosis (without bleeding), aching, itching, eye irritation, chronic sense of being cold and constant daily night sweats but no fevers, incessant weight gain despite no changes in diet or exercise, positive TCRGR in the blood, lactose and oral iron intolerance, vitamin D deficiency, mild diffuse pulmonary inflammation of uncertain cause, mild osteoporosis, chronic gastroesophageal reflux disease. Elevated 24-hour urinary prostaglandin D_2, elevated neuron-specific enolase, and a "Shelly" pattern to her plasma free catecholamines.

A 34-year old government worker with chronic gastroesophageal reflux disease, intermittent rash, idiopathic hip pain, chronic mild eosinophilia. Mildly elevated tryptase, CD117$^+$CD2$^+$, KIT-D816V-negative duodenal mast cells.

A 34-year old woman with the rare blood disease of paroxysmal nocturnal hemoglobinuria well controlled on the extremely expensive drug eculizumab, odd infections such as mastitis and parvovirus B19, persistent left upper abdominal quadrant pain, years of morning sore throat, nightly wakings with nausea and soaking sweats, chronic waxing/waning tingling of her bilateral toes, episodic distal weakness for no clear reason, constant constipation, waxing/waning diffuse migratory aching of both large and small joints, frequent presyncopal episodes, asymptomatic gastritis positive for H. pylori. Significantly elevated urinary N-methylhistamine and prostaglandin D_2 plus increased mast cells in a colon biopsy, but negative serum tryptase and marrow exam.

A 51-year old nurse with a plethora of ailments since childhood including idiopathic rapid weight gain in the few years (especially the last year – more than 100 lbs.!) prior to her gastric bypass at age 47, chronic fatigue, malaise, presyncope, diffuse muscular and joint aching, right thigh burning sensation, chronic cold sensation about her face, inability to correct chronic hypokalemia despite multiple medication adjustments, episodic diffuse migratory rashes and pruritus, profuse night sweats, episodic tingling/numbness in her face, fingers, and toes, a bad reaction recently to a horsefly bite, "dryness"-type irritation in her eyes, polydipsia, poor memory, episodic migratory edema that tends to principally affect her feet, lips, and tongue, frequent presyncopal (and even occasional syncopal) spells, anemia of chronic inflammation, iron deficiency of uncertain etiology given absence of detectable bleeding and normal oral iron absorption prior to her bypass, history of Graves' disease (failed multiple medical regimens, then ablation, then replacement therapy, strongly positive IgG anti-phospholipid antibody and a modestly elevated IgM anti-prothrombin antibody but no actual clotting suggestive of antiphospholipid antibody syndrome. Persistently 2-fold-normal plasma histamine and a fluctuating (but at times as high as 4-fold-normal) serum chromogranin A, and a significantly increased number of mast cells seen on CD117 immunohistochemical staining (66 per high power field) of a colonoscopic biopsy.

A 50-year old male long-term acute leukemia survivor, fatigued but not achy, frequent upper respiratory "infections," anemia of chronic inflammation, now with a persistent, substantial, inexplicable elevation of creatine kinase. Slightly elevated 24-hour urinary prostaglandin D_2, slightly elevated serum prostaglandin D_2, slightly elevated chromogranin A, and a "Shelly" pattern to his plasma free catecholamines.

A 40-year old male six-year survivor of widely metastatic medullary thyroid cancer with waxing/waning nausea, diarrhea, bilateral breast tenderness and mastorrhea, eye irritation, episodic visual blurriness, occasional diplopia, diffuse arthritis, dyspnea, aching, diffusely migratory tics, non-specific bilateral leg neuropathy, hyperglycemia, hypokalemia, relative hypernatremia, hypertension, elevated AST/ALT, low PTT, moderate to severe thrombocytopenia, mild anemia, lymphopenia, anasarca, and MRSA abscesses. Repeatedly seven-fold-elevated urinary prostaglandin D_2, plus a six-fold-normal chromogranin A (the latter of which might have been coming from the thyroid cancer, but not the former).

An elderly man with myeloma and many other problems myeloma couldn't possibly explain.

A middle-aged man with anti-phospholipid antibody syndrome (APABS) and many other problems APABS couldn't possibly explain.

A young man with iron-supplementation-refractory iron-deficiency anemia and many other long unexplained problems.

A middle-aged woman with iron-supplementation-refractory iron-deficiency anemia and many other long unexplained problems.

Another middle-aged woman with iron-supplementation-refractory iron-deficiency anemia and many other long unexplained problems.

An elderly woman with hydroxyurea-controlled hypereosinophilic syndrome without any of the mutations typically seen in that disease, and with many other chronic problems very difficult to attribute to HES.

A middle-aged woman, whose kidneys failed in her early teens for no identifiable reason, lost two transplanted kidneys over the next decade for no identifiable reasons, with chronic pancytopenia and many other long unexplained problems.

A woman with anti-phospholipid antibody syndrome and many other problems not possibly attributable to APABS.

A man with polycythemia vera (PV) who then developed APABS and many other problems impossible to attribute to PV or APABS.

A middle-aged woman with well-controlled essential thrombocytosis (ET) and a rafter of mild symptoms impossible to attribute to her ET.

A middle-aged woman with a lifetime's worth of idiopathic intestinal tract and other problems and eventually enough weight gain to go to gastric bypass which led to weight loss but no impact on any of her other problems which couldn't be attributed to her weight to begin with.

A middle-aged woman with an idiopathic hypercoagulability and a rafter of other problems impossible to attribute to her clots.

An asymptomatic man long treated for polycythemia vera but now found to be negative for the JAK2 mutation.

A middle-aged man with severe autoimmune thrombocytopenic purpura, refractory to all but the very latest drugs, with a rafter of other problems impossible to attribute to ITP.

A middle-aged man with a quarter century's worth of an uncountable number of heart attacks and strokes of unidentifiable cause and a rafter of other problems impossible to attribute to any known clotting disorder.

An elderly woman with well-controlled essential thrombocytosis and chronic idiopathic headaches and a rafter of other problems impossible to attribute to ET.

And those were just the ones I saw in January 2009 in whom I suspected MCAS, and then proved it in the next few months. (You can well imagine, too, that I was realizing I had been "missing" this diagnosis all along throughout all of my training and my 13 years of post-training practice to that point. My diagnostic failings weren't my fault, of course. They were simply the product of my ignorance – a blissful ignorance I had been sharing with all other doctors present and past. How could I have known about something that hadn't been taught and hadn't even come forth yet in my specialty's journals? But there was no denying, as I thought back to various "mystery" patients I had seen over the years (and failed to definitively diagnose), that MCAS likely was the key issue in many of them.)

My goodness. So many different presentations, so many different problems, all sharing the same odd, rare side issue? What was going on here? Was it odd? Was it rare? And was it a side issue? In other words, was it normal mast cell activation as a reaction to other diseases? Or was it something more fundamental?

What was more likely? Was it more likely that Shelly had not only a rare form of PV that was negative for the JAK2 mutation (2% of all cases is the percentage that's usually recited) but also an odd form of mastocytosis so rare it wasn't even described yet in the literature? Was it likely that she was really that special a person, that uniquely unlucky a person? Or was it more likely that she had not two problems but rather one problem that was biologically capable of causing all that had gone awry in her?

Obviously, in our universe, the odds favor one cause over two or more – the simpler solution over the more complex solution. And this, dear reader, is the essence of that bit of pith that's been known for the last 160 years as Occam's Razor.

Sir William of Ockham was a philosopher and logician in early 14th century England who espoused the notion that assumptions should be posited only when necessary. In other words, you're probably straying from the truth of a matter if you have to make up more stories than necessary to explain the matter. The "razor" comes into play from the sense that one ought to strive to trim away unnecessary parts of an explanation.

Sir William actually never referred to his insight as Occam's Razor. (Note Ockham became Occam over the centuries thanks to the fungibility of English spelling.) It was another Sir William – Sir William Hamilton, a Scottish logician and educator – who coined the term about 500 years later. But Ockham was far from the first to espouse this maxim of simplicity. A similar principle can be found in the writings of many earlier philosophers including Thomas Aquinas and John Duns Scotus (13th century), Maimonides (12th century), Ptolemy (2nd century), and even Aristotle (4th century BC). Later expressions, too, of the Razor can be found in the writings of other luminaries such as Isaac Newton and Albert Einstein. The Razor has been key in some of the greatest scientific discoveries including Dalton's atomic theory, Einstein's special theory of relativity, and Planck's theory of quantum mechanics. The "grand unified theory" sought by physicists to explain our entire universe, if ever found, will be the ultimate demonstration of the principle of the Razor.

It's important to understand that the Razor doesn't say the *simpler* of two explanations is the more likely, nor does it say that the more *popular*, more widely *believed*, or easier to *understand* explanation is the more likely. It doesn't even say that one explanation is necessarily more likely than two or more. All it says is that if one explanation can account for at least as much of the observed truth of a situation as two or more explanations, then it's more likely that the one explanation is closer to the true explanation than the two or more explanations.

Physicians have long taught their medical students that Occam's Razor is integral to the art of diagnosis. (And, to be sure, it applies in, and is taught in, many other disciplines, too.) But somewhere along the way in the course of medical training and practice, many of us lose sight of it. I know, because I sure did and I can also see it in the many notes my many colleagues write on their many patients with very long medical problem lists. The fact is, in a busy medical practice, it's much easier to forget about Occam and just unthinkingly accept, in spite of the contrary odds, that the patient really is so unlucky as to have acquired 10, or 20, or 50 problems, all developing independently of one another. Or perhaps somewhere in the backs of our minds we subconsciously understand that such patients really aren't so unlucky and likely do have a unifying diagnosis – but our training and experience haven't afforded us knowledge of that diagnosis, and we simply do not have the time to figure it out.

It's an open secret that most physicians around the world are paid for two services, and two services only. For one, we are paid to see a patient. It does not matter if we help the patient or not; regardless, we are paid for the act of having seen a patient. And for the other, we are paid to perform procedures on patients. Again, it does not matter if the procedures help the patients or not; regardless, we are paid simply for having performed the procedures.

In an ideal world, we would be paid in accordance with how much we have helped the patient (i.e., what the "outcome" is), regardless of whether our administered intervention were simply talking to the patient, or prescribing a medication, or ordering a diagnostic test, or performing a procedure, etc. But nobody has yet figured out how to quantify how much "help" has been provided a patient in any given doctor-patient encounter. And perhaps it's something that simply cannot be quantified. To be sure, the patient, the doctor, and the payer likely will have different notions about how much the patient has been helped in any given encounter. Upon whose notion of how much the patient has been helped should the physician's compensation be based?

Lacking any method for fairly quantifying how much a patient has been "helped," all we've been able to figure out is a very rudimentary accounting for how much a patient has been "served." We note on our bills whether we have seen the patient in the office or in the hospital, we identify one of about three or four categories of roughly how much time was spent in the encounter (maximum is about one hour), we note which procedures (if any) we performed, and we note which diagnoses we addressed. That's it. In the vast majority of doctor-patient encounters throughout the world, that's all that determines how much we get paid for having served the patient. And, unlike lawyers, we don't get paid for a single minute of time we put in on a patient's behalf once we're out of eye contact with the patient.

Thus, lacking any incentive to spend more time thinking about a unifying solution to the patient's 50 problems, it shouldn't surprise anyone that most physicians, facing waiting rooms and hospital wards full of patients needing their attention, take the easier route of attending to just the tiny slice of the patient's full problem set that constitutes his or her "chief complaint" at the time of the encounter.

I often begin my presentations on MCAS by showing the classic cartoon in which several blind men are contemplating the elephant before them, each trying to deduce the nature of the whole beast from the small part – a tusk, a leg, a trunk, a tail – before him. The analogy to the modern era of dominantly subspecialized medicine is inescapable: each physician sees – for reasons we'll address in a later chapter – little more than the one particular perspective of the patient that's most comfortable for that physician by dint of training and experience (and I'll be the first to note that I was, and still am, one of those physicians). (I should also note that a few of my patients, in view of that aptly metaphorical graphic, have taken to calling themselves "The Elephant Club.") In this vein, I'd like to spend the next several chapters highlighting what MCAS looks like from each of its many perspectives.

Chapter 5: Who is MCAS? Demographic Considerations

MCAS is epidemic.

Early research on the epidemiology of MCAS is suggesting that as many as 14-17% of the general population is affected. That's one out of every 6-7 individuals. Look around you right now. If this early research is correct, then if there are at least five other people in sight, odds are at least one of you has MCAS.

MCAS does not discriminate with respect to age.

Symptoms can initially appear at any age, but most commonly it is as an adolescent or child, sometimes even as an infant or neonate, at which symptoms first appear.   Due to the non-specific nature of almost every symptom of the disease, though, the diagnosis virtually always goes unsuspected in childhood and adolescence – and for a very long time thereafter. In fact, let's be honest: MCAS has been recognized only so recently that it must be the case that most MCAS patients have gone to their graves with it never having been diagnosed. But don't blame the doctor for missing it. Even if one sets aside the fact of the general lack of awareness of MCAS in the medical community, there's also the fact that kids inevitably get sick from time to time. Does every sniffle mean MCAS? Every tummy ache? Of course not. But *chronic* sniffles or tummy aches, or headaches, or rash, or aches and pains, or fatigue – especially *chronic* symptoms in *multiple* systems which *can't be explained* by routine testing and which *don't respond well* to standard treatments – *might* be signs of MCAS.

MCAS is chronic.

By the time they are diagnosed, most MCAS patients have been chronically ill for decades. In fact, as I alluded above, because of (1) the multisystem presentation in most patients, with symptoms in different systems often presenting at different times, and (2) the general lack of awareness of MCAS in the medical community, most MCAS patients live their entire lives without diagnosis, or even suspicion, of the root issue underlying the plethora of problems (many of a generally inflammatory nature) that they often acquire.

No system in the body is immune to MCAS...

...not even the immune system. MCAS patients often are regarded as inexplicably chronically multisystemically ill, perhaps recognized by astute physicians as likely having an underlying systemic inflammatory syndrome, though they don't fit the pattern of any well-known such syndrome, with typical diagnostic testing often yielding negative or "borderline" results (the latter are more dangerous than the former, as they often lead to treatments that incur costs and side effects but don't usually help much), or perhaps results which are mild to severe in their degree of abnormality but soon inexplicably, spontaneously normalize. For example, I have seen MCAS patients who have undergone serial allergy tests which sometimes show them to be "allergic to everything" and at other times (with no changes in environment or treatment) show them to be allergic to nothing, obviously a source of great vexation for their allergists.

MCAS is a chameleon that confounds diagnostic testing and treatments for other diseases.

Though their presenting symptoms in any given system are most commonly subtle to moderate in degree, occasionally MCAS patients will present severe abnormalities (which may have emerged acutely, subacutely, or chronically) in one system or another (e.g., end-stage renal failure, refractory diarrhea, etc.), with "exhaustive" diagnostic testing failing to reveal a specific etiology. In fact – and as another reflection of its heterogeneity – MCAS can present with polar opposite abnormalities in different patients (e.g., gastrointestinal dysmotility principally manifesting as diarrhea in one patient vs. constipation in another patient, or bone marrow abnormalities principally manifesting as too many red blood cells in one patient vs. severe deficiency of red blood cell production in another patient).

As noted above, and unsurprisingly (for obvious reasons), MCAS patients often respond incompletely, or even outright poorly or intolerantly, to therapies targeted at their superficially apparent ailments. Many therapies, too, are targeted at inconstant abnormalities – for example, allergy desensitization shots for patients who on one allergy testing show allergy to "everything" while on another allergy testing show allergy to nothing – and, again, unsurprisingly respond incompletely, or even outright poorly or intolerantly.

Conversely, because MCAS often exacerbates and complicates other diseases (which may or may not be due to MCAS), standard treatments for such other diseases often demonstrate confoundingly less benefit than would be expected.

If Disease X doesn't usually produce Symptom Y, then maybe Symptom Y in Patient Z isn't due to Disease X no matter how much care has been invested in treating Disease X in Patient Z.

Some MCAS patients have definitively diagnosed inborn or acquired ailments (e.g., sickle cell anemia or obesity) which come to be blamed by many of their physicians for most or all of their symptoms even though it is difficult to explain many of these symptoms based on careful consideration of the biology of the inborn definitively diagnosed ailment. When a patient – particularly a patient with chronic multisystem polymorbidity, generally of an inflammatory theme – presents for evaluation (whether urgent/emergent or routine), it is important for the physician to consider whether the presenting symptoms are *typical* for the definitively diagnosed ailment or not. If not, it is important to consider the possibility that a co-morbid (and potentially underlying/unifying) illness may be present.

For example, the sickle cell anemia patient who presents with rash and unusually severe fatigue and diffuse joint pain instead of his usual "sickle cell crisis" pattern of just back and thigh pain is probably not having a sickle cell crisis or, at most, is having a different-than-usual sickle cell crisis that's almost certainly being triggered by something going on in the patient other than sickle cell anemia. Similarly, a severely fatigued patient with morbid obesity whose weight plummets from 400 lbs. to 150 lbs. following gastric bypass surgery, but whose fatigue doesn't improve one bit, probably has some cause for the fatigue other than the obesity, and perhaps that other cause is also the cause for the obesity.

The severity of MCAS often permanently "steps up" to a higher baseline level following severe stress.

MCAS patients often can identify a specific point in their lives – a month, a year, sometimes even a specific date – at which their general health took a distinct turn for the worse. Such points commonly follow – typically by days to weeks but sometimes by several months or mere hours – acute events of either significant psychological or physical stress (e.g., death of a family member, or vehicular trauma) or of significant new antigenic exposure (e.g., travel or relocation). If they have recognized the temporal association between trigger and illness, such patients not uncommonly are quite convinced – even "invested," sometimes for socioeconomic reasons – that the trigger was the cause of the illness. However, careful review of the patient's history virtually always reveals symptoms of MCAS to have been present long before "the turning point" – again, often dating back at least to adolescence and perhaps even to childhood or infancy. (I have long tried to teach my trainees that history is the hematologist's – indeed, any physician's – best friend. If the doctor can take a careful enough history, in most such instances he will come out of the exam room having a pretty good idea what's causing the patient's problems. Unfortunately, taking a "careful enough" history is a very difficult thing to do in today's health care systems – which is why modern health care systems are themselves impediments to diagnosing MCAS. We'll talk more about why the system is a big part of the problem in a later chapter.)

Most people will put up with virtually anything if they don't see any choice.

History, history, history. It may be hard in today's health care systems to take a "careful enough" (life-long!) history, but doing so really is imperative in the evaluation of not only a patient thought to possibly have MCAS but also any patient presenting a diagnostic mystery (including the diagnostic mystery of why a patient with a definitively established diagnosis isn't responding appropriately to standard therapy for that "definitively established" diagnosis). History taking must include a *complete* review of systems as well (something most doctors do less and less as they subspecialize more and more), as many MCAS patients have been so ill for so long that they have come to accept various aspects of their illness as a baseline "healthy" (or at least "normal") state for them. It has to be recognized, too, that after extensive evaluations fail to identify a diagnosis, let alone effective therapy, some patients come to naturally omit certain aspects of their illness when providing their history yet one more time to yet one more physician. For example, I have seen many MCAS patients who simply stopped telling their doctors about their many episodes of syncope (passing out) and presyncope (nearly passing out). One of my patients had been suffering unpredictable syncopal episodes on virtually a daily basis for 20 years. Extensive evaluation and empiric treatment efforts in the first two years after symptom onset were unproductive. His doctors at the time told him they had nothing further to offer him. He made many adjustments to his life to be able to still function as productively as possible and to minimize his potential for injuries from these episodes – and he continued to suffer these episodes but never again mentioned the problem to any doctor or nurse he met because he knew it would be pointless and might even engender additional (expensive) testing for no good reason. The many other doctors he met after that never asked him about such a symptom (why bother taking time with such a question? the vast majority of patients would never answer "Yes"), and since he no longer had any reason to believe any doctor could help him with this problem, he never mentioned it. Eighteen years later, in the extensive review of systems I went through the first time he saw me, I asked him about syncopal episodes and he answered with a shocked, jaw-dropping "How did you know?" Another patient had suffered near-daily syncope for five years following the birth of her first child (certainly a stressful event!) but had been told by her obstetrician, upon symptom onset, that post-partum syncope was common (not true) and would resolve "in time," so she patiently endured five years of this life-altering symptom without mentioning it to any of her other doctors before it came to light again in the extensive review of systems I took.

Chapter 6: The Constitutional Symptoms of MCAS, or, "I Feel Like Crap and I Can't Put It Any More Specifically Than That"

A major challenge facing MCAS patients is that many "feel awful in general" but externally appear "OK" (if perhaps not the absolute picture of health). Many times, too, symptoms relatively reliably worsen at particular points in the day that don't correspond with when they can see their regular doctors.

The "constitutional" issues in MCAS cover a wide ground.

Temperature anomalies – more commonly subjective than objective – are common. Most commonly in this area, MCAS patients report a sense of being cold most or all of the time, but they also sometimes report "low-grade fever" (as in, "I used to run a baseline of 96.5F, but now I'm 98.5-99 all the time but nobody thinks it's a fever"). Only occasionally does the MCAS patient report a true fever per medical definition (≥ 100.5F) and/or frank chills.

Fatigue and malaise – to varying degrees at varying times on varying days but which in some patients can sometimes can be utterly disabling (to the point of being literally unable to get out of bed) – is one of the most common symptoms of MCAS. The fatigue and malaise can be so disabling so often as to render some patients unemployable. Yet, the path to financial assistance for such is difficult for many reasons, not the least of which is because, again, externally they often appear "OK." Many patients have found that keeping detailed diaries of their symptoms and disabilities, together with engagement of a lawyer specializing in disability, to be helpful in their process of applying for assistance.

Unprovoked sweats are common and occur more often at night (sometimes soaking bedclothes and linens), but sometimes they occur in the daytime, too.

Decreased appetite ("anorexia") and "early satiety" (a sense of gastric fullness earlier in the meal than would be expected given how much was eaten) are common.

Changes in weight are common, too. Sometimes they are weight losses, and sometimes they are weight gains – sometimes to extraordinary degrees, to the point of seeking gastric bypass or banding surgery. And sometimes there is an even more puzzling fluctuation between weight losses and gains.

Unfortunately, even when the weight gain pattern suggests an endocrine or metabolic disease has emerged, our health care financing system incentivizes expensive surgical intervention (i.e., treatment) and disincentivizes the office evaluations and specialized testing needed to accurately identify the cause (i.e., diagnosis). Some of my MCAS patients have suffered weight gains of more than 100 lbs. in just one year despite no change in diet or activity, and in some their gastric bypass or banding surgeries either didn't help at all or helped only temporarily in taking the weight off – and didn't, of course, help any of their many other symptoms. There may be a role for gastric bypass or banding surgery in some weight-gaining variants of MCAS, but given that I have seen some weight-gaining MCAS patients then lose significant weight upon gaining control of their MCAS, it's not clear to me that gastric surgery is a necessary intervention in all morbidly overweight MCAS patients.

Here's an example:

> Marsha, a 70-year old overweight widow and retired career-long office manager, was referred in April 2011 for further evaluation of iron-deficiency anemia initially found at a routine check-up with her primary physician two months earlier. She initially said she had been asymptomatic at that time (though a very different truth soon emerged). She had not noticed any bleeding. Her local hematologist started her on oral iron supplementation, but this immediately made her persistently nauseous. She also began developing intermittent chills and waxing/waning exhaustion. Three weeks later she was given intravenous iron supplementation and acutely tolerated the infusion well, but her severe nausea relapsed the following day and had continued (along with the chills and exhaustion) to wax and wane ever since. EGD (with biopsies) had been performed but had not revealed any abnormality. She also said that until the nausea developed, her appetite had been good, though she noted regretfully that she had never lost any weight after a lap-band procedure in 2008. Her past history was also notable for a long history of difficult-to-regulate hypertension, depression since 1990, hypothyroidism, obstructive sleep apnea since 1995 (treated with chronic positive airway pressure (CPAP), chronic atrial fibrillation (which a cardiologist had noted in 2004 was refractory to multiple medications and was causing increasing (eventually daily) spells of marked dizziness, fatigue, and palpitations and which was eventually treated that year with ablation, yielding an immediate, sustained, complete response in these symptoms), diabetes mellitus type 2, cholecystectomy in 2003 (for chronic nausea, which immediately resolved with the procedure), lap-band surgery in 2008 for obesity (though unfortunately with no improvement), GERD for at least 10 years (interestingly, it appears the GERD and the atrial fibrillation initially developed around the same time, and she has been on nightly Nexium ever since), hyperlipidemia (controlled on a statin drug), and narrow-angle glaucoma which improved with laser treatment.

> Marsha's review of systems was interesting for a range of active issues that went well beyond her presenting complaints. Most interestingly, she noted that on January 1, 2011 (what stressor or exposure did she suffer on New Year's Eve?), she acutely suffered an outbreak of an

intensely pruritic, "measles-like" rash that lasted all day, with her scratching yielding "streaks like I had run through a briar patch." She went to an urgent care facility on that holiday and was prescribed the H_1 blockers diphenhydramine and hydroxyzine, which promptly resolved the problem, but in February the same problem again spontaneously returned. Her primary physician started her on the H_2 and H_1 blockers famotidine, hydroxyzine, and fexofenadine, which again quickly resolved that incident, but the symptoms continued to irregularly recur without apparent provocation. She also describes noting at these times a skin finding that sounded like dermatographism. She also noted she was continuing to use the "prn" (as needed) Atarax on a regular basis because the rash and itching would quickly relapse if she stopped this medication. Although she denied problems with fevers, sweats, headaches, irritated eyes, nasal sores, mouth sores, dysphagia, chest pain/discomfort, palpitations, vomiting, diarrhea, constipation, tingling/numbness, urinary issues, or presyncopal/syncopal spells, she endorsed frequent chills and a sense of feeling cold much of the time, chronic coryza that worsens with relapses of her pruritus, a low-grade chronic throat irritation that's new in the last few months and which makes her want to frequently clear her throat, a new chronic mild hoarseness, mild dyspnea on (minimal) exertion, waxing/waning fatigue/malaise that at times is extremely intense, chronic mild dependent edema, relatively new easy bruisability, relatively new slowness of healing, and new (since December 2010) occasional episodes of cognitive dysfunction which she hadn't noticed herself but which she was aware of because her daughter has taken recently to telling her at times that she "wasn't thinking straight.

There were multiple cancers but no known hematologic or rheumatologic issues in Marsha's family history. Her daughter suffered refractory GERD, which wasn't yet helped by the gastric bypass surgery she had recently undergone. She denied any tobacco or illegal substance use or alcohol abuse.

Marsha had developed a new allergy to medical tape in the last few months; it quickly caused an itching rash similar to what had spontaneously appeared about her skin since January 2011. She also noted that contrast dye during her cardiac catheterization in 2004 (during which no significant CAD was found, per the old cardiology notes) quickly caused a widespread break-out of pruritic rash, but she subsequently has tolerated contrast dye OK with premedication of unknown type.

Examination found an obese woman in no distress. Blood pressure was 150/67 and weight, at 101.4 kg, was up 3.4 kg since November 2010. She had scattered small bruises and abrasions of origin uncertain to her along with small patches of macular erythema (all of which she said was new in the last few months). There was a tiny bit of edema in the bilateral forelegs and feet, and on a light scratch test on the upper back, mild dermatographism quickly emerged and was long sustained.

Old labs from 2004 included borderline anemia with minimal microcytosis (decrease in red blood cell size), otherwise completely normal CBC, and a mildly elevated glucose at 163 mg/dl. (Another thing that was interesting about her CBC was the normality of one of the numbers on the CBC, the "RDW" (red cell distribution width). The RDW is a measure of the variability in size in the red blood cells, and it should be normal when the bone marrow is monotonously pumping out red blood cells (of whatever size the marrow is genetically programmed to pump out), but the RDW edges upward as the earliest sign of any disorder in red blood cell production such as from iron deficiency. So this patient's small red blood cells with a normal RDW suggested a lot more that her marrow was programmed to make small red blood cells rather than the alternative that it was producing small red blood cells due to iron deficiency or some other acquired abnormality.)

My assessment at the time was thus: "She may be anemic and the ferritin may be low (though without knowing that her MCV [mean corpuscular volume, or average red blood cell size] is significantly low, it's hard for me to conclude with any confidence that this is an iron-deficiency anemia), but there's no apparent blood loss here (nor is there history to suggest a GI or GU malignancy that might be causing blood loss), and even if an iron deficiency due to malabsorption can be demonstrated here, there's no way such a problem alone could be causing the full extent of the problems here. Although I don't think a colonoscopy in a 70-year old woman is unreasonable, I will be surprised if an explanation for her (presumed) iron deficiency – let alone all the rest of her problems – is detected by that procedure. There's also the issue that the degree of fatigue/malaise she describes (along with its waxing/waning nature) is far beyond what would be expected in somebody with a Hgb of nearly 10 g/dl. Overall, given the full range of problems here, I get much more a sense of a systemic inflammatory syndrome of some sort than an isolated iron-deficiency anemia. Actually, the specific natures of the problems here are such that what I most suspect is actually going on at the root of all of this 'weirdness' (not only of late but perhaps underlying most or all of her problems going back for 10+ years) is a systemic mast cell disease, much more likely mast cell activation syndrome than systemic mastocytosis."

Testing for MCAS was sent (also, an oral iron absorption test was checked, which showed significantly reduced absorption) and H_1/H_2

histamine receptor blocking was empirically increased from once daily to twice daily.

Marsha returned a few weeks later to learn that her plasma histamine level had been found to be significantly elevated at 20 nmol/L (normal 0-8), and her chromogranin A level was 2,075 ng/ml (normal 0-50). Interestingly, too, her anemia and microcytosis had completely resolved. However, her symptoms were no better, and a subsequent trial of lorazepam didn't help, either. Oral cromolyn did provide some measure of symptomatic improvement, but low-dose quercetin proved to be the most helpful drug for her, immediately resolving her fatigue and malaise, nausea, diarrhea, and anorexia.

Another constitutional issue that's common in MCAS is itching ("pruritus"), and it usually afflicts different parts of the body from one episode to another, although sometimes the itch is maddeningly persistent in one particular area of the body in which there is absolutely no abnormality apparent on physical examination or imaging of any type, or even on biopsy. Sometimes the pruritus is "aquagenic," meaning it is triggered by exposure to water, and when that happens, it's far more often hot than cold water that sets it off.

Most doctors and nurses begin encountering early in their careers a range of patients with unusual extents of "sensitivities" to a wide variety of provocateurs (drugs, foods, environs). In my experience, MCAS patients definitely have a predilection for suffering odd, and prolific, sensitivities. The oddness includes not only reactivity to unusual substances but also reactivity to common substances to which there ordinarily wouldn't be expected to be any reactivity (for example, acetaminophen, or levothyroxine, or food or hair coloring). And yet, they sometimes maddeningly confound their allergists by demonstrating negative skin patch allergy testing – or, even more confounding, skin patch testing that *alternates* back and forth between positive and negative, often despite no significant intervention to cause such changes.

Chapter 7: Rashes, Ridges, and a Permanent Bad Hair Day: Integumentary Findings in MCAS

The body's "integument" – its outer covering, essentially, including skin, hair, teeth, and nails – is obviously a crucial barrier, a defense line, providing our vital internal tissues major protection from assaults from the environment (e.g., trauma, infection, heat/cold, etc.). And since the principal job of the mast cell, ever since its origins several hundred million years ago, is to serve as a sentinel of bodily assault and to sound the right alarms at the right volumes, in the right places, and at the right times, it should be no surprise that one of the more common places mast cells situate themselves is in the skin (the hair and nails, of course, don't contain any cells, though their roots at the skin do) – and therefore, if your mast cells go awry, it also should be no surprise that there will be consequences for the integument.

"Belle" was quite a sight. Somewhat mentally simple, morbidly obese, and spending her days in an adult day care program at age 49, she was cared for at nights and on weekends by her sister. She had been suffering blood clots – curiously in the arms and neck, mostly venous but also one arterial stroke, but not in the legs – for at least 15 years. The clots had never resolved on heparin or warfarin, and if she missed even a single dose of her high-dose enoxaparin, it seemed the clot in the left neck would immediately get worse and that side of the neck would start swelling. She was fatigued, occasionally short of breath, occasionally coughed, and occasionally had aches and pains scattered about her chest and various joints in no particular pattern. Aside from her obesity, the only notable finding on exam was what seemed to be some sort of a soft tissue prominence in the upper left chest; she said this was the area that became more prominent if she missed an enoxaparin dose. She also had extensive bruising all about the abdominal wall where her enoxaparin shots were administered.

Given that her abnormal clotting had begun at a relatively young age, my fellow and I wondered if Belle had an inborn hypercoagulable state, though we also wondered about an autoimmune issue. We sent off the appropriate labs and also obtained an ultrasound of the curious soft tissue prominence.

Belle returned a month later. The ultrasound had shown chronic left internal jugular and subclavian vein clots but no acute issues, and the extensive battery of labs we had run had shown no inborn hypercoagulable state and no autoimmune issue, but there was no question she was inflamed: her sed rate and C-reactive protein were quite high. We ordered T-cell-receptor gene-rearrangement (TCRGR) studies looking for any hint of a T-cell lymphoma (compared to B-cell lymphomas, T-cell lymphomas can present in much weirder ways and have more of a propensity to involve the skin – though she obviously couldn't have had a T-cell lymphoma her whole life) as well as some additional esoteric testing on the peripheral blood for inborn hypercoagulable states. We also requested a rheumatology consultation.

Belle returned again after another month. The TCRGR was positive, but there was no other evidence of lymphoma. The additional hypercoagulability testing showed a couple of inborn states associated with modestly increased risk for clotting, but there was no way these abnormalities could account for anywhere near the extent of abnormal clotting she had suffered.

This was now nearly a year after my first diagnosis of MCAS, and I was becoming suspicious that perhaps this, too, was another variant presentation. I asked for MCAS diagnostic screening.

Belle returned a month later, and many of the MCAS tests were positive (though the tryptase was only slightly elevated, nowhere near what's needed to diagnose systemic mastocytosis). Next, according to the textbooks, would come a bone marrow biopsy, which was going to be difficult given her size. I wanted to wait first for the rheumatologist's opinion.

She returned a month later. The rheumatologist had found no rheumatologic issues in her. We made plans for the marrow biopsy.

When Belle returned yet another month later, she underwent the marrow biopsy, which was difficult for me (her bone cortex curiously proved extraordinarily difficult to drill through – might this have been the osteosclerosis of mast cell disease?), but she breezed through it without any discomfort at all.

She returned a couple months later. The previous symptoms persisted, and she also was now showing a diffuse eruption of very itchy "bug-bite" sores about much of her body. Her marrow had appeared normal on every test except flow cytometry, which had shown two very tiny populations of abnormal mast cells, one co-expressing CD117 and CD25 ("CD117$^+$CD25$^+$") and the other co-expressing CD117 and CD2 ("CD117$^+$CD2$^+$").

There was no question Belle had MCAS. It was time for treatment. I started her on antihistamines (diphenhydramine and famotidine). I also had her seen that same day by one of our dermatologists for her new skin eruption, but no specific diagnosis was made and no biopsy was obtained. She was instructed to keep the affected areas clean and was prescribed a steroid cream.

She returned a month later obviously feeling and looking better. Her fatigue, breathing, aching, itching, and skin sores were much better.

Extensive bruising continued just as before, though. I asked her to try increasing the diphenhydramine.

She returned after another couple of months. There had been no further improvements, but she was more tired. The odd, persistent soft tissue prominence at the base of the left neck and in the left upper chest was a bit more prominent than usual, and I asked for a repeat ultrasound. I asked her to try substituting loratadine in place of diphenhydramine.

Belle returned after another couple of months. Fatigue was improved. Itching and skin sores remained largely in remission, but the extensive bruising continued. The repeat ultrasound at the previous visit had shown no improvement in the chronic left internal jugular and subclavian vein clots. It was time to try a different anticoagulant, so I switched her from enoxaparin to fondaparinux.

She returned yet again nine months later (much later than I had ordered), saying that everything had been stable (no better, no worse) on fondaparinux for the first few months, and then she had been admitted to her local hospital for a seven-week stay for pneumonia and heart and kidney failure. She also noted marked worsening of a problem that had long been with her but to a much lesser degree, the presence of mildly painful subcutaneous "knots" or "nodules" of all sizes and distributed irregularly and sparsely all about her body, often centrally within a bruised field (many of which were not the sites of fondaparinux injections).

I was concerned that her inadequately controlled mast cells were the principal factor underlying her severe episodic troubles with infection, and I felt it necessary to try much more aggressive mast cell stabilization. Cromolyn, I thought, would be insufficient, as it is not absorbed. I started her on low-dose imatinib.

She returned a month later reporting substantially better energy and substantial regression of her nodules and bruising. We kept the imatinib dose the same.

She returned after another month. Her subcutaneous knots were gone, her bruises were gone (even though she was still on fondaparinux), her energy level was much further improved, she was increasingly getting around without her walker, and she was socializing much more at the adult day care program.

She returned three months later. All improvements were sustained. She was now eating three regular meals a day without still feeling hungry. She was even beginning to lose some weight.

I tried to transition her from fondaparinux to aspirin at this point, but she proved intolerant of aspirin (not uncommon in MCAD), and ultimately I switched her anticoagulation to dabigatran without further incident. Meanwhile, her subcutaneous nodularity and bruising have remained in complete remission. She has been regularly dancing in her day care program for the last four years.

Around the time I was figuring out what was going on in Belle, I began having an e-mail dialogue with another patient (who I eventually saw a year or so later) who had been diagnosed with "Dercum's disease" but who also had many other problems that Dercum's disease couldn't explain and which, as she had learned from reading on the Internet, were much more consistent with MCAD.

What on earth was Dercum's disease? A little bit of reading discovered that it was yet another syndrome of unknown cause (first identified by a neurologist, Francis Dercum, at Jefferson Medical College in Philadelphia in 1892, and going by several other names, too, including adiposis dolorosa, Anders' syndrome, and Dercum-Vitaut syndrome) which, according to the National Human Genome Research Institute, "is a rare condition characterized by multiple, painful fatty lipomas that occur chiefly in post-menopausal, obese women of middle age. The lipomas are located primarily on the trunk and on the extremities close to the trunk. Unlike ordinary lipomas, there is also pain that can be severe and sometimes debilitating. Dercum's disease is a chronic condition and tends to be progressive. This syndrome consists of four cardinal symptoms: (1) multiple, painful, fatty masses; (2) generalized obesity, usually in menopausal age; (3) weakness and fatigability; and (4) mental disturbances, including emotional instability, depression, epilepsy, confusion and dementia." Further reading found that its onset is "insidious," that the pain is out of proportion to what one would expect from the physical exam, and that the patients often describe a body-wide pain, sometimes specifically citing that all of their fat (not just their lipomas) hurts.

Did Belle have Dercum's disease? Is Dercum's disease yet another variant of MCAS? I don't know. Maybe. All I know at this point is that if they did have Dercum's disease, low-dose imatinib sure seems to work well for it, at least in my limited experience with Belle and a few others since who have presented to me, and therapeutically responded, in similar fashion. This is another research project for the future.

At a minimum, Belle was just one example of the Wacky Wide World of Weirdness that mast cell activation disease can cause in the skin. Here's another one:

"Delores" first came to me about four years after Belle. Delores clearly didn't like the several-hour drive (even though she was chauffeured by her caretaker), but she came to see me anyway because nothing that had been tried for her weird, diffuse, intensely itchy rash had helped. Her local hematologist/oncologist, meanwhile, couldn't find an explanation for her persistently mildly elevated white blood cell count, and even though the rash had caused him to suspect a mast cell disorder, the tryptase level he had checked was normal, so (per any doctor's standard training) it couldn't be a mast cell disorder and he felt an explanation was still needed.

When I took the full history of all the problems she had ever had, this 79-year old woman had to go all the way back to adolescence, when thyroid problems of some sort were diagnosed. She had had parts of thyroid gland removed in her teens and again in her 20s, by which time she had been diagnosed with Hashimoto's thyroiditis, an autoimmune disease of the thyroid. She told me the second thyroid surgery caused nerve damage leaving her with permanent partial laryngeal obstruction. She also suffered "cystitis" (bladder inflammation) of unknown cause frequently in her 20s. Other surgeries along the way included a tonsillectomy and adenoidectomy, hysterectomy, and a face-lift. Significant osteoarthritis began developing in mid-life involving her spine, hands, and large joints in the upper and lower extremities; by the time she came to see me, she had long been using a motorized scooter for virtually all mobility including within her house. She also developed type 2 diabetes mellitus in mid-life, and though it had been well controlled, she also had developed a peripheral neuropathy which was attributed by default to the diabetes because no other cause was apparent.

She had slowly but steadily gained weight since her third and last pregnancy (how often might the stresses of pregnancy and delivery lead to escalation of MCAS?), and she was diagnosed on a sleep study at some point in her late 60s as having obstructive sleep apnea. Unfortunately, she was intolerant of CPAP and had slept ever since the sleep apnea diagnosis with oxygen via nasal cannula, which she felt helped her somewhat, though she still was waking every morning with a headache.

Her son chimed in, too, recalling his mother complaining about multiple "urinary tract infections" over the last few years. Delores then added that the pattern of these "infections" was odd: urine dipstick testing was negative for infection on several occasions even when she felt like she had an infection, and sometimes dipsticks were negative but cultures then showed "mild" infection which did not respond to an initial course of an antibiotic and required a second course of a different antibiotic before the symptoms would resolve. She also noted new urinary incontinence in the last year and said she currently had to urinate about every two hours.

As for the rash, Delores said it had been going on for a couple of years, consisting of both patches of pruritic macular erythema as well as intensely itchy clusters of "bug-bite" ulcerations and "sores" despite absence of any known insect attacks. She denied any significant travel or other concerning exposures.

She had been thoroughly evaluated by a local hematologist/oncologist recently for about a year's worth of minimal elevation in the white blood cell count. The only other abnormality found on blood testing was a persistent, mild elevation in a general class of immune system antibody called immunoglobulin A (IgA) and a marked elevation in the erythrocyte sedimentation rate ("sed rate"). He entertained the possibility of mastocytosis, but a serum tryptase level was normal at 7 ng/ml.

She denied fevers, chills, sweats, irritation of the eyes or mouth, visual problems, chest pain/discomfort, palpitations, trouble swallowing, nausea, vomiting, or enlarged or tender lymph nodes. However, she endorsed feeling cold all the time, chronic fatigue, diffusely migratory aching, diffusely migratory itching (not necessarily coincident with the aching), the above-noted morning headaches, chronic irritation of the nose and throat, chronic shortness of breath on minimal exertion, reflux, diarrhea alternating with constipation, the above-described rash, edema in the legs, presyncopal events about once or twice a quarter, and the above-noted urinary issues.

The son who accompanied her also had Hashimoto's thyroiditis and was on thyroid hormone supplementation. Another son, too, had been diagnosed as hypothyroid and was also on thyroid hormone supplementation. The patient also said her father died of hypothyroidism in his 30s. In addition, her own mother had had arthritis and her maternal grandfather had had arthritis and eczema. She had never smoked, abused alcohol, or used illegal substances.

Her medications already included loratadine and diphenhydramine once a day, assorted vitamins, triamcinolone cream (which wasn't helping the rash much), and occasional ibuprofen. Allergy-wise, celecoxib (a special type of non-steroidal anti-inflammatory drug (NSAID) for those who can't tolerate standard NSAIDs; of note, part of the celecoxib molecule is similar to the "sulfa" part of sulfur-based antibiotics, to which many people, especially MCAD patients, are allergic) had caused hives after just one pill, and prednisone had caused hallucinations.

Exam found an obese woman in no distress, pleasant, cooperative, fully alert and oriented, mobilizing via wheelchair. She required her son's assistance to (weakly) transit from wheelchair to exam table and back. There was no apparent weakness or lethargy in her conversation or in movements of her arms; it was just in moving her legs and whole body that the weakness really became apparent. Key findings were her comfortable general appearance at rest, scattered small bruises, obesity, slight swelling in the legs, edema, the lower extremity weakness – and the diffusely scattered patches of rash were obvious, with the two different components as described above scattered about different areas of her skin. There also were areas about her neck and waistline that seemed to be dermatographic responses to clothing and jewelry, and on a light scratch test on her upper back and abdomen, mild dermatographism (erythroderma only, no hives) promptly emerged but largely faded after about 1-2 minutes.

I ordered my usual set of screening labs for MCAS (though I noted her ibuprofen and omeprazole use might interfere with the testing) and asked Delores to increase her loratadine to twice daily and add famotidine, also twice a day, to her regimen.

She returned four months later reporting an "80% improvement" in her rash and itching, plus her sense of feeling cold all the time, headaches, nasal and throat irritation, diarrhea alternating with constipation, reflux, and edema had all moderately to markedly improved. Her presyncopal spells were a lot less frequent, too. That all said, her shortness of breath was unimproved, and her urinary problems and fatigue had worsened. On exam, the rash was moderately better and the edema was gone, but everything else appeared the same.

The initial labs had indeed come back all normal except for a slight elevation in chromogranin A, but that could have been due to her omeprazole. I asked Delores to repeat the testing.

She returned eight months later. Her rash and itching had largely relapsed in spite of continued antihistamines. She was using more diphenhydramine, her local physician had added a benzodiazepine to her regimen, and she was much more sedated than before. She had had a sleep study repeated and was told she did not have obstructive sleep apnea. On exam, her rash of "bug-bite" sores had completely relapsed.

The repeat testing done eight months earlier turned out to be positive on multiple fronts. Based on earlier experiences with this sort of a rash, I started her on low-dose imatinib.

She returned two months later obviously much more energetic (though still using the wheelchair for mobility) reporting that the itching had stopped almost immediately after starting imatinib, and the rash started disappearing a day or two later and was almost completely gone by the end of the first week. She said her fatigue and excess sleeping were unimproved, but on exam, aside from her greatly improved skin, she sure didn't look nearly as fatigued as she had previously appeared. She said her aching, too, had improved somewhat.

Delores continues on low-dose imatinib.

Troubles with skin, hair, nails, and teeth are common in MCAS.

All manners of rash are seen. The skin lesions of urticaria pigmentosa (UP) and telangiectasia macularis eruptive perstans (TMEP). The redness (erythema) of flushing. Migratory patches of erythema. Small cherry-red spots called telangiectasias. Prominent venous patterns called livedo (or livedo reticularis). Acne-like "folliculitis" lesions. Patches of small open sores. The list goes on. There also often are patches of sores with scabs on them, and when the patient is asked how they came about, there often is the answer, "Well, it just became a little bumpy and swollen and itchy there one day, and I picked at it until the skin opened a bit and some fluid came out, and now it's healing, but it seems to be taking a long time to do so" – which brings up the fact that one of the end effects of mast cell disease's impact on the immune system is impaired healing. (Actually, a type of rat has been bred in the laboratory to have no mast cells at all, and when such a rat is subjected to a wound, the wound doesn't heal. Not delayed healing. No healing. And there has developed over the decades plenty of other evidence, too, that normal mast cell activity is integral to normal growth and development in all tissues.)

Hair (especially on the scalp) often becomes brittle and dry, and patients often go through cycles of increased hair thinning and loss. However, even though the patient can tell she's suffering a lot more hair loss than normal, the general appearance (to others, anyway) is usually one of a full head of hair, so this is yet another manner in which MCAS patients are handicapped by *appearing* normal while in truth suffering abnormalities in a wide range of body organs and systems.

The nails become brittle and weak and don't grow normally. They often acquire longitudinal ridges, and sometimes there are cycles in which small white spots appear on the nails and then disappear. Janeway lesions (small short dark vertical lines that appear fairly suddenly in one nail or another, eventually disappearing as the nail grows out) sometimes appear in one or more nails, too, likely a sign of subclinical arterial clotting.

MCAS patients also often cause their dentists fits because of how much dental and periodontal deterioration occurs, even when the patient has always been good about attending to dental hygiene. Teeth "crumble" years prematurely. As with just about every aspect of MCAS, we are far from knowing the particular abnormal mast cell mediator "soups" that cause each of these problems.

Chapter 8: A Sight for Sore Eyes: Ocular/Ophthalmologic Findings in MCAS

We'll take a break in this chapter from a detailed case presentation because, in my experience, (1) virtually everybody with MCAS has some eye-related issues (not surprising given that back in the 1970s it was determined that there are about 5,000 mast cells per cubic millimeter of conjunctival tissue (i.e., the insides of the eyelids), and (2) virtually nobody with MCAS has a life-alteringly serious eye-related issue. (Note, though, there's some inherent bias in that statement because people with serious eye problems go to the ophthalmologist, not the hematologist/oncologist, so I guess it's possible that – just as in every other specialty – the ophthalmologists deal with some (or many?) "idiopathic" diseases driven by mast cell activation but don't recognize that that's what's driving them. But that's purely hypothetical, and I'll be the first to admit I've never really discussed MCAS with an ophthalmologist.)

Without a doubt, the single most common ocular/ophthalmologic symptom in MCAS is eye irritation. Patients usually don't report frank pain in their eyes but instead describe a waxing/waning "burning," "sandiness," "dryness," or "grittiness" in their eyes that's likely an inflammation of the conjunctival tissues. This usually doesn't affect vision except that closing the eyes often briefly provides a mild degree of relief. Some patients have already found that medicated eye drops such as the H_1 receptor blocker olopatadine, or cromolyn, or ketotifen, help these symptoms without realizing that they're targeting mast cells with these medications. Relief from these and other medicated eye drops is quite variable from one patient to the next. Thus, it's not at all clear whether it's histamine or some other mediator(s) being released by ocular (or other) mast cells that are causing this irritation in any given patient, and it might well be different mediators causing the same or similar symptom in different patients.

The second most common eye-related complaint I've encountered is brief, unprovoked episodes (typically a minute or two, sometimes shorter, sometimes longer) of loss of visual focus. This virtually always affects both eyes at the same time.

The third most common eye-related complaint I've encountered in my MCAS patients is blepharospasm, a trembling of the upper or lower eyelid. It bothers some patients to the point of asking their ophthalmologists to inject the affected area with the pharmaceutical form of the paralytic botulinum toxin, but this treatment sometimes causes temporary or permanent paralysis of other facial muscles resulting in cosmetic issues worse than the original problem, and in my experience, even if the blepharospasm is improved, it relapses within weeks to a few months. One hint that blepharospasms, at least in some patients, may be due to aberrant mast cell reactivity is that some patients (in my experience) note substantial or even complete improvement in this irritating symptom upon relocating to a new area or residence.

Inflammation – usually sterile, but sometimes infectious – can also occur in the whites of the eyes (the "sclerae"). Occasionally I also see unprovoked hyphemas (small bleeds) in the sclerae, making me wonder whether there has been a release of heparin by ocular mast cells (see more discussion in this vein in Chapter 10 about the sinonasal findings in MCAS).

Although I see no reason why inflammation in other eye structures (for example, the iris, the uvea, the retina) couldn't also occur as a consequence of MCAS, I haven't yet seen such cases, again likely because they'd go to the ophthalmologist, not me.

Chapter 9: Do You Hear What I Hear? Otologic Findings in MCAS

If you'll recall that the principal job of the mast cell is to serve as a sentinel against bodily insults and therefore the cell tends to site itself primarily at the body's environmental interfaces, then you shouldn't be surprised to learn that issues with ears and hearing are common in MCAS.

"Dwayne," a long-married, and congenitally deaf, 73-year old, was referred to me by his astute psychiatrist for evaluation for mast cell disease after extensive prior evaluation had failed to identify any causes (let alone a unifying cause) for the tinnitus (ringing in the ears; yes, it was news to me that the deaf could suffer tinnitus but, as I learned, that's not all that uncommon), tremor, and anxiety that had been plaguing him since shortly after surgery at age 71 for his enlarged (but non-cancerous) prostate.

Unlike most MCAS patients, Dwayne had had a pretty limited medical history. No reason for his congenital deafness had ever been figured out, but it hadn't stopped him from having a pretty full life including marriage (to a deaf woman), kids (whose hearing was fine), and a full career at an automotive plant. His appendix was taken out in childhood, and in his later years he developed some chronic low back and left hip pain of unclear origin, along with elevated cholesterol and symptoms of an enlarging prostate (e.g., increased difficulty urinating) that led to pretty standard surgery for this problem in 2009.

The surgery worked well, at least initially, with greatly improved urination, but a month later, weirdness emerged. This man who had never before had any psychiatric issues suddenly found himself beset with chronic anxiety – sometimes even to the point of frank panic attacks – and paranoia. And then, a month later, on came a constant, motor/jet/whistle-like sound bilaterally (I'll henceforth call this "tinnitus" for the sake of simplicity) which plagued him from the moment he woke in the morning to the moment he finally fell asleep at night. The tinnitus waxed and waned to some degree, but on average it was severe enough that it was Dwayne's #1 problem. Plus, around the time the tinnitus came on, he also developed a tremor all about his upper body (especially his head and ears) that would get triggered upon virtually any physical stimulus to his body (e.g., patting him on his back, jarring his elbows, even just walking). And every time the tremor was set off, the tinnitus would acutely worsen. He told me, too, that around that time he also developed a new, very poor tolerance for positional changes, immediately feeling presyncopal upon virtually any change in upper body position.

Unsurprisingly, these problems led to quite a bit of evaluation by otolaryngologists, neurologists, and psychiatrists. No causes for any of his new problems were found, and his physicians inasmuch openly admitted in their notes that a unifying diagnosis was completely unclear. There was no sign of stroke, of any disease of chronic neurologic deterioration, of any ear disease, or of any psychiatric issue that could come anywhere close to explaining all that was going on with Dwayne. He was tried, at various times, on antihypertensives (beta blockers), antidepressants (selective serotonin reuptake inhibitors), and anti-epileptic drugs, all to no avail. A benzodiazepine, lorazepam, seemed to limit somewhat the frequency at which his anxiety would escalate into panic attacks – but that's a pretty standard benzodiazepine effect. Nevertheless, his symptoms had essentially bound him to his home.

When I took his review of systems, he denied any problems with fevers, sweats, pruritus, irritation of eyes or nose or mouth or throat, significant visual deterioration or anomalies, dyspnea, chest pain/discomfort, palpitations, vomiting, diarrhea, urinary issues, or frank syncope. However, he said he felt cold much of the time and also suffered occasional slight headaches, frequent dry coughing with a choking sensation, marked gastroesophageal reflux (which also turned out to be brand new since his prostate surgery but at least was well controlled with a proton pump inhibitor (omeprazole)), occasional slight queasiness or nausea, frequent constipation (but also occasional mild fecal incontinence, even though he denied diarrhea), and what sounded like a somewhat pruritic-like paresthesia that migrated between his left foreleg and right foot. Another key finding was that in the half-year or so before coming to see me, he also had begun suffering roughly weekly episodes of unprovoked presyncope.

My initial physical examination of Dwayne was notable for his obvious deafness, borderline systolic hypertension, obvious presyncope upon virtually any motion of his upper body, and a very odd acute triggering of upper body tremor (most pronounced in the head, especially the ears) upon my palpation of just about every part of his body, though the reaction was definitely more pronounced on palpation of the upper aspects of the body compared to the lower aspects. He also acutely became mildly flushed with these tremors. He obviously was uncomfortable during these periods. When I stopped palpation, his reactions reliably settled down within a minute or so. Interestingly, too, when I lightly scratched his upper back, moderately bright dermatographism immediately emerged and was still present when I last checked the area several minutes later.

Labs showed a mild elevation in his plasma prostaglandin D_2 level, and his plasma heparin level was 250% above the upper limit of normal.

His chromogranin A level was elevated, too, but his proton pump inhibitor could have caused that.

The "total package" was quite consistent with MCAS (likely triggered either by the stress of surgery or by exposure to one of the agents used by the anesthesiologist), so I proceeded to try to treat him as such.

Unfortunately, just as had been seen with his trials on beta blockers, SSRIs, and anti-epileptics, he proved resistant to antihistamines, ketotifen, oral and otic cromolyn, quercetin, imatinib, and montelukast – but doxepin, at a relatively stiff dose of 50 mg twice daily, proved to simmer down his tinnitus and tremor enough that he was finally able to resume some semblance of his former "activities of daily living."

I'd like to tell the story of another deaf MCAS patient, too, to illustrate perhaps even better than with Dwayne's story how challenging it can be for these patients (as if their hearing impairment isn't challenge enough) and yet how much better they can get.

"Margerie" was a 50-year old disabled divorced deaf and legally blind woman referred to me in July 2012 by the same astute psychiatrist who, for the first time in this patient's long series of medical evaluations, seriously pondered the full scope of the patient's illness and wondered whether a mast cell issue might be a unifying diagnosis for her. (For those of you wondering, yes, all of the encounters I've had with my deaf or hearing-impaired patients have been facilitated by certified interpreters. It's not only the sensible thing to do; it's also been the law since 1973 (the Rehabilitation Act) for those receiving federally funded health care, and since 1990 (the Americans with Disabilities Act) for all other health care recipients in the U.S.) Unfortunately, despite the presence of the interpreter, the patient's cognitive dysfunction was immediately apparent and made for a difficult, prolonged initial evaluation. (I certainly couldn't blame any of her previous physicians for not taking the inordinate amount of time needed with this patient to get anywhere close to a full history and physical examination.) As best as I could gather from her and a small sheaf of records that had been sent by the psychiatrist, she had been healthy until needing knee surgery for uncertain purposes at age 8, and then somehow glaucoma developed in both eyes at age 12. By age 13 she needed nasal surgery for refractory epistaxis (keep this in mind when you read Chapter 10 about the sinonasal findings in MCAS), followed around age 20 by an appendectomy and a tubal ligation at age 21.

Somewhere around this time is when Margerie's husband at the time threw her down a flight of stairs. Bilateral sensorineural hearing loss (severe on the left and "mild-severe" on the right) developed in 1999 (around age 37) for unclear reasons. Somehow she managed to continue working as a department store sales clerk until 2007 (age 45), when she suffered her first event of acute "wooziness" and "falling out" (i.e., what sounded like a syncopal episode) while on the telephone one day trying to change a medical appointment (like that's never been a stressful event for anybody). She denied any other particular stress in her life at that point. She also noted that a waxing/waning stinging discomfort had developed in the right leg at some point prior to 2007. Her syncopal episodes continued to occur fairly often, sometimes as frequently as five times a month. She also was suffering what sounded like presyncopal episodes roughly once or twice a week. She reported substantial weakness in both legs, and though she could still walk with much effort (and with the assistance of bilateral foreleg braces), she said that frequently, soon after standing, her legs would just suddenly "give out" and she would fall.

Extensive evaluations had concluded Margerie had either a seizure disorder or a conversion disorder as the cause for these seemingly neurological issues, but I could find no records documenting any clear seizure activity. She had had another one of these attacks in February 2012 and was hospitalized for a few days. She said she felt a sharp pain in her head and the right side of her body fell numb as this attack was coming on. As best as I can tell, no clear cause of the attack was determined. Despite all of her afflictions, her psychiatrist noted she had been relatively high functioning until recently and had even tried to return to technical college in 2011, though those plans were foiled upon suffering another syncopal attack.

On review of systems, Margerie denied irritation of the eyes/nose/mouth, dyspnea, dysphagia, palpitations, GERD, alopecia, unusual dental deterioration, or any bleeding problems except for the epistaxis problem at age 13. However, she endorsed frequent subjective fevers, occasional chills, feeling cold much of the time, unprovoked unpredictable episodic profuse right axillary sweats that began in 2012, frequent headache, chronic waxing/waning fatigue, diffusely migratory aching, diffusely migratory pruritus, irritation in the throat (most frequently a "choking" sensation), unprovoked unpredictable non-anginal left anterior axillary discomfort that seemed to often get interpreted by her other physicians as left chest pain, frequent nausea and occasional vomiting, diarrhea alternating with constipation, diffusely migratory rash, diffusely migratory edema, cognitive dysfunction, insomnia, diffusely migratory tingling/numbness, left axillary tenderness, and easy bruising.

She denied any known hematologic or rheumatologic issues in the family history but for a sister with lupus. Family cancer history included a maternal aunt who died of breast cancer in her 60s, a brother with an unknown type of cancer for which he received a stem cell transplant, and another brother with an unknown type of cancer. Her mother, a smoker, died of lung cancer at 53. The patient herself had never used tobacco products or illegal substances and denied any history of alcohol abuse. She had been unable to work since the first syncopal event in 2007.

Unsurprisingly (given the mysteries of her multisystem unwellness), Margerie was taking a variety of medications including butorphanol, carisoprodol, celecoxib, hydrochlorothiazide, hydroxyzine, a mild narcotic, lamotrigine, and gabapentin. She reported many allergies: steroids caused palpitations, penicillin caused hives, CT contrast dye caused dyspnea, azithromycin caused abdominal pain, acetazolamide caused syncope, brimonidine caused dyspnea, cyclobenzaprine made her "hyper," tomatoes and celery caused a rash, and bananas caused nausea.

Exam found a woman initially appearing in no distress but obviously chronically ill with regard to mental slowness (or was it difficulty she was having seeing the interpreter's signing?), the bilateral foreleg braces, and her need for a wheelchair for mobility across any distance further than a few steps. She was accompanied by a friend who did not appear to know any sign language, and the patient's own abilities in "speaking" and understanding sign language were poor. She seemed to be reasonably pleasant and cooperative and was initially alert and was basically oriented, though obviously her insight into the medical details of her problems was very limited. She was weakly ambulatory, needing my assistance to steady her. She was wearing dark sunglasses. Vital signs were notable only for mild systolic hypertension. Other than her near complete deafness and obviously limited vision, the rest of the exam was unremarkable (not even any dermatographism) – until I asked her to try to walk. Almost immediately after I helped her stand and then walk three paces from the exam table to the wall and turn around and walk back and sit down, her left arm became paralyzed and tingly and crampy, and she was only just beginning to regain some motor control in the arm by the end of the visit. Around the same time this problem came on, though, she also "zoned out" and, though still awake, was unresponsive to questioning for about a couple of minutes. (Was this the spells of dystonia and cataplexy I eventually began seeing in some other MCAS patients? More in Chapter 18.) Absolutely no seizure activity was observed, and no post-seizure ("postictal") behavior was observed. There was just the faintest sweat ("diaphoresis") appearing on her forehead around this time.

Prior lab testing included normal routine blood counts, chemistries, thyroid function tests, and urinalyses. Extensive imaging of all parts of her body were notable only for fusions at multiple cervical spine levels "with residual moderate stenosis" and "large left C2-3 herniation." The only bloodwork of note was a very high anti-thyroid peroxidase antibody (1,067 (normal 0-34)), high anti-thyroglobulin antibodies at 133 (normal 0-40).

I doubted she had a seizure disorder (let alone a conversion disorder), and I also doubted that any cervical spine issue by itself was causing all that was going on in her. There were copious suggestions of a systemic inflammatory disorder, including many details particularly suggestive of mast cell activation.

I'll spare you the details of her visits over the next few months and simply summarize by saying that with twice-daily loratadine, famotidine, celecoxib, and quercetin, she has become completely functional again, walking without any difficulty, and has been discharged by her psychiatrist as no psychiatric issues are apparent. Her problems with sweats, pruritus, rash, presyncope, nausea, and diarrhea are all virtually eliminated, and syncope and vomiting in fact have been eliminated. She still has a few mild residual issues with occasional gastroesophageal reflux and now constipation instead of diarrhea (something I've seen happen in many diarrhea-afflicted MCAS patients who see improvement with aspirin or other NSAIDs), and she is beginning to become concerned about weight gain. She has not been able to find a primary care physician, noting the local primary care physicians she has approached have refused to accept her because of her MCAS diagnosis. (She's been repeatedly told "I don't know anything about that" and "That's too complicated.")

With the above two stories as context, I should state that in general the dominant otologic issues in MCAS patients continue the theme of generally non-infectious inflammation. Episodes of otitis externa ("painful" or "itchy" helices and/or canals) are fairly uncommon, while otitis media is more common, especially in children. In patients who suffer this manifestation of mast cell disease, the otitis media often seems oddly frequent in spite of no demonstrable cellular or humoral immune deficiency (with the underlying mast cell disease going unrecognized), and it often seems oddly refractory to antibiotic therapy, though in retrospect this is unsurprising since MCAS-driven inflammation is typically sterile.

MCAS patients also can suffer alterations in hearing (dysacusis). In the same fashion in which MCAS, depending on the particular pattern of aberrant mediator expression in the individual patient, can "push" a system to one extreme in one patient and to the opposite extreme in another patient, MCAS patients can suffer hearing loss, tinnitus or hyperacusis, and, rarely, but as illustrated by Dwayne's case, both hearing loss and tinnitus. While otitis seems to be the more common childhood otologic issue from MCAS, dysacusis – particularly tinnitus – seems to be the most common otologic issue from MCAS in adulthood. Tinnitus (which can be unilateral or bilateral or alternating) may be due to release of inflammatory and/or other neuroexcitatory mediators by aberrant mast cells in the vicinity of the acoustic-sensing hair cells in the semicircular canals or the fibers of the auditory nerve. Similarly, the audiologist often finds sensorineural hearing loss of unclear origin. Hearing loss presumably is due dominantly to the otosclerosis (of the tympanic membrane and/or the inner ear bones) which has been demonstrated in patients with mast cell disease, though degenerating canal hairs or auditory nerve function theoretically are other routes to hearing loss. (Interestingly, in contrast to most gain-of-function *KIT* mutations in mast cell activation diseases, loss-of-function *KIT* mutations have been demonstrated to be at the root of piebaldism, an inborn syndrome of deafness, hypopigmentation, and megacolon.)

Often, too, MCAS patients will report an intermittent or chronic, waxing/waning sensation of "fullness" in one or both of their ears, perhaps reflecting swelling from inflammation in the inner ear or Eustachian tube.

Other than identifying obvious otitis externa or media (which often is erroneously assumed to be, and treated as, infectious in origin) or dysacusis, otologic evaluations typically are unrevealing as to the *cause* of the problem; occasionally incidental findings (e.g., cerumen) are noted, but the otolaryngologist has difficulty attributing the described otologic symptoms to the exam findings.

Chapter 10: The Nose Knows: Sinonasal Findings in MCAS

I'll take another break in this chapter from telling you in detail about a specific case because, somewhat ironically, I really haven't had a patient (yet!) whose dominant issue with MCAS has been in the sinuses or nose. I say "ironically" because sinonasal issues actually are very frequent in MCAS, which shouldn't be at all surprising given that some of the highest concentrations of mast cells normally found in the body are in the nose and sinuses, which of course are environmental interfaces. So sinonasal symptoms are frequent in MCAS, but just not nearly as life-altering as some of the other symptoms.

What are the sinonasal symptoms of MCAS? For the most part, just as one would expect in somebody suffering an environmental allergy (which of course is often a mast-cell-driven issue): congestion (stuffiness), post-nasal drip (into the throat) and coryza (external nasal dripping), and sometimes nasal and sinus irritation and closed or open sores. In some patients the sinonasal edema from MCAS actually does lead to obstruction of the nasal passages, or of the passages from the sinus cavities into the nasal passages, and such obstructed spaces then become breeding grounds for infection, but usually the sinonasal inflammation in MCAS – just as is the case with MCAS-driven inflammation anywhere else in the body – is of a sterile, rather than infectious, nature.

Unsurprisingly, though, in many patients the symptoms of sinonasal inflammation are interpreted – despite absence of fever – as signs of infection and are treated not only with decongestants and H_1 antihistamines but also antibiotics. Many patients wind up receiving extended and/or multiple courses of antibiotics, and when the episode eventually winds down a few weeks after it began, it's assumed by doctor and patient that it was the latest antibiotic tried, or the extended duration of antibiotic therapy, that finally got the better of the resistant strain of bacteria that must have been causing such a terrible rhinosinusitis. Or, perhaps, that just happens to be when the flare of mast cell activation causing a bout of sterile (i.e., of non-infectious origin) rhinosinusitis naturally began to wind down.

Of course, as has often been discussed in the medical and popular literature for more than 20 years now, the indiscriminate use of antibiotics for these sorts of upper respiratory tract infections ("URIs") has contributed to the emergence of ever scarier strains of multi-antibiotic-resistant bacteria now causing an increasing amount of morbidity and mortality. Current guidelines from an assortment of professional societies exhort doctors to not prescribe antibiotics for most URIs in most patients, but it shouldn't be surprising that in a busy practice, when it might take 3-5 minutes for the doctor to explain to the patient why he's not going to prescribe an antibiotic and to brook the dissatisfaction and counter the inevitable protests from his paying client, vs. the 15-30 seconds it would take to issue a prescription – and when the doctor will get paid the same amount for either approach – the prescription will often win out. (This is just one more example of how our current health care financing system is geared to deliver poor care. Much more on this subject – particularly as it impacts those with MCAS – later.)

To defend the physician, though, I should add that it's not easy to use absence of fever as a definitive marker of the absence of infection. Although in the appropriate clinical context the presence of fever is a relatively reliable indicator of infection, infection nevertheless can be present without fever in a wide variety of clinical situations. All of that said, even if sinonasal infection is present, the current guidelines to withhold antibiotics for most URIs are appropriate (relying instead on the patient's own immune system to eventually resolve the problem) despite their relative impracticality in a busy practice operating within the incentives/disincentives structure of our modern health care financing system.

Another sinonasal issue occasionally seen in MCAS is idiopathic epistaxis (the medical word for nosebleed), with or without associated sinonasal inflammatory issues. Idiopathic epistaxis is a problem that's particularly well known to otolaryngologists (ear-nose-throat, or "ENT," doctors), of course. Sometimes the epistaxis is frequent and/or severe enough to spur not only cauterization, which may or may not resolve the problem, but also consultation with a hematologist to try to identify a systemic abnormality in the patient's coagulation system. What's generally not recognized, though, is the potential for MCAS to be at the root of this problem through (abnormal) release of the natural anticoagulant heparin by the relatively large number of mast cells embedded in the linings of the nasal passages, where there also happens to be a particularly rich network of blood vessels so that cold inhaled air can be warmed somewhat before passing into the lungs. It shouldn't be surprising that if one mixes a rich network of blood vessels with blood vessel fragility induced by inflammation, and then one pours heparin into the mix, there might be some bleeding as a result.

Those with medical experience will recognize heparin as an anticoagulant drug (typically refined from bovine and porcine intestinal tissue) but may not be aware it's a natural product of the human body. As best as we presently know, heparin is made by only two types of cells in the human body, the basophil and the mast cell. In fact, heparin was the very first mediator product of the mast cell to be discovered (back in 1939), but the amount of heparin that gets released by (usually localized) mast cell activation phenomena almost never is enough to cause any abnormality in the partial thromboplastin time (PTT) test that's used to monitor whether enough of the pharmaceutical heparin is being administered to achieve the desired systemic anticoagulation effect. Thus, even if the patient comes to the hematologist to be evaluated for a systemic coagulation problem, the PTT determined in the standard way (from blood collected via routine systemic blood draw) will be normal and it is unlikely that any thought will be given to the possibility that intense *local* heparin release in the sinonasal region

92

might be contributing to the epistaxis. I think it would be an interesting study to compare the PTT and heparin level in blood collected from the vigorously bleeding noses in patients with idiopathic epistaxis against the blood collected from those same patients at the same time via standard blood draws.

Chapter 11: Mouthing Off About Mast Cell Disease: Oral/Pharyngeal Findings in MCAS

My first encounter with the oral findings in MCAS, of course, was the case of burning mouth syndrome (BMS) in Marlene, presented in Chapter 2.

In the course of all the reading I had done over the 3-1/2 years it took from her first visit to me until I discovered Marlene's underlying MCAS, I had learned BMS was first described in the literature about half a century ago. Unsurprisingly, these patients quickly get routed to dentists and oral surgeons (and sometimes even oral pathologists), who I'm sure usually make good attempts to identify any of the known causes of BMS, a disease unknown to most doctors outside of those in the oral field even though it's not a rare disease: a general U.S. population health survey undertaken by the NIH in the early 1990s found 1% of respondents reported chronic oral burning. (Who knew? And, I can't imagine what led some NIH researcher to propose including that question on the survey, but kudos.) But no clear cause is identifiable in most BMS patients, who then languish for years, perhaps even the remainders of their lives.

So, after making the diagnosis in Marlene and seeing her good, rapid response to MCAS-targeted therapy, I called an oral surgery colleague and asked whether he had any BMS patients. His answer was predictable: "Absolutely – and they're very challenging patients. I can't figure out what's wrong with them, and I can't figure out how to help them. Nobody can." So I said, "I've got an idea about what may be going on in them. Why don't you send me a couple?"

A couple turned into three, four, five… I published an article describing the first three, but I've now seen more than a couple dozen whose histories fit the MCAS profile, who demonstrated elevated mast cell mediator levels (different patterns in different patients, to be sure), and who all responded well to MCAS-targeted therapy (again, different therapies proved to be helpful in different patients, another attestation to the substantial heterogeneity of MCAS). These results, of course, are just "anecdotal" and don't come anywhere close to proving that MCAS underlies most or all cases of BMS in which the other classic causes of the disease can't be found, but they are intriguing results nonetheless.

The oral findings in MCAS continue the theme of inflammation that's usually sterile but occasionally is aggravated by superimposed infection. Symptoms and other findings include pain (often "burning," as in Marlene), sores and ulcers, white patches termed leukoplakia, fibrosis (scarring), another inflammatory tissue reaction pattern called lichen planus, throat discomfort (or "irritation" or "tickle") often leading to intermittent dry cough, proximal dysphagia (difficulty swallowing, from a real or perceived obstruction high in the throat, which might actually be episodes of edema in the throat), globus (persistent sensation of material or obstruction in the throat without actual dysphagia which, again, might actually be episodes of edema in the throat), and excessive pharyngeal mucus production.

Understanding of the mast cell-driven roots of the oral findings is substantially challenged by the absence of increased oral tissue mast cells in the vast majority of MCAS patients with oral symptoms. This fact, of course, is what caused such a substantial delay in diagnosing the root cause of Marlene's BMS – and it's what's kept BMS an enigma in most patients since the first cases were described in the literature about half a century ago. Oral tissue biopsies in most BMS patients have been maddeningly normal, unsurprisingly leading to psychiatric diagnoses (e.g., psychosomatism, depression) in many. There are some BMS patients in whom evidence of other specific causes (e.g., the idiopathic autoimmune disease Sjögren's syndrome, or *Candida* fungal infection) can be found, but clearly, what has to be going on in cases of BMS in which no cause other than MCAS can be found is that one or more mediators being released by aberrant mast cells either in the oral tissues (or potentially elsewhere) are either inflaming oral epithelial tissues (seems less likely given the normal biopsies) or activating oral sensory nerves to cause the sensation of pain.

The oral symptoms in MCAS often improve partially to dramatically with mast-cell-directed therapy of one sort or another, but the throat discomforts of various sorts – likely due to edema and/or inflammatory mediators being released by mast cells in the pharynx (or possibly elsewhere) – sometimes are much more challenging to effectively treat. Patients with globus and excessive pharyngeal mucus production have been particular vexing.

"Darla" was referred to me in late 2010 for further evaluation of a mild decrease in her white blood cells count ("leukopenia"), but this 61-year old woman's chief complaint was quite removed from the reason for referral: she had been producing thick mucus from her upper airway incessantly for the past 3-1/2 years, and extensive diagnostic efforts and empiric interventions to date were all in vain. Her past medical history included bronchiectasis, gastroesophageal reflux disease with hiatal hernia, allergic rhinitis (with failed desensitization and immunization therapy), hypertension, cholecystectomy, chronic sinusitis, and a minimal, remote history of smoking, but she told me she had always been healthy up until the mucus problem began (fairly acutely at that). Exposure to hot or cold foods, or hot environments, also seemed to trigger flares of this problem. Associated problems included chronic sinonasal congestion with a lot of post-nasal drip, frequent throat clearing, chronic throat irritation, waxing/waning but overall pretty persistent hoarseness, and proximal dysphagia.

Darla had undergone very extensive evaluations by pulmonary and ENT physicians and even underwent a type of significant surgery for gastroesophageal reflux disease (GERD) called a Nissen fundoplication which she thought helped her GERD symptoms "somewhat," but nevertheless the primary "mucus" problem never abated one bit. Multiple endoscopies hadn't shown much beyond fairly persistent redness ("erythema") at a place in the voicebox ("larynx") called the posterior arytenoids. She denied fevers, chills, headaches, itching, irritation of the eyes/nose/mouth, chest pain, nausea, vomiting, diarrhea, rashes, edema, or cognitive dysfunction, but she did note moderately frequent soaking night sweats, occasional shortness of breath, wheezing, constipation, and tingling in the toes, occasional aching in the bilateral knees, and frequent abdominal bloating and gas. There was no significant social or family history except that her daughter has just been diagnosed with multiple sclerosis. She thought there was a mold/mildew problem in her trailer, but she couldn't afford to do anything about it. Medications were mainly symptom-directed respiratory drugs. She denied any known medication allergies but said she had been found to be allergic to dust, pollen, mold, and mildew.

Exam was notable for a voice that simultaneous sounded hoarse and nasal sinus-congested, and she frequently manifested a junky cough (though without any actual sputum/mucus production that I could see). Darla was obviously uncomfortable from this. She had a new minimal diastolic hypertension. Most of her teeth had been removed because "they were bad." There was no coryza or post-nasal drip seen, and no obvious oral or pharyngeal lesions. Lung exam was unremarkable. There was no visible edema or rash, but on a light scratch test on the upper back in this African-American woman of relatively light skin tone, it was easy to see that bright dermatographism briskly arose and was long sustained. The rest of her exam was unremarkable.

Lab review showed stable mild-moderate leukopenia dating back a year (the oldest available data) and stable mild normocytic anemia in the 10-11 g/dl range. A very wide battery of other tests for endocrinologic, inflammatory, infectious, respiratory, gastrointestinal, and malignant diseases had all been negative. The erythematous arytenoid has not been biopsied.

I noted at the time, "I highly doubt a primary hematologic abnormality in the marrow and instead suspect the anemia is a reactive anemia of chronic inflammation, and the leukopenia/neutropenia is either benign ethnic leukopenia/neutropenia (doubt) vs., again, reactive to the chronic upper airway inflammation. Her review of systems, too, includes a few hints of a chronic systemic inflammatory disorder, yet there is no classic such disorder that well fits the particular combination of findings here. Although I guess atypical presentations of sarcoid, Wegener's granulomatosis, or other autoimmune disorders or any of a large number of uncommon infections technically are all possibilities, it's quite likely that if any of these were her problem, her other excellent pulmonary and ENT physicians would have figured this out by now. Overall, then, I find myself wondering whether a mast cell disease is what's really at work here, almost certainly not systemic mastocytosis but rather a mast cell activation syndrome; many aspects of her illness fit the profile well."

Screening tests for MCAS were sent and she began twice-daily loratadine and famotidine. She returned a few weeks later saying her mucus production was improved somewhat, but as her other physicians had also started her in the same interval on guaifenesin and assorted vitamins and steroids, I couldn't say whether the antihistamines were helping. Her chromogranin A level had been found to be double the upper limit of normal, and I also learned that biopsies taken during an EGD done elsewhere in September 2008 had found "chronic esophagogastritis."

Addition of aspirin (325 mg twice daily) to her regimen helped her feel better in general and helped further decrease her hoarseness and mucus production. Additional blood testing had found elevations in Factor VIII and norepinephrine, and re-testing of the September 2008 biopsies found up to 47 mast cells per high power field, not aggregated (as would be required to meet the definition of mastocytosis) but definitely increased over normal.

Darla's other doctors tried her on additional courses of steroids as well as montelukast and some other medications, all to no avail. Her symptoms soon relapsed back to baseline. That said, it was also becoming apparent that she was becoming substantially non-compliant with her medication regimen, but I couldn't tell whether that was due to the cost or the complexity of her regimen or some other factor.

Subsequent trials of cromolyn (oral and then nebulized), lorazepam, imatinib, doxepin, hydroxyurea, and N-acetylcysteine didn't help, and she wasn't able to access a prescribed trial of ketotifen, but, again, it also was difficult to figure out how compliant she was with any of these medications. I was next going to have her try omalizumab when she was lost to follow-up.

I have since encountered a couple of other patients who report excessive mucus production as their chief complaint and in whom I found evidence of MCAS – but have not yet been able to find helpful therapy.

Chapter 12: The Consequences of a Dysfunctional Clean-Up Crew: Lymphatic Findings in MCAS

The body's lymph nodes, as well as the spleen (essentially, the body's largest lymph node), are major parts of the immune system, and given that the mast cell is not only part of the immune system but also produces a wealth of mediators that influence immune system function, it shouldn't be surprising that the lymph nodes and spleen – responsible for "cleaning up" from the breakdown of other cells (both human cells and foreign microorganisms) in the body – often are affected in MCAS.

Enlargement of the lymph nodes is seen in a sizable minority of MCAS patients, and just as MCAS itself principally manifests waxing/waning inflammation migrating about the body, so, too, do the lymph nodes – in different parts of the body, over time – wax and wane in size. Rarely do they markedly enlarge (as might be seen in lymphoma or major infection), and rarely do they continuously enlarge (if they do, lymphoma needs to be ruled out). There might be modest enlargement of the nodes in the right side of the neck in the spring, but then by summertime those nodes will have shrunk and no longer be palpable and instead there might be modest enlargement of the nodes in the left groin – and then by wintertime those nodes may have resolved and a CT scan or ultrasound (done to keep an eye on long-present mild enlargement of the spleen) may show new mild enlargement of intra-abdominal lymph nodes – and once again no change in the mildly enlarged spleen. Sometimes the changes in node size occur much more quickly, too.

Sometimes the enlarged nodes in MCAS are painful, or at least tender to the touch, and sometimes they're completely asymptomatic.

Enlargement of the spleen is also seen in a significant minority of MCAS patients. Usually it is stable over the long term, and usually it is so modest that the enlargement cannot be appreciated on palpation of the left upper quadrant of the abdomen. Thus, usually it's discovered by scanning done for one purpose or another – though sometimes that purpose is the left upper quadrant abdominal discomfort that is also commonly seen in MCAS patients even if there is no other abdominal discomfort and even if there is no enlargement of the spleen. I suspect such episodic left upper quadrant abdominal discomfort is due to periodic aberrant release of inflammatory mediators by dysfunctional splenic mast cells, but that's just a guess.

It's important to keep in mind, too, that the full spectrum of symptoms and abnormalities seen in any given MCAS patient is of course not coming exclusively from inappropriate mast cell mediator release. If only this extremely complex disease were that relatively simple! No, it has to be kept in mind that the mediators released by fundamentally dysfunctional mast cells – again, per the work by Dr. Molderings' team in Bonn (which no other team has yet even tried to replicate), thought to be due to assorted mutations in the mast cells – go on to cause inappropriate behaviors by not only other dysfunctional mast cells but also plenty of normal other types of cells including lymphocytes, neutrophils, eosinophils, and, yes, mast cells. Therefore, dysfunctional mast cells can wind up causing many different problems through both direct and indirect routes.

In any event, persistent enlargement of lymph nodes presents a real dilemma for the doctor. Is it benign or malignant? Most of the time, lymph node enlargement is due to benign reasons (most commonly, a reaction to infection), but either way (i.e., whether benign or malignant), what's the cause?

Deciding when to biopsy a lymph node is far more a medical art than science, but the biopsy of an enlarged node in MCAS often leads to even more confusion than was present before the biopsy, as what the pathologist usually will find is an "atypical reactive non-specific lymphoproliferative disorder" that doesn't look like a typical reactive lymph node but also doesn't look like a typical lymphoma. Sometimes there also will be an influx of another type of white blood cell called a histiocyte, leading to a reading of "sinus histiocytosis" in the lymph node. Thus, for all of these reasons, sometimes the pathologist will be tempted to declare that there's a lymphoma or a histiocytic disease (like Langerhan's histiocytosis) present – but the cautious pathologist usually holds back, as he can sense that "it's just not quite right" for making such diagnoses.

The situation gets even more complicated when the pathologist says there's no lymphoma present in the biopsy but the molecular or genetic testing that's usually done on the biopsy when lymphoma is suspected yields results consistent with lymphoma. Since the *sine qua non* of lymphoma diagnosis at present still remains the histologic interpretation of the biopsy (i.e., does it look like a lymphoma when viewed under the microscope?) rather than any molecular testing, all that can be recommended in such a situation is careful monitoring of such patients.

Of course, sometimes there really is a clear-cut lymphoma present, and when that happens, treatment that's appropriate to the particular type of lymphoma that's seen is warranted. This does raise the question, though, of whether there might be any utility to defining, as has already been done for mastocytosis, a subcategory of MCAS in which there is an associated hematologic malignancy. This is a useful subcategory of mastocytosis because there are clear guidelines that treatment of such a subcategory should involve treatment of *both* the mast cell disease *and* the hematologic malignancy, an approach that clear yields better outcomes than just treating the hematologic malignancy. I've also now seen a few patients who were initially found to have cancers with poor prognoses and who indeed did poorly with treatment but then, upon finding and successfully treating their MCAS, experienced a turnaround in their cancers. Clearly, mast cell disease of any sort can influence the development of cancer in at least some patients, and whether the mast cell disease is mastocytosis or MCAS, recognition and treatment of mast cell disease that co-exists with cancer is likely to be important for optimizing outcome from the cancer.

Let me illustrate the difficulties of dealing with lymph nodes in MCAS by relating the following case.

> Susan, a 70-year old accountant who had retired a decade earlier, had perplexed her dermatologists to the point of suspecting a mast cell disorder, thus leading to the referral to me in July 2013. We weren't long into the history before it was evident that, like many MCAS patients, she had a complicated, virtually life-long history of multisystem unwellness of a generally inflammatory theme. Mild asthma and roughly annual episodes of seemingly unprovoked syncope came on at age 7. By mid-adulthood she seemed to have "grown out of" the asthma, though not the syncopal episodes. No cause had ever been found. Somewhat more frequently, she also had long been suffering episodes of presyncope (both orthostatic (upon rising) and non-orthostatic) and nausea, and she had found that taking ginger helped quell these episodes. At age 13 she suffered a curious outbreak of hives which seemed to be associated with exposure to intense cold, but that problem was soon put to bed by better protecting herself from the elements as needed. Later in adolescence she developed a "poison oak" rash, which curiously continued to recur for the next three years even without apparent re-exposure; this improved each time with a course of a common steroid medication called prednisone.

> Susan's only two pregnancies, in her 20s, were unremarkable and also resulted in unremarkable deliveries of healthy babies, but around age 27 she began thinning and became nervous, jittery, and anemic. She says a thyroid disorder was diagnosed; it sounded to me as if it was more consistent with hyperthyroidism than hypothyroidism, but post-partum autoimmune thyroid disorders are not rare. Various medication trials proved unhelpful. Around age 29 nodules were newly appreciated on her thyroid and she underwent removal of one lobe of her thyroid, followed by removal of the other lobe (and lifelong thyroid hormone replacement ever since) around age 43 when nodules again became appreciable. She says neither operation found thyroid cancer.

> Around age 50 Susan was noticed to have developed intermittent microscopic traces of blood in her urine, and this had continued ever since without any clear diagnosis. Around age 52 a neurologist diagnosed her with exercise-induced migraine headaches. Somewhere around her 50s she also suffered a single curious episode in which her

right face acutely swelled; she says this resolved after two days of cetirizine (a non-sedating histamine H_1 receptor blocker). She wasn't quite clear about when her next set of troubles truly began, but roughly around age 60-65 she began experiencing a new fatigue, malaise, and insomnia – overall, a sense just that "something wasn't right." She also began noticing that her face began getting unusually red upon washing in the morning. Evaluation by a neurologist resulted in a recommendation for a tilt-table test, but the cardiologist she then saw found low serum sodium and chloride and recommended Gatorade rather than a tilt-table test. Gatorade, though, didn't seem to help either her malaise or her electrolytes and instead just made her feel full all the time; she couldn't even drink it in the afternoon because it would interfere with her sleep, which was already down to just 5 hours a night from her usual 8.

Despite the fatigue and malaise, Susan attempted to do her best and remained active at virtually her normal baseline, but then in May 2012 she hurt her back in a lifting accident. She soon went to a spine center. She says she was told the MRI showed only a "very small cyst," and she was given an injection of some sort and began a course of physical therapy, which helped somewhat. Curiously, soon into this course she began noticing a new intolerance for sun exposure, quickly developing "burning spots" about her extremities that felt and looked much like the "poison oak rash" she had recurrently suffered for a while as a teen. Soon after she began suffering this sun-induced rash, she was prescribed a course of prednisone but found the rash just steadily worsened in spite of the medication. She said the rash looked "just like lupus, the rosette pattern." Although, again, her face by this time had long been turning unusually red upon washing in the morning, she says she did not have the classic "malar rash" of lupus.

Her primary physician referred her to a dermatologist, who performed a skin biopsy looking for lupus, but when this came back negative, he obtained several more biopsies, all of which were again negative. Meanwhile, the seemingly sun-induced rash was slowly but steadily worsening about all of her body except for her face. Another trial of prednisone again didn't help, and then a trial of ranitidine and diphenhydramine made her sleepier than usual but otherwise also didn't help. The only intervention that would provide her relief was application of a cold pack to the burning rash. Over the next few weeks the rash seemed to modestly improve, but then she felt a raised lesion on her back. Her dermatologist felt this was different, biopsied it, and empirically started her on doxycycline. When the biopsy was reported to show Grover's disease, he changed her doxycycline to a steroid cream (this was now around August 2012), which she thought helped to tone down the rash somewhat.

Around this time Susan's endocrinologist switched her from generic to brand name thyroid hormone medication. A chest X-ray and an EKG were done and were unremarkable. At this point her gynecologist referred her to a urologist to investigate the intermittent microscopic traces of blood she had now had in her urine for about 20 years, but the cystoscopy procedure performed by the urologist was unrevealing. Meanwhile, as winter came on, it seemed that her sun intolerance was only worsening, but she stopped the steroid cream around the turn of the year. In October 2012 she underwent allergy testing (and noted that stopping her steroid cream to prepare for the testing led to her entire back quickly turning into a solid rash) which found minimal reactivity to titanium nitride, gold sulfamate, and a manganese compound of some sort. In January 2013 a follow-up MRI of her back was unchanged, but there was suspicion that the observed cyst might have been more extensive than apparent on the MRI and might have been causing her ongoing back pain, so she underwent surgery which discovered that the cyst "wrapped around some nerves." A laminectomy was done, with insertion of a titanium plate and screws. She says she had told the surgeon ahead of time about the recent allergy testing, but the surgeon assured her that implanted titanium hardware is well tolerated.

Susan told me she made a good recovery from the surgery, but then she also said that she had been newly very easy to bruise since this surgery, and soon after the surgery she also began noticing a "bumpy" rash on her scalp and feet; furthermore, she said her feet felt as if she were walking on rocks. She also began noticing tender small lymph nodes about the bilateral neck. (And you were wondering when lymph nodes were going to come into this story!) She saw an otolaryngologist, who performed a fine needle aspirate that was non-diagnostic. She saw another dermatologist who suspected an autoimmune skin disease called bullous pemphygoid, and to try to prove that he did another skin biopsy in April 2013, but this was again reported to be normal. Her allergist and first dermatologist began wondering around that time if she might have a mast cell or eosinophil disorder. A sedating H_1 antihistamine called cyproheptadine helped only a little.

Susan's dermatologist contacted me. I wasn't able to see the patient right away, but it sounded like it might be MCAS based on what he told me on the phone, so I recommended laboratory evaluation for MCAS followed by empiric initiation of twice-daily loratadine and famotidine.

At her initial visit with me, Susan reported the rash and burning/itching rapidly cleared after beginning these two medications, though a small scar-like lesion has been left behind at the sites of some of the previous lesions. However, she has noticed a pattern that the itching seems to be trying to relapse toward the end of each dosing interval. She also noted that while the skin about her scalp and feet had gotten much better, her easy bruising and tender adenopathy had continued. A right neck node had been fully excised two weeks before her visit with me. On a full review of systems, although she denied issues with sweats, mouth or throat irritation, nausea, vomiting, diarrhea, paresthesias, abdominal discomfort, GU or gyn problems, or dental issues, she endorsed a wide range of other chronic and/or intermittent, waxing/waning/episodic issues with feeling alternately hot and cold and being newly intolerant of being covered by a blanket, chronic mild headache, fatigue, diffusely migratory aching, diffusely migratory pruritus (including deep in her ears), irritated eyes, dry nose, a single episode of epistaxis in April 2013, easy bruising, occasional bleeding from the open skin lesions she had had until recently, intermittent mild shortness of breath, occasional non-anginal chest discomfort, palpitations, odd episodes of acute fluctuations of blood pressure up and down, mild gastroesophageal reflux, constipation (relatively new, and she attributed this to the pain medication for her chronic back pain), prior diffuse rash as above (now largely resolved), diffusely migratory edema, diffusely migratory adenopathy (small, sometimes mildly tender nodes scattered about various points about her bilateral neck and axillae), the above-noted microscopic traces of blood in the urine (very occasionally producing some barely pink-tinged urine), insomnia, episodic cognitive dysfunction (especially short-term memory and word-finding), mild alopecia, and newly yellow nails.

She knew of no hematologic issues in the family history. The only rheumatologic issues were a sister with lupus and a grandson with an odd rheumatologic condition of "dermatomyositis not involving the muscles." (Interestingly, I've also seen a few MCAS patients who have "odd dermatomyositis not involving the skin." When desperately searching for a diagnosis, physicians who see a pathology report stating that the microscopic appearance of biopsied tissue is "consistent with" a given disease, they usually will then (mis?)label the patient with that diagnosis even if the patient is not *behaving* as one would expect for that diagnosis, forgetting that it's always possible that there might be other potential – recognized and unrecognized – reasons for the tissue to look the way it does. I don't like to make a diagnosis unless the patient is *behaving* as one would expect for the diagnosis I'm assigning.) The patient had never smoked or had significant secondary smoke exposure. She had never abused alcohol and has never used illegal substances. Her only medications were loratadine, famotidine, levothyroxine, zinc, ezetimibe, a multivitamin, calcium, and occasional lisinopril/hydrochlorothiazide if her blood pressure went too high, and with regard to allergies/intolerances, she said statins all seemed to cause aching (she noted she was presently on a statin but tended to take it for only 2-3 days at a time before stopping it due to aching), erythromycin caused pharyngitis, and sulfa caused blisters.

Exam found a thin woman in no apparent discomfort at rest, pleasant, cooperative, fully alert and oriented, independently ambulatory (though in quite an achy manner), accompanied by her husband. Vitals were notable for a systolic blood pressure of 180, but she had not taken her Lisinopril/hydrochlorothiazide that morning. Key findings were her comfortable general appearance, absence of rash, minimal sparsely scattered bruising, 1-2 nodes lymph nodes roughly 5-10 mm in size in her bilateral neck but no other palpable adenopathy at any of the usual node-bearing sites (though the palpated nodes and all the other node-bearing sites are definitely tender on palpation), mild tenderness in her left mid-abdomen, no appreciable enlargement of liver or spleen, and trace edema in her legs. On a light scratch test on her back, moderately bright dermatographism immediately emerged and was fully sustained when last checked about 10 minutes later. Her husband told me that the tiny cherry angiomata I saw scattered about the trunk were all old, and I could also see the bits of scarring she had told me about at many of the sites of the rash that seems to have been cleared up of late with loratadine and famotidine, but otherwise I really didn't see any active rash.

Laboratory screening for MCAS showed mild elevations in the 24-hour urinary prostaglandin D_2 and, in the blood, Factor VIII and plasma free norepinephrine. Mild-moderate elevations in her eosinophil percentages over time were the only other notable findings in the blood.

The April 2013 right neck lymph node fine needle aspiration was read as "reactive lymphoid cells." When I saw her initially that day in July, the only interpretation available from the node that had been excised two weeks earlier was that the "flow cytometry" molecular testing was normal. Later that day, though, even before he had seen the node under the microscope, the chief pathologist called the otolaryngologist who had taken out the node to report that the special stains (CD1a and S100 and Langerin) on the lymph node were markedly positive in the many sinus histiocytes found in the sample, suggesting a diagnosis of Langerhans histiocytosis. The otolaryngologist immediately called the patient to report the diagnosis and to inform her that that's the sort of a diagnosis that I (as the hematologist) can handle. Shortly after the otolaryngologist made that call, though, the pathologist finally received from his technicians the section of the lymph node to be looked at under the microscope, at which point the pathologist recognized this was not Langerhans histiocytosis. His final report, instead, was just "reactive lymph node with sinus histiocytosis; the histiocytes are increased in numbers, present singly and in large groups, and occasionally display wrinkled membranes and grooves," and his final pathologic diagnosis was simply "dermatopathic lymphadenopathy" (i.e., an abnormal lymph node in association with the skin).

I noted in my assessment at the time that although a modest eosinophil disorder of some sort, or even a histiocytic disorder of some sort, might be entering the equation of late, the history overall was most consistent by far with a mast cell activation disorder, far more likely MCAS than mastocytosis. I also noted that in MCAS symptoms usually seem to emerge beginning in youth (though typically non-specific at the time) and escalate over time in a stepwise fashion soon following significant stressors, or novel exposures, of potentially any sort – and thus I wondered whether the lifting accident in May 2012 itself was the trigger for the escalation she had seen since, or perhaps the injection she was given shortly after the accident was the trigger, as spine center injections typically involve steroid/anesthetic mixtures and -caine anesthetics are well recognized provocateurs of mast cell disease in some patients.

The January 2013 surgery (and/or the accompanying anesthesia) might have been another trigger leading to the easy bruising seen since, as I suspected the cause of this bruising was aberrant heparin release from the misbehaving mast cells she likely has; this unifying, one-diagnosis scenario seemed to me to be more likely than the presence of a separate disorder (e.g., acquired von Willebrand disease) to cause the new bruising and bleeding. I also noted that mast cell disease of any type leads to increased risk of malignancy of any type (particularly hematologic), and thus it was possible that she might have MCAS as an underlying problem plus recent emergence of a malignant histiocytic disorder, but at present we didn't have pathologic confirmation of malignant histiocytosis, and I additionally noted that mast cell disease also can feature reactive adenopathy in quite a variety of odd clinical and histologic patterns that create diagnostic and management challenges. I have seen more than once before a situation of modest adenopathy which was worrisome for malignancy but which (1) the pathologist was reluctant to label as malignant because there were (typically subtle) aspects of the pathologic evaluation that were not consistent with what would be classically expected for the suspected malignancy, and (2) on follow-up never appeared to progress, or even spontaneously regressed.

Thus, in the absence of pathologic confirmation of malignant adenopathy, I was more inclined to suspect the adenopathy was reactive to the MCAS I also was suspecting had been her underlying issue for roughly the last 63 years. There literally was not a single aspect of her history which was inconsistent with mast cell disease, and while the diagnoses definitively made throughout her life were likely all valid, each of them accounted for only a portion of her issues, while MCAS could account for most or all of her issues.

Susan soon found that thrice daily antihistamines keeps control of her rash but not her blood pressure lability, her nocturnal tinnitus, dry skin, episodic ear pain, left tonsillar nodules, episodic imbalance, and episodic cognitive dysfunction (principally, memory and word-finding issues, the two most common cognitive issues I see in MCAS patients). She is now moving on to try other MCAS-targeted medications.

Chapter 13: "I Just Can't Catch a Deep Breath": Pulmonary Findings in MCAS

Given that mast cells tend to hang out at the body's environmental interfaces to best serve their defensive role, and given that the airways constitute a huge portion of those interfaces, it's not surprising that there are relatively more mast cells in the upper and lower respiratory tracts than most other places in the body (except possibly the gastrointestinal and genitourinary tracts) – and therefore it's not surprising that there are few MCAS patients who get away without any respiratory tract issues at all.

> "Trent" was a 55-year old, effectively completely disabled small business owner when he was first referred to me in February 2011 for further evaluation of low red blood cells (anemia) and low platelets (thrombocytopenia). Sure, that's what he was referred to me for, but it quickly became evident that he had a plethora of other problems – and as I was (re-)learning, it was far more likely that all of his problems were tied together somehow. Like many other MCAS patients, he recalled being chronically ill essentially ever since his earliest childhood memories (frequent "pneumonias" and "colds" and "sinus infections" and "lots of diarrhea" throughout childhood, adolescence, and adulthood), and he said he was also told by his parents that even as an infant he was quite colicky and frequently non-specifically ill. He said his parents were often upset with him about his illnesses and not uncommonly suspected he was faking it – an unfortunate parental reaction I've heard from many of my MCAS patients.

> In addition to the chronic respiratory and GI tract issues, in his 20s chronic diffusely migratory bone and joint and back pains set in (and had continued ever since), and in his 30s chronic headaches and fatigue set in (and had continued ever since). More recently, starting about a decade before his referral to me, Trent had begun suffering "gastroesophageal reflux disease" (GERD) which quickly proved itself to be utterly refractory to many manners of medical therapy and even surgery (laparoscopic Nissen fundoplication) in 2008. He endorsed a large number of additional symptoms as well, most of them following chronic, waxing/waning courses over the prior several to many years or even decades including fevers, chills, soaking sweats, diffusely migratory pruritus (he showed me photographs of a wide variety of skin lesions including some hive-like lesions and some bruised-welt-like lesions), bilateral eye irritation, blurriness of vision, nasal sores, sores on his tongue and gums, throat discomfort, hoarseness, cough, dyspnea, chest pain (in 2010 alone he presented to the ER five times for this), palpitations, dysphagia, "GERD," nausea, bloody and non-bloody vomiting, alternating diarrhea and constipation, urinary hesitancy and frequency, dysuria, rash, tingling and numbness in the fingers and toes, diffusely migratory edema, poor healing, cognitive

dysfunction, depression, unprovoked presyncopal episodes which had increased in frequency over the years and were now occurring essentially daily, two frankly syncopal episodes (the last one just a few months earlier), and panic-attack-like episodes including one just the day before his first visit to my clinic ("I thought I was going to die"). He had been receiving from a neurosurgeon what sounded like epidural injections that he thought were slightly easing his back pain. He said he was applying again for disability but had been rejected in the past. He said he was a workaholic in spite of all of his chronic problems until the totality of his issues finally rendered him disabled around age 50.

Trent's medical history also included hypertension, hyperlipidemia, and a pulmonary inflammatory condition of unknown cause called sarcoidosis in 1987 which had been treated by taking out the right upper lobe of his lung, at which time a relatively uncommon, typically low-grade but resistant infection called "MAC" (*Mycobacterium avium intracellulare*) was also diagnosed for which, 20+ years later, he was still receiving therapy from an infectious disease specialist. He also had suffered a "mini-stroke" (medically called a transient ischemic accident, or TIA) soon after the 2008 surgery for his GERD. He also had had nodules of tissue sprout about various aspects of his skin, which he said had been diagnosed by his dermatologist as lichen planus. He says he had been evaluated by more physicians, and had undergone more tests, than he could count, but no clear explanation for his cornucopia of problems had ever emerged. He was a very light smoker in his 30s and had quit around his mid-40s. He had never abused alcohol or used illegal substances.

There was a lot of cancer in Trent's family history. His paternal grandmother had died of liver cancer at 72. His maternal grandfather had died of bone cancer at 74. His mother had had rheumatoid arthritis and breast cancer and had died of liver cancer at 74. His father, a smoker, had had lung cancer and had died of brain cancer at 75. His paternal uncle died of kidney cancer at 56. There was no known family history of hematologic issues. His medications included pantoprazole, fluticasone, nebivolol, sucralfate, duloxetine, iron sulfate, loratadine, pregabalin, and oxycodone. The only allergic reaction he knew of was a rash to penicillin.

Examination found a thin, concerned man with mild systolic and diastolic hypertension. His diaphoretic appearance (which he said was quite chronic) nevertheless made him appear mildly acutely on chronically ill. The only other abnormalities on the exam were mild tenderness to palpation across the upper part of the abdomen and tingling and numbness across all the fingers and toes. Oh, and on a light scratch test on the upper back, bright dermatographism briskly emerged and was fully sustained when I last checked it 10 minutes later.

In reviewing his many labs on file dating back many years, I saw that his mild anemia and thrombocytopenia had emerged in late 2009. He had long had a minimal elevation in his "MCHC" (mean corpuscular hemoglobin concentration), one of the several parameters describing red blood cells on a complete blood count (CBC), and he had long shown a mild increase in the eosinophil percentage in his white blood cell differentials. There was no sign of iron deficiency. Extensive testing for rheumatologic and other pulmonary and infectious disease had all been negative. Interestingly, IgG and IgM levels were normal, but IgA was undetectable (though there was no way that primary IgA deficiency was causing anywhere close to the full range and chronicity of his troubles). Imaging of all sorts was unrevealing except for changes to his anatomy from his surgeries as well as acid-related damage to his lower esophagus. Endoscopies in '07, '08, '09 and '10 all fairly consistently showed a hiatal hernia and inflammation of the esophagus (esophagitis). Biopsies during these endoscopies all consistently showed either normal tissue or esophagitis but not cancer.

In my initial assessment I remarked, "Clearly, his anemia and thrombocytopenia have been reactive, not primary. The real question here is whether there is a single process that could be responsible for most or all of his morbidities. Congenital IgA deficiency might explain the lifelong history of infections and perhaps some of the GI issues but doesn't come anywhere close to explaining the full gamut of his problems. Similarly, pheochromocytoma and carcinoid could explain some of his issues (e.g., hypertension, diaphoresis, diarrhea), but these diagnoses come nowhere close to explaining the full range of his problems, let alone their marked chronicity. There also isn't any one infection that can explain all of this. Rather, I think what's probably going on here is a mast cell activation syndrome (MCAS) (much more likely than systemic mastocytosis). MCAS could explain not only the full range of problems (except, perhaps, a congenital IgA deficiency, though we have no way to know whether if his IgA deficiency truly is congenital) but also their remarkable chronicity." I ordered testing for MCAS and asked him to increase his loratadine to twice daily and accompany it with famotidine to achieve as full a histamine receptor blockade as we can presently achieve.

Testing showed moderate elevations in serum and urinary prostaglandin D2 as well as the less specific mast cell mediators Factor VIII and norepinephrine. I cautioned him that we had no way to predict which mast-cell-targeted medications would most effectively control his dysfunctional mast cells and that it would require a patient, persistent, methodical approach to trying the available interventions one by one. And indeed, it did take patience, persistence, and a methodical approach, and as of this writing we still haven't found any single hugely effective ("home run") drug, but in two years of trying (and discarding several medications along the way), he found that a regimen of antihistamines, ketotifen, celecoxib, lorazepam, montelukast, and low-dose hydroxyurea controlled his symptoms well enough that he now has significantly more good days than bad (whereas before virtually every day was a bad day) and he is sufficiently comfortable that, for the time being, he is not interested in trying any other medications.

The respiratory tract issues with MCAS include issues related to inflammation and edema all up and down the tract. Symptoms include sinonasal congestion, internal (post-nasal) and external nose drip, hoarseness and laryngitis, cough (much more commonly dry than productive), shortness of breath (medically called dyspnea). Wheezing (often diagnosed as asthma) appears to be less common than dyspnea.

The dyspnea is of a curious form, as most patients deny feeling "short of breath" and instead most commonly report, "I just can't catch a *deep* breath," but testing usually can't find anything wrong and physicians begin to wonder if the complaint is psychosomatic. It's obviously a real symptom, though, and my suspicion is that short-lived, migratory flares of edema, inflammation, and/or bronchoconstriction cause this symptom. Of course, flares of such an ephemeral nature almost certainly won't be present when the patient presents for scheduled pulmonary function testing, but even if they are present, they usually aren't severe enough, or affecting a wide enough extent of the respiratory tree, to cause abnormalities in pulmonary function testing. On X-ray and CT scanning, inflammation appears as "patchy ground-glass infiltrates," but most physicians interpret such a reading as indicative of pneumonia (i.e., infection) and give little thought to the possibility of sterile inflammation even if no fever is present.

Mast cells may even play critical roles in the development of chronic obstructive pulmonary disease (COPD) and interstitial pulmonary fibrosis, which usually lead eventually to death.

110

Chapter 14: Getting to the Heart of the Matter: Cardiovascular Findings in MCAS

A wide range of cardiovascular issues can afflict – and can *seem* to afflict – MCAS patients. Let's start with a typical "fake-out" case that also illustrates the extremes to which such patients sometimes need to go to get the treatments they know will help them. I'll follow that with another couple of cases that demonstrate real cardiovascular issues from MCAS, and then we'll wrap up the chapter with a general discussion of the cardiovascular issues in MCAS.

> "Gladys," a 54-year old nurse, was referred by her allergist in October 2012 for further evaluation of suspected mast cell disease. Like most such patients, she reported an extraordinarily complicated, essentially lifelong history of unwellness. She had been a "preemie twin" (her twin sister unfortunately died around the time of birth) and dated her history with illness back to her days as a toddler, observing she was "always" a "sickly" child suffering frequent attacks of asthma and frequent respiratory "infections" often requiring hospitalization. She also noted she had always found it "easy to get colds and respiratory and GI viruses" since childhood. The worst of the respiratory issues seemed to spontaneously resolve around age 4, though she had continued the rest of her life suffering occasional acute onset of dyspnea (especially when exposed to smoke). She also noted frequent ear infections throughout childhood and adolescence but otherwise was well until problems with frequent "urinary tract infections" began around age 21 and had continued to the present – though she said only about 50% of these "infections" had actually shown positive cultures, even when she had substantial urinary-tract-infection-like (UTI-like) symptoms including bleeding, pain, malaise, and right kidney pain. She suffered bacterial meningitis at age 24 with her first pregnancy (conceived with the help of fertility drugs), but her daughter was born fine and had been healthy since. During her second pregnancy at age 26, she suffered a number of traumas including falling (for unclear reasons), death of her husband by electrocution, and then victimized by a motor vehicle accident that caused bleeding throughout the last month of pregnancy, but her son was born fine and had been healthy since. Soon after remarrying, her third pregnancy, at age 28, led to problems with toxemia and "heart issues" throughout (including episodes of her distal extremities and face turning blue, acute dyspnea, and palpitations), but no diagnosis was made, no treatment was given, and another son was born healthy except for supraventricular tachycardia requiring ablation at age 16. All pregnancies were delivered by C-sections.

Gladys then moved a few states away and soon started suffering severe malaise, dyspnea, and palpitations for which she was hospitalized and diagnosed with ventricular ectopy. She then soon suffered a left leg deep venous thrombosis and pulmonary embolus requiring anticoagulation with warfarin for a year. Her ectopy proved refractory to multiple medication trials but eventually "settled down" with flecainide.

Next, waxing/waning aching in the distal extremities (especially the legs) developed and was diagnosed (without biopsy) as "fibrous myositis." Endometriosis was also diagnosed. She underwent hysterectomy at age 30. Fibroid tumors were found throughout the peritoneum, and she was determined to need right ovarian torsion surgery, but the left ovary was accidentally resected first, and then a month later she had the right ovary resected. She subsequently had yet another procedure for lysis of adhesions (for ongoing abdominal pain), and then an appendectomy, but abdominal pain and constipation nevertheless persisted (at least until around 2009).

Since her 30s Gladys had also noticed "irritable bowel" symptoms and frequent attacks of sneezing (up to 18 sneezes in a row) while eating. She also had begun suffering spontaneous ligament and tendon tears.

After six years in her new home, Gladys moved back to the town she had come from and soon (after walking into a glass door) needed surgery for a herniated C5-6 disc whose primary pathology she dated back to age 22, when she was kicked in the neck by a psychiatric patient. At age 34 she underwent a right partial mastectomy for a suspicious lesion, which proved to be benign.

At age 38 she again moved several states away and did well except for continued "UTIs" and "colds" and "respiratory and abdominal stuff." At age 42 she again moved a few states away and continued suffering "UTIs." She continued using diclofenac for "arthritis" and "fibrous myositis" in her hips and hands and legs, as if she failed to take it, her pain prevented her from even getting out of bed.

At age 45 she moved once again and soon underwent cholecystectomy for her ongoing attacks of abdominal pain. After the surgery, she noted the attacks continued, "just not as bad" – but her irritable bowel symptoms in general actually seemed to worsen. A C4-5 spine fusion was needed (unclear cause), and she also incurred a stress fracture in the right foot simply upon stepping off a curb. She also tore a right foot tendon.

At age 52, during a visit in May 2010 to her primary physician, Gladys was prescribed a combination pill of simvastatin and extended-release niacin for hypercholesterolemia, took a single dose, developed a rash, then took another dose about 1-2 days later and immediately developed a sensation of "bee stings" about her skin and severe diarrhea and malaise and dyspnea, palpitations, diffusely erythematous rash ("I looked like a lobster"), and diffuse tremor. Evaluation in the emergency room (ER) led to treatment with epinephrine, famotidine, diphenhydramine, and methylprednisolone, which "turned it around," but she was admitted anyway (for three days) for continued wheezing and was discharged still feeling unwell. She had required frequent ER visits ever since for similar reactions from assorted foods (such as shrimp at a Japanese restaurant) or medications (such as naproxen or an epidural injection for a ruptured disc). It was questioned whether she was reacting to lidocaine, so she was switched to bupivacaine (with premedications) for subsequent injections and appeared to tolerate it OK. She also suffered an episode of *Salmonella* urosepsis (severe urinary tract infection) requiring home IV antibiotics for two weeks via a peripherally inserted central catheter (PICC), and she thought the otherwise unidentified premedications she got with PICC placement helped her feel the best she had been in a long time.

No, we're not done yet with Gladys' story – not even close. She had suffered "constant" back pain since 2009 due to ruptured and bulging discs. In 2011 she suffered two episodes of acute onset of edema, chest discomfort, and dyspnea upon sun exposure for which she took antihistamines and felt better within 48 hours. She was empirically started on standing H_1/H_2 antihistamines after her third ER visit for anaphylaxis and felt that after a year of this treatment her daily diarrhea has decreased and she had had "only" 2-3 hospitalizations for malaise and hypokalemia (low potassium). She always felt "hyper" throughout her body with diffuse sensations of "crawling," "bee stings," and palpitations and dyspnea. Hydroxyzine had helped insomnia. Oral cromolyn caused "bad edema" and dyspnea. Niacin was found to be a trigger, too. She complained about diffusely migratory waxing/waning bone pain without any clear trigger. In September 2012 she suffered spontaneous onset of a "bad" diffuse pruritic (itchy) erythematous (red) folliculitic (pimply) rash; her dermatologist thought it was due to mast cell disease and recommended nightly hydroxyzine, which helped the pruritus and rash, but when she noticed symptoms were relapsing in the mid-afternoon, she started taking a second dose in the late afternoon and noticed this helped even more. She repeatedly said, "I now have a life" with these medications, but she was not always well and was looking to achieve further improvement.

On review of systems, although she denied fevers, feeling cold much of the time, irritation of the mouth, vomiting, enlargement or tenderness in the nodal areas, or syncope, Gladys endorsed chills, feeling hot much of the time, soaking sweats, diffusely migratory pruritus, headaches (worse since 2009), chronic fatigue, diffusely migratory muscle/bone/joint pain, irritation of the eyes (her optometrist told her she had the driest eyes she had ever seen, along with corneal and scleral ulcers, and she now was regularly using eye drops to help with these problems, but evaluation for Sjögren syndrome had been negative, and besides, Sjögren syndrome couldn't possibly explain all that had gone on in her), episodic difficulty focusing her vision, irritation of the nose, coryza, light epistaxis, easy bruising, occasional "hemorrhoidal" rectal bleeding, irritation of the throat with constant throat clearing and frequent dry cough ("it drives my husband crazy"), dyspnea, chest discomfort/pain, palpitations, slight proximal dysphagia, GERD, unprovoked nausea, diarrhea alternating with constipation (though much less constipation since 2009), diffusely migratory rash, diffusely migratory edema, episodic diffusely migratory tingling/numbness and burning paresthesias and fasciculations and tremors, restless legs, insomnia, waxing/waning alopecia, onychodystrophy, new dental cavities since 2009 despite a lifetime of good dental hygiene, cognitive dysfunction, virtually daily episodes of presyncope (not always postural), and a 50 lb. weight gain since 2009 possibly due to decreased exercise since her dyspnea impedes exercise.

There were no known hematologic issues in the family history. Her mother, now deceased, had osteoarthritis and survived some sort of a rare type of cancer in her duodenum in her 50s. There have been no issues with tobacco, alcohol, or illegal substances.

Her current medications included atenolol, butalbital/acetaminophen/caffeine (Fioricet), cetirizine in the morning, cyclobenzaprine, diclofenac, epinephrine autoinjector (but had never used it), esomeprazole, conjugated estrogen, fexofenadine, flecainide, hydroxyzine (afternoon and evening), potassium, ranitidine, tramadol, and triamterene/hydrochlorothiazide (Maxzide). She anaphylaxed to lidocaine, naproxen, niacin-simvastatin, and azithromycin, and she noted codeine caused her nausea and morphine caused her pruritus. The last time she had IV contrast (without premedication), she felt hot and noted some dyspnea but didn't anaphylax. Nevertheless, this had been listed on her chart as causing anaphylaxis and she had been cautioned to henceforth always get premedicated before taking IV contrast.

Exam found a slightly plump but otherwise outwardly healthy appearing woman. Vitals signs were notable for a blood pressure of 163/83 (her highest in about a year). Key findings included her comfortable general appearance, some dental fillings, slight diaphoresis (sweating), mild scattered bruising, resolving diffuse sparsely scattered rash of small (< 1 cm) ulcerative skin lesions, and just the slightest trace of distal bilateral lower extremity edema. On a light scratch test on the upper back, mild dermatographism immediately emerged and remained fully sustained when last checked 10 minutes later.

Labs on file were notable for moderate hypercholesterolemia (223-532 mg/dl, upper normal 200) and moderately severe hypertriglyceridemia (244-1759 mg/dl, upper normal 150), minimal transaminitis, mild hypoproteinemia and hypoalbuminemia, three normal tryptases in 2011-2012, mildly elevated chromogranin A (105 ng/ml, normal 0-50), and negative extensive evaluations for pheochromocytoma, carcinoid, and a variety of other autoimmune diseases and neuroendocrine cancers except for an elevated plasma free norepinephrine at 889 pg/ml (normal 80-520). IgG, IgA, and IgM antibody levels were normal. Only about 25% of the many urine cultures on file showed unequivocal infection. CT scanning had shown marked hepatic steatosis (fatty infiltration of the liver). Cardiac function was normal on echocardiogram. Bone densitometry in 2005 was normal.

My assessment at the time was that "this is about as classic a presentation of mast cell activation syndrome as one can see. Every single thing that has ever happened to her is potentially attributable to mast cell disease (even including the hyperlipidemia – she's not the first MCAS patient I've seen with severe hypertriglyceridemia which virtually normalizes on effective MCAS treatment – and the elevated chromogranin and norepinephrine, which are known mast cell mediators (though obviously not completely specific for the mast cell)). Tryptase is almost always normal (to perhaps slightly elevated) in MCAS, as this is not systemic mastocytosis, a disease of mast cell proliferation which almost always drives elevations in tryptase."

I pursued additional testing for levels of mediators more specific to mast cell production than chromogranin and norepinephrine, and the first round of testing found elevated plasma histamine (13 nmol/L, normal 0-8), but the prostaglandin D_2 testing at that point was compromised by her use of diclofenac, an NSAID. She did a second round of testing after having abstained from NSAID use for a week, and this time not only was the plasma histamine again elevated (same level as before) but also the serum, and spot and 24-hour urinary, prostaglandin D_2 tests were all about 50-150% above their upper limits of normal. While enduring this testing and waiting for results, though, she had continued having "bad days" just as often as "good days," with problems including a flu-like syndrome (despite getting the seasonal flu vaccine 7-8 weeks earlier), a "regular" cold, a true urinary tract infection, bilateral middle ear inflammation that was treated as if it was due to an infection, and an Achilles tendinitis. Meanwhile, she remained grateful that standing H_1/H_2 blocking therapy seemed to still be helping her stay out of the ER.

I noted that Gladys needed to move on to additional maneuvers to try to get better control over her disease, and NSAIDs and benzodiazepines often are inexpensive maneuvers to be tried next. (NSAIDs help by blocking the cyclo-oxygenase 1 and 2 (COX1 and COX2) enzymes that are necessary for prostaglandin production, and benzodiazepines not only engage inhibitory mast-cell-surface benzodiazepine receptors but also neural receptors that can help decrease stress that can result in CNS release of mediators (such as corticotropin releasing hormone) that can trigger mast cell activation.) However, she had anaphylaxed to naproxen and suffered the same effects, though to a lesser degree, with diclofenac and tolerated those effects on an ongoing basis because she knew that going without the diclofenac led to rapid relapse of "crippling" joint pain. Thus, I decided that before we necessarily resorted to adding a whole new class of drug (benzodiazepines) to her regimen, she should try tweaking her NSAID regimen by changing diclofenac to celecoxib since I had seen the COX2-only-blocking celecoxib be better tolerable in some MCAS patients who react to classic COX1-and-COX2-blocking NSAIDs. She did not have any (known) sulfa allergy that would predict allergy to celecoxib. Some insurers require evidence of having "failed" at least two classic NSAIDs before going on to celecoxib, and she certainly couldn't tolerate naproxen, and clearly diclofenac was suboptimally effective for her disease and also caused symptoms, and she had been told by her allergist to never take aspirin, so I thought it reasonable to declare that she had failed 2+ NSAIDs and ought to be approved for celecoxib. We briefly discussed the slight cardiac risks with celecoxib and I wrote the prescription.

Gladys returned several weeks later reporting the switch from diclofenac to celecoxib was very positive, as all of the anaphylactoid and GI side effects (abdominal pain, cramps, diarrhea) and anxiety the diclofenac used to cause had completely resolved, while the one positive effect she had been gaining from the diclofenac – control of her otherwise "crippling" joint pain – had been controlled very well by celecoxib at just 100 mg twice daily. She noted ongoing occasional reactions to environmental provocations such as a new type of perfume she had opened recently, but she had learned to aggressively take diphenhydramine for these reactions, and this strategy was working very reliably for her, usually settling down her reactions within minutes to a few hours. She even reported having recently had a reaction recently which at first she was certain was going to require a trip to the ER (based on her past experiences) but this time settled down quickly with self-treatment at home. She was quite pleased with how she was doing.

Unfortunately, at her next appointment two months later, Gladys reported she had suffered a break-in at her home, causing anxiety and then chest discomfort. She thought that lorazepam likely would significantly contribute to settling her flare, but she could not access the drug via phone calls to her other doctors, and I was out of town, so she went to the ER with her complaint of chest pain. She requested lorazepam, but this was not given. She was recommended to undergo cardiac catheterization *and accepted this because the premedication regimen would include lorazepam.* She says that her flare symptoms dramatically settled upon receiving the premedication regimen, and the catheterization then was performed and – surprise! – reported to her as negative. She said she had been steadily improving since then and, except for some minor residual URI-type symptoms, she was almost back to her prior baseline. She additionally noted she had been instructed to double her atenolol to help better control her blood pressure, but this seemed to be causing new edema in the lower legs and feet at the end of the day and didn't seem to have helped her blood pressure. She requested a prescription for lorazepam to have on hand to assist with control of her flares. I provided this but reminded her of the importance of getting new symptoms promptly evaluated rather than assuming they're directly due to flares of mast cell activation.

Gladys is typical of MCAS patients who have chest pain that (appropriately) worries physicians about the possibility of angina or an actual heart attack (or, as it's medically called, a myocardial infarction or MI, resulting from obstruction of blood flow through the coronary arteries to the heart muscle) and yet has no obstructions in her coronary arteries. It's not known yet whether the chest discomfort in these sorts of situations is a result of a flare of inflammation or spasm of the chest wall or esophagus or lung or some other thoracic structure, but it's not likely being caused by damage to muscle (chest, heart, or esophageal) since our blood testing has gotten pretty good for detecting muscle damage, and yet such patients usually don't show any signs of muscle damage.

To contrast, here's a case of how significantly – and yet oddly – MCAS can affect the cardiovascular system.

"John," a 48-year old former welder retired since age 30 when his first heart attack occurred, was referred to me in September 2008 regarding his apparent problems with excessive blood clotting, or what we medically call a hypercoagulable syndrome. He reported a principal problem of having had 9 heart attacks (in med-speak, "myocardial infarctions," or "MIs"), 10 coronary artery stent placements, a one-vessel coronary artery bypass about 4-5 years earlier (though the grafted vessel clotted off about a month later), and 5 strokes, 1 of which was so large that it was read on MRI as a tumor, prompting a neurosurgeon to explore that area of his brain, finding to his surprise it was a scar from the stroke. John's chronic problems included residual left hand numbness and minimal residual dysarthria (difficulty speaking) from his strokes, alleged near- deafness bilaterally (which he thought was due to auditory trauma from when he used to work in noisy environments, though he never seemed to have any difficulty hearing me), "arthritis" and "3 herniated discs" in his neck, chronic mild scattered bruising ever since being placed on the anti-platelet drug clopidogrel to try to keep him from clotting, a decade of chronic diffuse aches and pains in all of his joints along with numbness in his feet and hands, and problems with low blood sugars (in contrast to his siblings, who all had problems with high blood sugars).

John told me all of his problems dated back to the appearance at age 15 of enlarged lymph nodes through his neck and underarm areas (medically speaking, the axillae), accompanied by fevers, chills, profuse sweats, diffuse aches and pains, and anemia. A trial of the chemotherapy drug methotrexate did not help, and he underwent removal of his painfully enlarged spleen at that time, and though there was some debate as to whether the underlying diagnosis was Hodgkin's vs. non-Hodgkin's lymphoma, ultimately a precise diagnosis could not be made and he did not receive further treatment. He says his enlarged lymph nodes (which had not responded to the brief trial of methotrexate) went away on their own after the splenectomy and had never returned. Although he wasn't having any fevers, sweats, or weight loss that might have signaled return of lymphoma (which sometimes can trigger clotting), he said he had had irritable bowel syndrome for 20 years, consistently producing diarrhea 10-15 times daily in all that time; he said his last colonoscopy and EGD in early 2008 showed only a few benign polyps. He had been evaluated for Buerger's disease, which causes arterial obstruction, but that had turned out to be negative. He has complained of headaches at various times in the past. He also had been diagnosed with emphysema and said he got pneumonia very easily. He had undergone extensive evaluation in the past for his hypercoagulable syndrome by two hematologists I know and respect very much, but no diagnosis had ever been established.

John had smoked one pack of cigarettes per day since age 13. There was no history of alcohol abuse or illegal substance use. He said his job as a nuclear submarine welder had routinely involved exposure to radiation as well as asbestos. His father had hypertension and asbestosis, and heart disease was rampant throughout his mother's side of the family; his mother died at age 52, allegedly due to diabetes-related coronary artery disease (CAD). Four sisters had diabetes; one had autoimmune hyperthyroidism called Graves' disease. His maternal grandfather died at age 42 of a "massive stroke." His maternal great-great grandfather died of "large lymph nodes all over."

Exam found an outwardly healthy appearing man except for his smoker's voice, mild bruising scattered about the extremities, and minimal residual neurologic deficits in the left hand.

I reviewed every one of John's 15 years' worth of lab results on file. He indeed had undergone very extensive evaluations of his clotting system, but no hypercoagulable syndrome had ever been found, either inborn or acquired. Curiously, though, his prothrombin time (PT) and/or partial thromboplastin time (PTT) (two very common screening tests of coagulation system function) had been modestly abnormal (elevated) on some occasions which didn't correlate with acute presentations in which he would have been anticoagulated (different anticoagulants normally elevate the PT or PTT). Other subtle oddities abounded, too. His mean corpuscular volume (MCV, or average red blood cell size) was consistently modestly elevated through 2006. He has been consistently mildly anemic throughout 1997 and then again ever since 2002. He had had a fairly consistent mild elevation in his white blood cell count since at least 1993, but perhaps that was just due to his splenectomy. His red cell distribution widths (RDWs, measures of the variability in red blood cell size) had been consistently mildly elevated since 2004. The total amount of the IgM type of antibody had always been low in him, roughly half to two-thirds normal. Extensive blood studies looking for molecular traces of B- and T-cell lymphomas had been negative. Eosinophils were occasionally slightly elevated, but he also had frequently shown a moderate percentage of "reactive lymphocytes" on many of his blood counts. CT imaging in 1995 and 2005 showed persistent mild adenopathy at many places about his body. H. pylori gastritis had been found in 1993 and again in 1995. EGD and colonoscopic biopsies in the 1990s had found mild chronic inflammation in the small and large bowel and benign colonic polyps. Skin biopsy of a cyanotic right great toe in 1995 and again in 1996 found microvascular thrombosis both times. A skin biopsy in 1998 of an itchy back lesion found an "atypical lymphoreticular infiltrate."

I pretty thoroughly re-evaluated John for virtually every inborn or acquired hypercoagulable syndrome that hadn't already been checked out, but all the tests came back negative – around the time when I was figuring out my first few MCAS patients. I hadn't yet seen MCAS-induced clotting (not that I was aware of, anyway), but I was rapidly learning that MCAS can affect many other systems in the body depending on which mediators the given patient's dysfunctional mast cells would produce, so given that some of these mediators clearly had interactions with the clotting system, why wouldn't the clotting system, too, be involved in the clinical presentation in at least some MCAS patients?

And, indeed, subsequent testing for MCAS showed a significantly elevated chromogranin A level (178 ng/ml, normal 0-50), a significantly elevated urinary prostaglandin D2 level (399 pg/ml, normal 100-280), and an elevated plasma free norepinephrine (591 pg/ml, normal 10-520). I asked the pathologist to re-examine John's old GI tract biopsies for evidence of mast cell disease, but that additional testing was negative.

I set about reviewing John's old MI and stroke records in detail, and the story that emerged was not what I had expected. John had actually never been found to have any obstructions in any of his own arteries. In fact, his first few MI presentations really puzzled his cardiologists precisely because repeated catheterizations never showed any CAD. Finally, somewhere around the fourth MI, his cardiologists felt compelled to place a stent in the artery that the tests said should have been the occluded artery, and since that time he had undergone numerous stent placements – *and had always soon developed obstructions located exclusively in the stents*. As noted above, he also underwent a coronary artery bypass, and soon after the operation an obstruction developed in the grafted vessel.

Unfortunately, although H_1 and H_2 histamine receptor blockers and inhaled and oral cromolyn helped John a little bit with a range of his symptoms, I never found a "home run" drug for him before he died in early 2011 from another MI.

In retrospect, I suspect his MCAS not only drove his baseline hypercoagulability but also led to abnormal reactions to his stents (ironically, most of them of the variety suffused with one immunosuppressive drug or another to try to prevent immune reactions) that provoked the intra-stent clotting.

So MCAS can affect thoracic structures to mimic a heart attack, and it can affect blood vessels to cause an actual heart attack, but what about the heart itself?

"Regina" was a 50-year old jewelry designer when I was initially asked to see her in the hospital in May 2011 while she was recovering from a strange case of heart failure, but her history of lifelong unwellness stretched back literally a lifetime. As far back as she could remember, she had been allergic to grass and shellfish and "could never play outside" and to the present could not "touch a Christmas tree." She had had waxing/waning diffusely migratory pruritus since childhood. She had always been "sensitive" to most medications. She had reportedly suffered a seizure at age 2. She had suffered seemingly unprovoked episodes of what sounded like hives about her fingers since childhood. She said she had suffered asthma as a child, but this resolved by adolescence. She had been dealing with irritation of both of her eyes as well as "constant" coryza and a "constant lump in my throat" "my whole life."

Regina also noted she had suffered frequent unprovoked palpitations "my whole life." At age 16 she was in a bad motor vehicle accident causing extensive orthopedic trauma including bilateral femur fractures. She was in the hospital for 8-1/2 months and had great trouble healing from surgeries including *Staph* infections "that would not heal." She had been markedly fatigued, waxing/waning, ever since that accident and also had carried a diagnosis of post-traumatic stress disorder (PTSD) ever since that accident.

As if all of that history wasn't bad enough, she then suffered a second severe motor vehicle accident at age 37. Her right leg was again crushed, requiring implantation of several plates, and she had very limited flexion remaining in the right knee. She also accumulated multiple vertebral disc problems with this second accident.

Then, believe it or not, in 2008 (at age 47) she suffered a third car accident. Regina told me none of these accidents was her fault (i.e., she didn't lose control of her car). She said she had been in constant back pain for many years; "I don't know what it's like to have a day and not be in pain," she told me. She had long sought care at a spine care center for her back problems and even underwent a rhizotomy (selective spinal cord nerve root destruction) there in 2008 to try to control the pain (after which surgery, curiously, she gained another 35 lbs.), but then, because it was becoming too difficult to travel to their facilities, she began seeing a new pain management physician locally in December 2010.

Regina told me she got a series of "16 steroid shots" in her back from that physician over the course of several weeks that resulted in marked abdominal bloating, hoarseness, facial edema, and dermatologic changes such that her "skin didn't feel right." Then, in February 2011, she joined her family at a restaurant and ate a roast beef sandwich, and though the rest of her family was fine, a few hours later she developed severe non-bloody vomiting and diarrhea that quickly led to an ER visit and hospitalization for dehydration, during which 5-day stay she also was newly diagnosed with diabetes mellitus type 2 and diverticulitis. She again got out of the hospital for five days but then had to be readmitted for nine days, this time for a new diagnosis of congestive heart failure. She was out of the hospital again for 2-1/2 weeks, then acutely developed an odd type of chest pain (brief (2-10 minute) episodes of severe "grabbing" central chest pain) and returned to the ER, was hospitalized, and was soon transferred to the cardiology service at my hospital, where she stayed for a week and was diagnosed with severe systolic heart failure of uncertain cause (on assorted testing, both atria and ventricles were enlarged and left ventricular ejection fraction was 8% (normal is 50% or higher), but no scar or infiltrative process was found; cardiac catheterization was not done, but cardiac MRI suggested no arterial or venous disease of any sort). Since discharge, she had been suffering "severe" fatigue ("sleeping all the time" but also staying up most of every night), and felt overwhelmed, depressed, and as if she couldn't feel anything. She also felt more like an "it" than a woman; "my femininity is gone."

Past medical history also included endometriosis for which she underwent surgery not too long before her first pregnancy at age 30 (presented breach, delivered a daughter by C-section). She then underwent another pregnancy two years later, delivering a son. She was diagnosed with obstructive sleep apnea in 2008 and, though CPAP initially was helpful, she soon became intolerant of it and had largely given it up.

On review of systems she denied problems with fevers, queasiness/nausea/vomiting, rash, or neuropathy (except her left leg as described above), but she endorsed a wide range of other problems including feeling cold ("freezing") virtually all the time for the past several months (following, oddly, a very long prior history of feeling hot virtually all the time), chills, unprovoked (often at nighttime) soaking sweats since 2009, relatively new problems with frequent headaches, waxing/waning visual acuity over the last year or so, development of sores in her mouth whenever she was nervous, onset of malaise whenever she had to wear pink-colored clothing, seasonal allergies, proximal dysphagia, "grabbing" chest pain (for which she had used furosemide and sublingual nitroglycerin three times since she was discharged), relatively new GERD, weight loss since discharge, intermittent right hearing loss for 2-30 minutes, frequent crying, "constant" urethral burning since a urinary catheter was placed during one of her recent hospitalizations, newly constipated since discharge (which she attributed to her medication regimen), diffusely migratory waxing/waning aching ever since her first accident at age 16, fairly frequent, unprovoked episodic cognitive dysfunction and panic attacks since her car accident in 1997, and frequent episodes of "vertigo" for many years now (always seem to be orthostatic in nature). She denied frank syncope. She noted that very tiny macular hyperpigmented areas had been newly appearing scattered all about her skin over the last several months. She had "always" had a problem with "rotting teeth" in spite of what she felt was good attention to dental hygiene since childhood. She said her periods had recently abruptly stopped.

Regina's father had been ill for the last 10 years of his life with diabetes, heart disease (requiring a four-vessel coronary artery bypass), and a *Staph* infection requiring revision of the sternal incision for his coronary artery bypass; already a double-amputee from gangrene, he eventually died a day before a planned hand amputation for gangrene. Her mother had never been ill, but a maternal uncle (a smoker) died of metastatic lung cancer. This uncle's son had been afflicted lifelong by eczema, and this uncle's daughter had just delivered a baby "covered" in eczema. A maternal aunt had diabetes. Her maternal grandmother had suffered two episodes of septicemia, one in labor in her first pregnancy, which led to loss of the baby, the other a fatal episode allegedly related to diabetes. Her daughter was healthy, but her son had an enlarged heart.

Although she had suffered heavy secondary smoke exposure from her father as a child, she herself had never smoked, nor had she ever abused alcohol or used illegal substances.
She was on many medications, of course, and the details really aren't relevant to the point of this story. In addition to the above-noted environmental allergies, she said sulfa and azithromycin made her throat close, and aspirin and ibuprofen gave her "welts."

Exam found an overweight, slightly pale woman in no acute distress, obviously mildly awkward and painful about the low back, hips, and legs in (nevertheless independent, unassisted) ambulation. Aside from her mildly chronically ill general appearance, key findings included deteriorating teeth, mild epigastric tenderness, and the previously noted chronic left leg neuropathy. The right knee was chronically fixed in a semi-extended position. On a light scratch test on the upper back, mild-moderate dermatographism quickly emerged and was nearly fully sustained when I last checked it 10 minutes later. She also tried to point out some small subcutaneous masses she had felt developing in the abdominal wall, but I couldn't appreciate them.

Labs obtained in the hospital included a mildly elevated plasma histamine level (10 nmol/L, normal 0-8), an elevated Factor VIII level (275%, normal 50-150%), and a top-normal spot urinary prostaglandin D_2 level (even though it had not been chilled upon collection). A repeat urinary prostaglandin D_2 level, properly chilled, was clearly elevated at 466 pg/ml (normal 100-280).

I'll spare you the long story of her various medication trials. Suffice to say, on H_1 and H_2 antihistamines, clonazepam, and montelukast, her heart function quickly recovered to normal (59%), her heart failure medications were successfully stopped, and pretty much all of her chronic symptoms either improved significantly or completely resolved. By late 2011 she was telling me she was steadily losing the excess weight she had tried in vain to lose for many years, she was (newly) feeling happy, and was "thrilled" to be on the "go, go, go" all the time. "I can't remember the last time I felt this well." Her cousin, too, told me that everybody in her family had been amazed at her improvement.

Interesting coda: a year later many of her symptoms began relapsing soon after she switched to a new hair coloring product. She initially didn't want to part with the new product because of the youthful look she thought it provided her, but finally in spring 2013 she gave it up, and over the next month all of her symptoms again remitted. (Anybody beginning to see the potential connections between "multiple chemical sensitivity" syndrome and MCAS?)

Probably the most common cardiovascular issue I see MCAS cause is episodes – usually without any apparent provocation – of presyncope, which of course is never reported as such by the patient. Patients instead use terms like "lightheadedness," "dizziness," "weakness," and "vertigo." Sometimes (fortunately, not often, and only in a small minority of patients who suffer presyncopal episodes) an episode becomes so severe as to cause frank syncope (i.e., actual loss of consciousness).

Many MCAS patients with presyncope come to be diagnosed with postural orthostatic tachycardia syndrome (POTS), particularly the hyperadrenergic variant of POTS. It remains to be determined by specific study what portion of the POTS patient population (hyperadrenergic or otherwise) harbors MCAS.

MCAS patients also often report lability – again, usually without any apparent provocation – in pulse or blood pressure. Same thing with palpitations, which many times leads to continuous cardiac monitoring (a "Holter monitor" study) which usually doesn't find any significant cardiac anomaly.

The chest pain from MCAS usually is not in the typical pattern seen with anginal chest pain from coronary artery obstruction, but make no mistake about it, MCAS in some patients can drive the development of substantial vascular abnormalities, both arterial (e.g., aggressive atherosclerosis or aneurysms) and/or venous (e.g., hemorrhoids).

Congestive heart failure (CHF) is a common medical problem (almost always of unknown cause), and it very commonly causes edema (swelling), but edema from mast cell activation follows a very different pattern than edema from congestive heart failure. Edema from CHF usually is "dependent" – fluid collects in accordance with gravity, and this edema often responds to drugs which increase urine production ("diuretics"). Edema from MCAS, on the other hand, usually manifests a confounding pattern of showing up in random places at random times – today it might be in the left foot on waking in the morning, later today the left foot may return to normal and edema will then show up around the left eye in the evening, and then by tomorrow morning the left periorbital edema will have resolved but at mid-day right hand edema develops. And the edema from MCAS often does not respond to diuretics but will respond to extra doses of mast-cell-targeted medications.

In CHF, heart function is easily demonstrated to have decreased, while in MCAS heart function usually is normal.

Cardiologists are beginning to learn that two odd acute cardiologic phenomena often are associated with mast cell activation. Takotsubo syndrome is an uncommon (about 1-2% of cases) acute heart failure syndrome in which the "apex" portion of the heart's left ventricle takes on an odd, balloon-like shape. Testing at the time of presentation often mimics what would be expected from obstruction of one of the heart's main coronary arteries, the left anterior descending coronary artery, but no obstruction is seen on cardiac catheterization. Interestingly, a significant stressor (emotional more common than physical) shortly precedes onset of the syndrome in about two-thirds of cases. Norepinephrine levels commonly are elevated in takotsubo syndrome, but the source of such elevations is unclear.

Kounis syndrome, or "allergic angina," is an acute coronary syndrome which acts just like angina (or frank myocardial infarction) due to coronary artery obstruction because it's in fact due to coronary artery obstruction – just not "the usual" coronary artery obstruction. Instead of atherosclerotic plaque accumulation, the coronary artery obstruction in Kounis syndrome is caused by spasm of a relatively plaque-free artery, and it's becoming increasingly clear that such spasms are due to mast cell activation. Kounis syndrome has recently been described in cerebral arteries, too, causing strokes, and in mesenteric arteries, causing a variety of abdominal problems.

It is possible that John's MI and stroke presentations might have been Kounis syndrome in action – and it's possible that Regina's heart failure might have been takotsubo syndrome in action, though we can't say for sure since we didn't have access to her initial echocardiogram when she was first hospitalized for heart failure. Of course, MCAS might be capable of causing other, non-takotsubo-like heart failure syndromes, too – perhaps even the garden variety "idiopathic" CHF. Time (and much more research, of course!) will tell.

Chapter 15: Well, We're In a World of S**t Now: Gastrointestinal Findings in MCAS

The introduction to Chapter 13, about pulmonary findings in MCAS, could be applied virtually unchanged to this chapter, too: "Given that mast cells tend to hang out at the body's environmental interfaces to best serve their defensive role, and given that the gastrointestinal (GI) tract constitutes a huge portion of those interfaces, it's not surprising that there are relatively more mast cells in the GI tract than most other places in the body (except possibly the respiratory and genitourinary tracts) – and therefore it's not surprising that there are few MCAS patients who get away without any GI tract issues at all."

"Ellen," a 22-year old college senior (who had had to switch majors due to workload limitations imposed by her illness) was referred to me in April 2013 for further evaluation of suspected mast cell disease. Although the records from her other physicians all stated her illness began only 2-3 years earlier, the patient and her mother were quick to tell me she had been sick literally her entire life. Her mother noted Ellen had been afflicted by unusually severe problems with reflux right from birth, and as time went on, she had suffered virtually incessant difficulties with nausea, vomiting, abdominal cramping, diarrhea (but never constipation), and many days of missed school because of these problems. Her uncountable number of medical evaluations were consistently non-diagnostic. These problems continued all the way through high school and beyond (she missed nearly a year of high school and so far had missed two semesters at college from her illness).

As childhood and adolescence progressed, many other problems began emerging, too, and it was all so complicated that neither Ellen nor her mother could really recall the specific timeline of which symptoms emerged when. All in all, it amounted to troubles with diffusely migratory patchy red rash, marked dermatographism, frequent severe presyncopal spells (clearly both orthostatic and non-orthostatic) (but never frank syncope), sensitivities to an ever-widening array of foods, flushing episodes, frequently recurrent episodes of burning/tearing/pulsating pain predominantly centered in one particular location in the right mid-abdomen and another particular location in the upper medial aspect of the left lower quadrant, migraine headaches and dysmenorrhea ever since menarche, marked mood swings, anxiety attacks, a wide variety of medication sensitivities (e.g., all birth control pills made her sick, low doses of sedatives caused extreme sedation, nitrous oxide exposure at the dentist caused her to become violent, and other unknown general anesthetics also caused excessive sedation in her exploratory laparoscopy two years earlier for suspected (but disproven) endometriosis), diffusely migratory joint pains, chronic fatigue and malaise (often to a disabling degree), excessive sleepiness alternating with insomnia, night sweats, chills, and occasional urinary tract "infections." She had poor appetite (without weight loss) and poor GI transit, with regurgitation of food eaten several hours previously. Work-up had included negative extensive GI evaluations, negative extensive evaluation for porphyria (her mother says she and her own father (i.e., the patient's maternal grandfather) had acute intermittent porphyria), negative findings for celiac disease and pancreatitis and pancreatic insufficiency, and negative extensive imaging including ultrasound, CT, and MRI.

Finally, in late 2011 Ellen's gastroenterologist (who had been learning to "smell" MCAS from other patients he had sent me for otherwise inexplicable GI issues) performed yet another EGD, obtained random biopsies of the otherwise completely normal-appearing upper GI tract and had the biopsies specially stained looking for increased mast cells. Indeed, a modest increase (up to 24 per high power field) was found in a duodenal biopsy. Serum tryptase was normal. A blood test for a rare condition that can cause abdominal and other problems, hereditary angioedema, was negative. She had been referred to a local hematologist a year before she saw me for further evaluation for possible systemic mastocytosis, but a bone marrow aspiration and biopsy done on her first visit there was unrevealing (though the flow cytometry report didn't specifically comment on whether the specific testing needed for mast cell disease (co-expression of markers $CD117^+CD25^+$ or $CD117^+CD2^+$) had been sought or performed). She underwent evaluation by a porphyria specialist a few months after that, with negative findings, and then in early 2013 (while suffering another severe upper respiratory "infection" – or was it just another flare of sterile inflammation driven by mast cell activation disease?) she was referred to another hospital's GI service for further evaluation, again with no additional significant findings or recommendations. She then was referred to me.

On a full review of systems, although Ellen denied irritation of the eyes/nose/mouth/throat, tinnitus or other hearing deficit, epistaxis or other easy bleeding/bruising, coryza, dyspnea, dysphagia, or chest pain/discomfort, she endorsed (in addition to the items already mentioned above) subjective fevers, feeling cold all the time, diffusely migratory aching, diffusely migratory pruritus, episodes of blurred vision (especially with her presyncopal spells), hypersensitivity to strong fragrances (e.g., lotions, coffee), palpitations, "constant" gastroesophageal reflux, abdominal bloating but no other edema, diffusely migratory tingling/numbness paresthesias distally in all extremities, waxing/waning enlargement (adenopathy) and tenderness (adenitis) of lymph nodes in the bilateral cervical and inguinal areas, episodic cognitive dysfunction, mild hair loss, and weakening nails. She said it took her a month to recover from *E. coli* and *Salmonella* infections contracted during a family trip to Egypt in 2010. She also had undergone knee surgery in 2010 following an accident.

Besides the above-noted porphyrias, the hematologic, oncologic, and rheumatologic aspects of the family history were notable only for rheumatoid arthritis in the maternal grandmother and two episodes of breast cancer in the mother in her 40s after a bout with uterine cancer in her 20s. She had never used tobacco products or illegal substances of any type and only rarely used modest amounts of alcohol.

Ellen's only medication was the mildly helpful anti-nausea drug promethazine at a mere 12.5-25 mg when necessary. Despite all of her medication "sensitivities," she denied any medication "allergies." She was certain that while even low doses of diphenhydramine were excessively sedating for her, this medication also helped her problems with itching and abdominal swelling, though not any of her other GI issues. NSAIDs taken occasionally did help her aching somewhat.

Exam found an outwardly healthy appearing young woman in which the only notable finding was that on a light scratch test on the upper back, dermatographism began emerging immediately and just steadily worsened, with frank welting then adding on top of the red tracing in the skin about 3-4 minutes in. The brilliant reaction was only continuing to intensify when I last checked it 10 minutes after the scratch. I also noted modest dermatographism at all clothing pressure points.

All of her past, obviously extensive laboratory evaluations were unremarkable.

Ellen fit the MCAS profile perfectly, so I asked her to submit blood and urine specimens for mast cell mediator testing and then begin an H_1/H_2 histamine receptor blockade with twice-daily loratadine and famotidine.

She returned several weeks later reporting that the histamine receptor blockade had definitely helped her feel better, with decreased itching, dermatographism, gastroesophageal reflux, nausea, paresthesias, and palpitations. She was newly able to exercise and was running, and her appetite had increased "from none to normal." However, she said there had been no improvement in her abdominal bloating and gassiness and headaches and migratory adenitis, and she thought her chronic anxiety was somewhat worse, almost panic-like at times, along with more emotional lability.

Ellen is now seeking further improvement with trials of other MCAS-targeted medications.

And, at the other end of the age spectrum, there was "Judy":

Judy was 73 years old and had been referred to me in October 2009 for further evaluation of her anemia. She knew virtually no details of her medical history, and it was a challenge gathering records, but I eventually pieced the story together. She related a chief complaint of a six month history of feeling fatigued (though I eventually determined that this complaint, like most of her other complaints, had actually been going on for many years), suffering a chronic tingling/numbness and weakness throughout her left leg (from the foot to the groin), episodic left upper abdominal quadrant discomfort, and perhaps a mild degree of anorexia. She initially said she had been feeling fine prior to the onset of this illness. The episodes of abdominal pain lasted about 15 minutes; there were no identifiable inciting, aggravating, or alleviating associations. Her left leg hurt more as she did more with it. It caused a limp. She thought the leg and abdominal difficulties had worsened a bit since onset, but the fatigue was unchanged; her husband, though, thought the fatigue, too, had worsened. She denied fever, chills, sweats, weight loss, itching, rash, chronic eye or throat irritation, respiratory or chest discomfort (she did note occasional past episodes of bronchitis with wheezing), pain anywhere other than the abdominal pain and leg discomfort, or changes in bowel or bladder habits or products. She denied any particular problems with infection, bleeding, or clotting. She had frequent mild end-of-day edema in her feet.

Her past history (as I eventually put it together) included hypertension, diabetes mellitus type 2, hypercholesterolemia, hypothyroidism, GERD that responded well to a proton pump inhibitor (Prevacid), left kidney cancer in 2008 treated solely with radiation therapy, stable minimal chronic kidney disease, a 2006 episode of chest pain (three days following a cataract extraction and intraocular lens placement) that was interpreted as a myocardial infarction (i.e., a heart attack) (though cardiac catheterization showed no CAD), a cholecystectomy in 1985 due to abdominal pain, a hysterectomy also done the same year as a consequence of a bladder operation for some sort of a tumor, and an upper and lower endoscopy in April 2009 (which found only a hiatal hernia), followed by an octreotide scan (negative) that had been ordered because she was found to have a significantly elevated chromogranin level (45 ng/ml, normal 0-5).

Judy retired in 1989 from a long-time position as an assistant schoolteacher. She had been pregnant three times, and her three children were healthy. One sister had died of colon cancer at age 43, another sister died of colon cancer at age 42, another sister survived colon cancer at age 58, and three living sisters all had rheumatoid arthritis. She had never abused alcohol or used tobacco or illegal substances of any sort.

Her medications included amlodipine, atorvastatin, benazepril, metoprolol, hydrochlorothiazide, levothyroxine, lansoprazole, insulin, and one baby aspirin a day. Judy had no known allergies.

My exam found an overweight woman in no apparent distress at rest, independently ambulatory but with a moderate limp resulting from an obviously painful left leg, and severe systolic hypertension (repeatedly around 200, though her husband noted it was usually normal at home and only got that high at medical appointments), obvious left upper quadrant tenderness to modest palpation, mild numbness in the left thigh, and left straight leg raising constrained to about 60 degrees due to thigh pain.

Other than a mild anemia (hemoglobin 10-11 g/dl) that had been stable for almost a decade, Judy's labs were mostly unremarkable including long-stable minimal elevations in creatinine and glucose that had long been well controlled. The only standout test was the chromogranin A level, but the octreotide scan that had been done (based on an expectation that such a high chromogranin A level must reflect a neuroendocrine tumor such as carcinoid) was negative.

It was most definitely a complicated situation, especially given her past history of left kidney cancer (was this the source of the left-sided abdominal pain?) and her neurological issues, so I ordered restaging CT scanning for her cancer and lumbosacral spine MRI for her left leg troubles, plus blood and urine testing for mast cell disease, carcinoid, pheochromocytoma (which might explain her very high blood pressure), and an assortment of other rheumatologic and thyroid issues.

A few days after the initial visit, I received some additional records. So much for Judy's history of everything being OK until just six months earlier. A May 2007 initial consult report from her local gastroenterologist noted she had had abdominal pain for several months. It would start in the left flank, radiate to the umbilicus, last for about 30 minutes, be relieved by a bowel movement, and occur roughly weekly. She also reported worsening constipation and GERD controlled with a PPI. Additional complaints included excessive nighttime urination, a waxing/waning rash she had had for years, elbow and right shoulder pains, and intermittent mild ankle edema. Past history included benign colonic polyps in 2003, a duodenal neuroendocrine tumor called carcinoid removed endoscopically in 1998, gall bladder surgery for stones, history of idiopathic pancreatitis with no recent episodes, previous frequent nausea with no recent episodes, hysterectomy (but no oophorectomy), history of rheumatic fever, hypertension, "previous" congestive heart failure, CAD with stable effort angina, history of renal artery stenosis, and insulin-dependent diabetes mellitus. A May 2007 CT scan found a 15 mm left kidney upper pole solid mass "suspicious for a small renal cell cancer." In June 2007 her gastroenterologist performed upper and lower endoscopy, finding insignificant gastric polyps and a "small" submucosal polyp in the second portion of the duodenum, which proved to be a carcinoid. A follow-up endoscopy done in March 2009 found only a small hiatal hernia and multiple "insignificant" gastric polyps. However, that's when he ordered the chromogranin A level, which returned at nine times the upper limit of normal, and that's what led to the confusingly negative octreotide scan.

At follow-up a few weeks later, Judy unsurprisingly reported no improvement. Her fatigue prevented her from standing up in the kitchen for any extended periods; she said that for more than a year she had had to mop her kitchen floor while sitting down because of her fatigue. The leg neuropathy was no worse than before. The MRI had found some mild disc disease. I suspected it wasn't enough to be causing her left leg symptoms, but I offered her a referral to the neurosurgeon, which she declined.

More significantly, a repeat chromogranin A level had now come back 55-fold elevated above the upper limit of normal. Carcinoid is notorious for causing elevations in chromogranin A and another marker called 5-HIAA, and carcinoid had already been found in one intestinal polyp, so did her high chromogranin A level mean she had other sites of carcinoid in her? Could she have so much carcinoid as to cause such a high chromogranin A level and yet still have a completely negative octreotide scan? And could carcinoid cause all that had been going on in her?

No, carcinoid really couldn't cause all that had been going on in her. And it was highly unlikely that she had enough carcinoid to produce such a high level of chromogranin but not enough to light up an octreotide scan. Oh, and her 5-HIAA level was normal, too.

This couldn't be carcinoid. But what else could cause such a high chromogranin A level? A proton pump inhibitor (PPI) drug can cause some elevation in chromogranin A, but her level was significantly higher than would be expected from a PPI effect. An H_2 blocker can do it, but she wasn't on one. High chromogranin A has been associated with prostate cancer, the one thing I could be absolutely certain she didn't have. Kidney failure can cause some elevation in chromogranin A, but she had only a very minimal degree of kidney failure, so that wasn't the explanation. Heart failure can do it, but despite an alleged past history of heart failure, she clearly didn't have it now. (And, other than a few specific viruses that had never been found in her, what would cause heart failure that would come and go like that?) Certain other neuroendocrine tumors can cause high chromogranin levels, but if she had such a tumor, again, all the scans and scopings of various sorts should have shown something.

All that was left to explain Judy's chromogranin A level and the full set of her symptoms was mast cell disease, but given the confounding factor of the carcinoid that had been found and her PPI use and the minimal kidney disease, I needed some additional points of evidence besides the chromogranin A level.

I had the pathologist take another look at her "insignificant" gastric polyps, and sure enough, there was a mild increase in her mast cells. The gastroenterologist even went back in and took some additional biopsies, and the pathologist again found the same thing.

It really did look like mast cell disease tied it all together. Since she was already tolerating low-dose aspirin, I asked her to try increasing it, but at any dose above two baby aspirins (162 mg) twice daily, she developed too much heartburn to bear and had to return to just one baby aspirin per day.

I asked her to start twice-daily loratadine and famotidine. She returned several weeks later reporting that although her irritated eyes, cough, rash, edema, bilateral lower extremity cramps, and constipation were unimproved, her left upper quadrant discomfort, dyspnea, and arthralgias were markedly improved, and her fatigue, too, had significantly improved in that she used to have spend the entire afternoon back in bed after doing a little bit of housework in the morning, but now she was finding she only had to spend about two hours resting in the early afternoon.

I asked her now try increasing her aspirin, and though she never was able to tolerate more than 162 mg twice daily, at that dose all the rest of her problems resolved, including her leg discomfort. She was very pleased with her greatly improved energy level and said she now could easily sweep and mop her floors and still had energy left to spare.

As I write this, it's now four years later, and her improvements have all been fully sustained. Repeat chromogranin A levels remain markedly elevated, and repeat octreotide and CT scans remain completely negative.

The GI issues in MCAS include pain, discomfort, and inflammation of any or all components from the mouth to the anus and the solid organs, too (e.g., the liver and pancreas). "Refractory GERD" (suffered by tens of millions in the U.S. alone) and "irritable/inflammatory bowel syndrome" (similarly) are very common. Episodic queasiness, nausea, and vomiting (sometimes "cyclical," as in "cyclical vomiting syndrome") are common. Diarrhea and/or constipation (usually maddeningly alternating) are common. Malabsorption, too, is common (one study suggest it's present in up to a third of cases) and may be either a general protein/calorie malnutrition and/or malabsorption of selected micronutrients such as assorted vitamins and minerals.

Weight can rise or fall, sometimes a result of edema and sometimes a result of changes in fat tissue. Weight gain seems much more common than weight loss, but sometimes the weight maddeningly fluctuates repeatedly up and down – all without change in diet or activity. Sometimes the weight gains are frighteningly large and lead to all manners of complications as well as gastric bypass or banding surgery without any stopping to consider what metabolic issues must be going on to cause such a problem. Such surgery sometimes is successful at achieving sustained weight reduction, but often, after initial reduction, the weight frustratingly starts rising again.

Chapter 16: How To Piss Off Urologists: The Infectionless Urinary Tract "Infections" of Interstitial Cystitis and Other Genitourinary Findings in MCAS

As with the respiratory and gastrointestinal (GI) tracts, the genitourinary (GU) tract is a major point of interface between the human body and the surrounding environment, so one should expect to (normally!) find more mast cells in these tissues than in many other tissues. Thus, one should expect to find symptoms of mast cell disease more often in the GU tract than in many other body systems – and, indeed, that does appear to be the case.

Just as in the respiratory and GI tracts, the symptoms of mast cell disease in the GU tract are most commonly those of inflammation, and sometimes fibrosis (which, in truth, is just another aspect of inflammation that's not usually recognized as inflammatory), in one segment of the tract or another. In my experience, painful urination (medically called "dysuria") is one of the most common such symptoms, and because physicians are conditioned in their training to associate dysuria with infection, many times MCAS patients who are having flares of disease in their GU tracts are assumed to have a urinary tract infection (UTI) even though routine urinalysis and urine culture show little to no evidence of infection. Instead, what's likely going on is sterile inflammation, which admittedly can have many potential causes but often comes from a flare of mast cell activation. When this happens in the bladder, it's known as interstitial cystitis (IC), and urologists are increasingly coming to understand that in many cases IC is a mast-cell-driven illness.

> "Fiona," a 52-year old graduate student (yes, some people do get started on that sort of thing later in life than usual, and I say kudos and more power to them), came to me from several states away to be evaluated for the mast cell disease she had come to suspect was causing her panoply of problems. She reported an extraordinarily complicated, life-long history of multisystem unwellness, much of it of an inflammatory theme. Her history of illness dated literally from infancy, as her parents told her that she was "always" sick as a baby. She exhibited projectile vomiting to breast feeding, but this did not improve with a transition to formula. She allegedly suffered mumps twice and chicken pox twice during childhood. A smallpox vaccine at age 7 "didn't take," as evidenced by the lack of a scar on her arm. A tonsillectomy at age 9 had to be postponed four times due to Strep pharyngitis. (The tonsillectomy didn't appear to help any of her problems.) She missed many weeks of school each year with illnesses including pharyngitis, adenopathy, "itchy eyes," sinonasal congestion, and "stomach pains" (exacerbated by "everything" she ate). Menarche at age 14-1/2 was "horrible," causing "terrible" cramps, severe bleeding, and persistent irregular periods. Presyncopal episodes first emerged around this time, too, and seemed related to

hypoglycemia. Migraine headaches emerged at age 19 and hadn't left her since.

Fiona felt great throughout her first (and only) pregnancy at age 21 but suffered assorted complications during the forceps delivery including what sounded like a tailbone fracture and ligament tears which eventually led to uterine prolapse which in turn ultimately resulted in a hysterectomy at age 28. (Her son, too, had most of the problems the patient had suffered over the years.) She also had been on "arthritis medications" (NSAIDs) of various sorts ever since age 22 (rofecoxib back when it was available, but more recently meloxicam, though she had stopped it a week before the visit to prepare for anticipated lab testing, and she said it had been a "terrible" week without the meloxicam).

At age 23 Fiona suffered relatively acute onset of diffuse adenopathy and was initially suspected of having lymphoma, but then the adenopathy suddenly, spontaneously resolved. With the exception of a left tympanic membrane rupture at age 30 due to spousal abuse and a chronic breast discharge (galactorrhea per previous medical records) dating back to age 31, she said she had a few good years after the hysterectomy, but then in her mid-30s urinary problems emerged including urinary frequency and dysuria (she estimates about 70% of her many urine cultures were negative), leading to a diagnosis of interstitial cystitis (IC). Diffusely migratory soft tissue aches/pains emerged around this time as well, as did a worsening of her longstanding seasonal allergies and a worsening of her migraines. Testing for connective tissue diseases was negative, and she was given a diagnosis of fibromyalgia. Trials of tricyclic antidepressants helped her migraines somewhat but otherwise only caused a weight gain of 40 lbs. and made her feel "like a zombie." (She later switched to topiramate, which provided better control over her migraines.) She went on trials of infusion of heparin and lidocaine into her bladder for her interstitial cystitis symptoms; these treatments helped somewhat, while a trial of pentosan didn't help at all.

In her 40s Fiona's diffusely migratory aching only further worsened. New food allergies emerged, and degenerative joint disease in the cervical spine advanced to a point where she switched from her previous regular aggressive exercise regimen to yoga. Seasonal allergies steadily worsened, though a combination of montelukast, fexofenadine, and two inhalers in the spring and fall did help. At age 41 she underwent cholecystectomy for biliary dyskinesia after three years of right upper quadrant abdominal pain; ultrasound had been unrevealing, but a special ("HIDA") scan showed a "less than 3%" ejection fraction. At age 45 she figured out she had an allergy to dairy products (symptoms of pruritus and coughing).

As her 40s rolled on, all of Fiona's symptoms seemed to steadily worsen. She separated from her husband at 47 and divorced at 50. A "Fuchs corneal dystrophy" was diagnosed at age 49 and was causing sufficient problems with night vision that she underwent a bilateral partial corneal transplant. Around this same time (i.e., in 2009) she developed a "horrible" renal colic (either a stone or infection), was prescribed ciprofloxacin in the ER, slept for three straight days, and then suffered "constant" bladder spasms for the next six months. Her urologist started her on solifenacin in 2009 for her bladder spasms, and this helped some, but overall her health was just continuing to deteriorate, and food allergies were worsening. Two attempts at infusion of DMSO into her bladder left her feeling "poisoned" with "hangover and flu [and it] almost killed me." She then found that oral aloe vera helped her interstitial cystitis somewhat, and a low-potassium/low-acid diet also helped somewhat. A primary physician tried to change her Topamax to a beta blocker, whereupon she "almost died" with what sounds like severe presyncope and cognitive dysfunction; these problems improved when she was switched back to Topamax.

In her early 50s Fiona's diffusely migratory aching ("body pains") had further worsened (especially multi-level spinal pain), and chiropractic, massage, and acupuncture treatments had been unhelpful. She underwent steroid/anesthetic injections at multiple levels for about 18 months, found they helped a bit at first, but then they actually seemed to worsen the pain and she stopped them. A possible diagnosis of Ehlers-Danlos Syndrome (EDS) was then considered, and she was referred to a local expert in this who she said confirmed she had Type III and started her on physical therapy. Meanwhile, her "GI issues" had only further worsened, and she said she was now having very watery bowel movements about 15-20 times daily. Most recently she had begun developing diffusely migratory rashes and hives as well as worsening spells of edema, mostly about the face and throat. Through Internet-based dialogue with other EDS patients, she became aware of mast cell activation syndrome (MCAS), began reading more about it, and felt an evaluation for MCAS would be worthwhile. Her medical history also included a multinodular goiter, but it didn't seem that thyroid function had ever been significantly problematic.

On review of systems, although she denied problems with fevers, epistaxis, and vomiting, Fiona endorsed waxing/waning and/or episodic chills, feeling cold much of the time, headaches (though relatively well controlled on topiramate), diffusely migratory pruritus, soaking sweats (often at night), irritation of the eyes, episodic difficulty focusing her vision, hearing deficit (subjectively bilateral, though testing had shown this objectively only on the right) and tinnitus (only on the left), irritation of the nose, frequent coryza and post-nasal drip, easy bruising, slow to stop bleeding from incidental trauma, occasional tongue soreness, oral and esophageal ulcers, chronic sore throat, intermittent mild waxing/waning dyspnea ("I just can't catch a deep breath"), chest discomfort, palpitations, proximal dysphagia, gastroesophageal reflux, nausea, diarrhea alternating with constipation, diffusely migratory patchy erythematous macular rash (also an outbreak of scattered petechial-type lesions coincident with flares of many of her other symptoms), diffusely migratory edema, urinary frequency and dysuria, frequent vaginal yeast infections (though her previously reliable post-coital yeast infections had been well managed for the last year by post-coital prophylactic use of an anti-fungal drug), enlarged and/or tender nodes in most of the usual node-bearing sites, a variety of sleeping issues, cognitive dysfunction, excessive dental decay, alopecia, brittle/peeling nails, fluctuating weight and appetite, labile blood pressure, diffusely migratory (though typically distal) paresthesias, frequent presyncope, and a single episode of syncope when she was pregnant.

Strokes and heart disease ran in her family, but she knew of no hematologic or rheumatologic issues in the family history. Her mother survived breast cancers at ages 49 and 62, and her paternal grandmother survived colon cancer in her 80s, but her father, a lifelong smoker since age 10, died of emphysema. She was engaged to be married again. She smoked intermittently from age 18 to 40; at the worst it was still less than a pack per day. She had never abused alcohol. Her only history of illegal substance use was smoking marijuana on occasion in her late teens and early 20s.

Fiona had a long medication list, most of it irrelevant to the discussion here, but she noted that since beginning twice-daily cetirizine and ranitidine in September 2012, her rash and diarrhea had markedly reduced. Allergies include vomiting with clarithromycin, sulfa, and the sulfa-based celecoxib, headaches upon exposure to "blue dyes," hives upon exposure to norfloxacin, imaging contrast dye, oxycodone, methylsulfonylmethane, codeine, or hydrocodone, and unspecified reaction to metoclopramide. A reaction in July 2012 to CT contrast was quelled with prednisone and diphenhydramine, and she also found the prednisone helped her GI issues.

My exam of Fiona was notable for her pulse of 93 (technically in the normal range, but in truth higher than it should have been for a thin 52 year old at rest), diffuse slight clamminess to her skin, sparse scattering of small irregularly contoured patches of macular red rash, cherry angiomata where she thought she had a petechial rash, poor dentition (including several missing teeth), clear lungs (albeit with a single dry cough at one point on deep inspiration), mild mid-abdominal tenderness on deep palpation, and mild distal paresthesias. On a light scratch test on the upper back, moderately bright dermatographism quickly emerged and was fully sustained when last checked 10 minutes later.

With regard to her prior laboratory testing, suffice to say that she had been very thoroughly evaluated, but nothing diagnostic had ever been found, including a normal tryptase level. An abdominal CT in August 2009 showed thickening and distention of the second and third portions of the duodenum. An abdominopelvic CT in December 2011 showed hepatic cysts and a single renal cyst. Her only known GI biopsies on file were from April 2005, including a proximal transverse colon biopsy provocatively showing "mild non-specific active colitis with eosinophilia" and an ascending colon biopsy also provocatively showing "mild non-specific active colitis."

My initial assessment was thus: "As I initially noted, [Fiona] has suffered an extraordinarily complex, obviously multisystem array of polymorbidity, much of it of an inflammatory theme. Although I can envision many diagnoses that can account for assorted subsets of her problems, I know of very few illnesses that might possibly account for the entire range of these findings. Given the old maxim about common things occurring commonly – and we have been learning rapidly these past few years that mast cell disease is far more common than historically appreciated – I think it's far more likely that she has been suffering a mast cell activation syndrome (MCAS) her entire life, and far less likely that she has been suffering any of the variety of rare inborn autoinflammatory syndromes which virtually always cause such severe pediatric morbidity as to be diagnosed by pediatricians or geneticists relatively early in life. With regard to her EDS diagnosis, I note that EDS Type III is the only type of EDS which to date has defied all efforts to identify a root mutational defect, and given that I have a number of MCAS patients previously diagnosed with EDS Type III (among a number of other comorbidities, of course), what I suspect is going on here is chronic aberrant elaboration of a particular set of mediators (drawn from amongst the mast cell's repertoire of more than 200 such molecular signals) not only influencing virtually every other system and organ in the body but also influencing connective tissue development to yield the "hyperextensible" phenotype long associated with EDS Type III."

I asked her to submit to testing for MCAS, but as she didn't have a diagnosis yet, I didn't feel I could responsibly recommend any treatment beyond the antihistamines she was already using.

A few weeks later we had an answer in her elevated plasma prostaglandin D_2 level (123 pg/ml, normal 35-115), elevated plasma histamine level (9 nmol/L, normal 0-8), elevated serum chromogranin A (155 ng/ml, normal 0-95), elevated plasma free norepinephrine (1449 pg/ml, normal 80-520), and Factor VIII (205%, normal 50-150%).

I made recommendations to her local physician to begin trying MCAS-directed medications one at a time. The patient e-mailed me several months later:

Dr. Afrin,

Just wanted to drop you a quick note and let you know that I am doing Fantastic!!!! My life has changed!!! I am now on singular [sic], 2 maximum strength Pepcid, Claritin, lorazepam, all 2x per day and feel like the old me!!! I take 1mg of lorazepam at bedtime and .5 in the morning for the nausea but it really works well. If I start feeling "weird", headache, itchy, grumpy, I will take 25-50 of Benadryl and 40 mg of Pepcid and it always does the trick. I have only had to use my albuterol inhaler while I was sick and I noticed that adding Benadryl when I had a virus made me much more comfortable in general. I will add that to my "do this when you get a cold" list. Hopefully there won't be any more of those since when my mast cells are behaving, I rarely get ill. The cognitive issues are also slowly clearing but I think they are taking the longest to get back on track.

I am so happy to have my life back. I was ready to call it quits by the time I saw you.

Hmmm. So UTIs that don't behave like UTIs might indeed not be UTIs and instead might be IC – and IC might be a sign of something more fundamental than just a GU issue.

Here's another example:

"Barbara" was a 35-year old accountant when she was referred to me in March 2012. She, too, dated her chronic unwellness literally back to her earliest memories in childhood, noting she had never been without chronic malaise, fatigue, an assortment of "GI issues" (e.g., abdominal pain and alternating diarrhea and constipation), difficulty standing for extended periods, then onset around the time of menarche of chronic problems with severe headaches. She lived overseas from age 8 to age 11, but she is certain her symptoms began well before she moved there. Repeated testing for mononucleosis was negative until she tested positive for this during a "flare" of her assortment of symptoms while a senior in high school, though she cannot remember whether she had any adenopathy at the time. (Substantial adenopathy, especially about the neck, is a virtually inescapable accompaniment to the Epstein Barr virus infection of mononucleosis when it occurs at this age.)

In Barbara's late teens, problems with spontaneous vomiting (preceded by onset of significant headache just seconds earlier) and chronic nausea emerged, and she had been on 19 different PPIs since age 19. Though initially she never had "heartburn," now she noted that reflux reliably developed whenever she tried to taper off or stop her PPI du jour. Age 19 is also when she suffered a bout of *Clostridium difficile* colitis, and though this was treated, it soon relapsed and required re-treatment, and this is around the time when her chronic problems with diffusely migratory soft tissue and joint pains began.

At age 21 Barbara suffered a bout of severe diarrhea leading to hospitalization and colonoscopy with a diagnosis of severe colitis; no definitive cause was found, though she says some of her physicians attributed this to her oral contraceptives which had been started at age 15 to try to help (and which did help) her abdominal cramps. Even after she recovered from the colitis, alternating diarrhea and constipation continued, nausea and vomiting decreased but did not resolve, and headache and fatigue problems continued.

By her late 20s Barbara began having difficulty attending adequately to her work as an accountant. Postural orthostatic tachycardia syndrome (POTS) was diagnosed in 2007 using a tilt table test; she was started on various medications which she was still taking, but overall she thought that avoidance of her "triggers" of heat, cold, sun, stress, and exertion helped her control her symptoms more than her medications did. Such avoidance helped her feel somewhat better in that she was "not as completely exhausted" but still felt easily overtaxed and frequently experienced flushing.

Barbara's medical history also included a sweat gland problem of unknown cause called hydradenitis suppurativa, a spontaneously detached retina in 2010, alleged history of iron-deficiency anemia of uncertain cause, frequent urinary tract "infections" occurring both spontaneously and with any sexual activity but virtually always with negative urine cultures and a negative thorough urologic work-up to date (except for finding renal papillary necrosis), club feet at birth, and scoliosis.

Although she denied any irritation or sores of the nose or mouth, dental problems, edema (except in response to spicy foods and alcohol), enlarged or tender lymph nodes, or syncope, Barbara endorsed subjective fevers, chills, feeling cold much of the time, frequent headaches, diffusely migratory achiness, diffusely migratory pruritus, dry eyes, intermittent difficulties focusing her vision, frequent coryza and sneezing (antihistamine nasal spray helped quell this), easy bruising, chronic throat discomfort/irritation, subtle dyspnea intermittently at rest and more so on exertion, occasional proximal dysphagia, frequent non-anginal chest discomfort, frequent palpitations, reflux issues as above, chronic nausea and vomiting, chronic diarrhea alternating with constipation, polyuria, frequent urinary tract "infections," reactivity to alcohol and spicy food (both causing a rash of patches of dry scaly skin and facial edema and flushing which can last for up to 2 weeks), occasional insomnia, diffusely migratory tingling/numbness paresthesias (mostly in the distal extremities), episodic cognitive dysfunction, and presyncopal episodes several times daily.

Her father allegedly had both polycythemia vera and Hodgkin's disease (which he survived) in his 60s; he eventually died of heart disease. Her mother's side of the family was rife with rheumatologic issues. There was lung cancer and relatively early onset leukemia on her father's side of the family, though those who got lung cancer were smokers. There was no personal history of tobacco or illegal substance use, let alone alcohol abuse.

Barbara's current medications included the proton pump inhibitor esomeprazole plus a number of medications for her POTS including fludrocortisone, propranolol, midodrine, and L-methylfolate. She knew of no frank medication allergies; there were just the allergies to spicy foods and alcohol.

My exam found Barbara to be a somewhat pale, vaguely unhappy/tired/chronically ill-appearing woman with slight left upper quadrant tenderness to even modest palpation and, on a light scratch test on the upper back, bright dermatographism (erythroderma only, no hives) immediately emerged and was fully sustained when I last checked it again 20 minutes later.

The history reeked of MCAS, so I sent off "the usual" blood and urine testing and also asked the pathologist to retrieve and re-examine her 2007 GI tract biopsies with CD117 staining and an eye toward mast cell disease. Her 24-hour urinary prostaglandin D_2 level was about 50% above the upper limit of normal, and her chromogranin level A was elevated both on and off her PPI. Her old duodenal biopsy, too, showed a mild increase in mast cells.

Antihistamines quickly helped some of her symptoms (including her GU symptoms), but she still was in need of significant further improvement. She just as quickly proved unable to tolerate even low-dose aspirin (skin boils, bleeding, GERD, and nasal burning). A trial of lorazepam caused intolerable depression at the low dose of just 0.5 mg twice daily, and a trial of doxepin also proved intolerable (grogginess) after just 10 days at a very low dose. However, in September 2012 she began a trial of oral cromolyn and soon found that one vial (200 mg) four times daily worked best for her, relieving virtually all of the symptoms not already addressed by the antihistamines.

And, lest you think that the GU issues in MCAS are only found in women, here's a final story for this chapter demonstrating men to have "equal opportunity" for MCAS-driven GU issues.

"Mickey" was a 52-year old white male disabled airline pilot when he was referred to me in June 2009 by his primary physician for further evaluation of chronic painful mild splenomegaly. He started by telling me that in 2005, shortly after a bout of "food poisoning," he developed acute left-sided abdominal pain, which was initially diagnosed as a kidney stone. This pain slowly improved over the next several weeks, except that it never fully resolved and indeed had persisted ever since in a waxing/waning fashion. A CT scan performed early in the work-up of this problem found mild splenomegaly which immediately led to his being grounded from flight duty and being placed on disability; he has been told he had to be pain-free for at least six months before he could requalify for flight duty, but the longest he had been able to go without pain was about two months. When the splenomegaly was found, he was immediately referred to a local hematologist/oncologist who ran many tests (including a repeat CT in February 2009 showing stable to slightly reduced splenomegaly) but could find no explanation for his pain and splenomegaly.

On further history, many other complaints emerged, all of them new since the "food poisoning" episode in 2005. Mickey told me he had always been quite healthy previously and denied any prior chronic medical problems or major medical events. The left upper abdominal quadrant pain waxed and waned and was sometimes accompanied by nausea – and sometimes even non-bloody vomiting. The worst episodes of pain occurred roughly every 2-4 weeks; the pain was 8 on a 0-to-10 scale and left him curled on the floor in a fetal position. His family always wanted to take him to the ER when this happened, but he knew the pang would resolve after 5-10 minutes, and it always did just that. He endorsed early satiety and a 25 lb. weight gain since all of this began. He said his temperature often felt as if it were in flux, sometimes making him feel hot but more often making him feel cold, sometimes even with mild rigors. He endorsed near daily night sweats. He also noted episodic migratory edema, most often in the feet and/or hands. He noted an itchy red rash about his lower neck that had plagued him since his illness began and which, he said, had defied diagnostic and therapeutic efforts by multiple dermatologists.

Mickey had been chronically fatigued since the illness began, sometimes feeling as if he couldn't even get out of bed in the morning. He had acute-onset "spells," every few days to every few weeks, of lightheadedness accompanied by a flushed appearance. His eyes were chronically irritated, as if they were dry (he thought it might be from his contacts, but moisturizing solutions such as saline didn't seem to help at all). He said he has bad gastroesophageal reflux disease and had "learned the hard way" he could not do without ranitidine. He also had a "bad back" and "arthritis in all my joints."

His worst stiffness was in the morning; a "very hot" shower helped him loosen up. He was occasionally constipated but had not noticed any diarrhea. He had occasionally briefly had bloody urine these past few years with episodes of his "kidney stones," which were always on the left; except for those rare instances of bloody urine, his urine has never appeared an abnormal color, even when left standing. He said that at one point porphyria was suspected and testing was run and indeed hinted at the disease, but he says when his case was reviewed by a porphyria expert, the expert thought it was not likely he had porphyria.

Mickey had had much more difficulty recovering from minor infections, or healing from minor trauma, since the illness began. He also had noted occasional tingling/numbness in his toes, soles, and fingertips. He denied any respiratory issues, including no problems with wheezing. He said his family had noted to him that his mood had chronically changed since he got sick and that he was now often quite irritable, though he thought it was due to the chronic pain.

Mickey also told me he had had one summer, around age 11 or 12, when he spent much of the summer ill with central (not left upper quadrant) abdominal pain which was never diagnosed and which, at the end of the summer, spontaneously resolved and never returned.

His father survived a bout with prostate cancer; his mother lost a bout with breast cancer; a maternal aunt, too, may have had breast cancer. He had two healthy sons. He worked part-time as a retail store clerk, a job he took because he was getting "bored crazy" at home. There was no history of use or abuse of tobacco, alcohol, or illegal substances.

Exam was notable solely for tenderness to palpation across the upper abdomen, worst in the middle of this area (the epigastrium), together with a modest, red, mildly blanching rash about the full circumference of his neckline, but he never scratched at it. I also noted mild dermatographism.

My assessment at that initial visit was that "Chronic leukemias and lymphomas of any sort really don't fit the full picture here, nor do metabolic diseases leading to splenic infiltration. I can't imagine a solid tumor that could explain all of these findings. Porphyria doesn't fit very well, either; I suspect what was seen on his porphyria screening was a mildly elevated coproporphyrin or uroporphyrin fraction, which can be seen in virtually any stressful situation. And I can't think of a single chronic infection that would produce this particular clinical picture. Instead, this whole situation sounds fairly classic for mast cell disease of some sort, though I can't presently tell whether it's a qualitative/dysfunctional mast cell issue, i.e., idiopathic mast cell activation disorder, vs. the frankly proliferative classic systemic mastocytosis." (You can see from this how the terminology has evolved over time. Today, "mast cell activation disorder [or disease]" is the top-level term, encompassing not only mastocytosis but also the MCAS that I meant at the time in my use of the term "mast cell activation disorder.") To start, I recommended blood and urine testing for mast cell disease.

He was a hard one to diagnose, as three rounds of testing were negative, though there were doubts along the way as to whether the specimens were being handled correctly, and the first couple of tests were done when he was feeling relatively well. I kept thinking along the way about other potential diagnoses, and I did order some additional tests in other directions, but they were all negative and the overall picture kept fitting mast cell disease better than anything else. After three negative rounds of testing, I not only asked him to wait for a "particularly bad day" and then pursue a fourth round of testing, but I also referred him to the gastroenterologist for upper and lower endoscopy with blind biopsies. And indeed, on a bad day his urinary prostaglandin D_2 was found to be elevated, and though every single one of his GI tract biopsies was reported as benign on routine staining, almost all of them showed mildly increased mast cells on special staining. We finally had a diagnosis of MCAS.

He's had a complex therapeutic history since, but after about three years finally found a combination of antihistamines, low-dose dasatinib, and vitamin C got him feeling well again. He eventually re-applied for flight privileges, passed his flight physical, finished retraining, and is now back in the cockpit. For purposes of this chapter, I want to focus on one of the symptoms that had been plaguing him the worst, a waxing/waning, occasionally spasmodic deep pelvic discomfort that would sometimes progress up into the abdomen, usually on the left side, sometimes convincing him he must have a kidney stone, except that repeated evaluations for such were always negative. His urologist repeatedly found his prostate to be in a "state of spasm" but was never able to find a cause for it.

Mickey had learned early in his trials of various MCAS therapies, though, that lorazepam quickly relieved this discomfort. Unfortunately, it also reliably caused a headache. A trial of an alternative benzodiazepine, clonazepam, caused grogginess and didn't help anything. Trials of multiple other urinary tract-directed medications (e.g., phenazopyridine, silodosin, hydralazine, and even the mast-cell-directed pentosan) didn't help. Then, wondering if the fillers or dyes in the commercial lorazepam formulation he had tried might have caused his MCAS to react and produce a headache, I had him try an alternative formulation of lorazepam, custom-compounded with baby rice cereal, which he knew he could tolerate. A low dose of 0.5 mg clearly again helped his pelvic discomfort, but made him too groggy. Subsequently, though, he was very happy to report that a dose of just 0.25 mg of the compounded lorazepam, taken twice a day (and occasionally a third dose when facing an occasional flare of pelvic pain), did a great job controlling this problem. Eventually, though, as he arrived at his "final" regimen noted above, he found he no longer needed the lorazepam at all.

So, as you can see, MCAS can cause pain, discomfort, and inflammation of any or all segments of the GU tract. The inflammation is usually sterile, but the chronic inflammation and other immune dysfunction from MCAS can easily lead to true infections, too. There is increasing literature suggesting that mast cell disease can drive acute and chronic kidney disease and perhaps even kidney fibrosis (scarring).

Mast cell disease definitely can reduce libido and cause infertility, too. Interestingly, a prostaglandin D_2 breakdown product, 15d-PGJ_2, has been shown to generate and maintain fibrosis in the tubular wall of the testis. Mast cell disease has been associated with reduced sperm count ("oligospermia"), and in fact it's even been shown that, at least in some cases of oligospermia, mast cell blockers can treat this condition and result in pregnancy.

Chapter 17: Sticks and Stones May Break My Bones, but That Pain Doesn't Even Begin to Compare to What I've Got: Musculoskeletal and Joint Findings in MCAS

[Warning: This is going to be a long chapter, and most MCAS patients reading this will think that it is fitting given how common musculoskeletal and joint complaints are in MCAS.]

Alright, let's just jump right into a case:

> In his e-mailed request to see me, Bob said he hurt. More in his legs than other places, but he hurt all over, and it had been going on for a long time – years. And he was only 30 years old. He said he had been in a couple of accidents many years ago, had suffered some trauma in both of them. But the weird thing was that his pain seemed to get *worse* starting *a few months after* each accident, plus he began developing pain in areas that hadn't even seemed to be injured in the first place. He had been evaluated "by everybody," and "nobody had ever found anything." He was certain that none of his doctors believed he truly had the pain he knew he felt. Thanks to the Internet, he eventually began wondering whether he might have mast cell disease, and called on his own to schedule an appointment to see me despite the four-hour drive (each way) it would require.

> Of course, in the exam room it quickly emerged that there were other problems – *lots* of other problems – that Bob hadn't mentioned in his e-mail. When he first came to see me in the late summer of 2010, initially he dated the onset of his troubles at age 14, but on further questioning, it seemed that he had suffered throughout childhood a substantial number of traumas (all "accidental") sufficient to require attention in the emergency room and sometimes even hospitalization. He was quite certain none of these traumas were from parental abuse and that they all were related to sports or entertainment or other innocuous activities; many of the traumas involved fractures. Despite all the traumas and fractures, he believed he had healed promptly and well from each such incident.

> Then, at age 14, Bob suffered sudden onset of migraine headache, which had waxed and waned over time but to date had essentially never completely resolved. He said the headache had very consistently been blamed on chronic sinusitis but that no sinusitis treatment of any sort – and he certainly has tried an awful lot of them – had ever helped significantly or in a sustained fashion. For example, sometimes when his sinusitis and headache would flare, initiation of antibiotics would help a good bit, but only for 1-2 days, and then symptoms would resurge and sustain even while he continued and finished the course of the antibiotic.

By age 17 Bob was sleeping through many of his classes because the light in the classrooms sometimes triggered flares of his headache. Also at age 17 he was a front-seat passenger in a bad car accident that literally sent him crashing headfirst completely through the windshield. And as if that year wasn't already bad enough, a while later (still age 17) he suffered a collision on the baseball field which acutely caused what sounded like an abnormal heart rhythm (ventricular tachycardia) requiring resuscitation; his sternum was fractured in this incident, too. Later that year he was pushed by another student, lost his balance and fell, struck his head and lost consciousness.

At age 18 Bob was the non-fault driver of a car involved in another accident in which his head again struck the windshield (though at least he wasn't projected through the windshield that time).

After finishing high school, Bob worked as a manufacturing supervisor and later in an office position of some sort. However, he had been unemployed for many months by the time he came to see me, partly because of chronic right shoulder pain arising from an accident at the manufacturing job. He had suffered marked impact trauma to the right shoulder and low back (even though an MRI of these areas hadn't found any acute trauma at all). He eventually wound up having two surgeries to improve his right shoulder, but he was told nothing could be done for the low-back issue. He dated much of his present pain in his legs to that accident.

So that was Bob's history. His chief complaint at the time of his initial visit with me was persistent pain that was principally in the legs all throughout, up to about the mid-thighs, plus chronic right shoulder pain. He described the pain in his legs as a crampy, achy throbbing all throughout both legs. Interestingly, the benzodiazepines lorazepam and clonazepam had always helped this pain much more than pain medications of any sort, narcotic or non-narcotic, but this was found incidentally and his doctors did not want to prescribe him benzodiazepines for pain. He also noted migratory pain throughout pretty much all the rest of his body, too, including throughout the abdomen. He said he had had severe GERD for about a decade and frequently suffered non-bloody vomiting after eating. He said his GERD had been helped somewhat in the past by Nexium (an acid-inhibiting proton pump inhibitor); this was somewhat worse when he reclined, and he could feel the burning all the way from his stomach up into his throat. Spicy foods very reliably triggered his reflux. He said he underwent upper and lower endoscopy almost a decade earlier (about a year after the GERD came on) due to rectal bleeding, but the scopings didn't find anything. He reported he had had a constant, waxing/waning "brain fog" ever since onset of his headache. He had never noted a consistent provocation for his headache. He also noted episodic migratory swelling of his bilateral feet, ankles, and hands; sometimes his left ring finger was swollen badly enough that he could not remove his wedding ring. He also noted episodic swelling and tenderness in the left submandibular region.

That was the end of what Bob could think to bring to my attention, but the review of systems revealed far more. He had had fevers intermittently for about eight years, initially just subjective and "low-grade" but more recently frankly objective and increasing in amplitude (to 103 for six hours just the day before he saw me) and frequency (nearly daily by that point). He said often the fevers were accompanied by terrible whole body aching, and he occasionally had been hospitalized for this, though he didn't think a specific diagnosis had ever been identified. He had had frequent (nearly daily) unprovoked soaking sweats (typically at night) for about five years. He had increasingly been having either frankly rigorous chills or sometimes just a sense of being cold. He reported many years of mild episodic migratory pruritus, which he hadn't given much attention since this symptom had always been just about the least of his problems. He had long had intermittently "itchy" eyes. He periodically (perhaps once a month?) developed intranasal sores, but he denied epistaxis.

Bob denied any problems in his mouth, but for many years – and with increasing frequency, to the point where it was now happening every other day or so – he had been having acutely arising bouts of "throat itching – like there's a hair caught down there" which he would have loved to scratch but instead could only repeatedly cough and try to clear his throat. This was a frequent and chronic enough problem that part of his regular nightly bedtime routine was to prepare a glass of water at his bedside since he was confident he would need it to try to help clear his throat when the "throat itching" would come on.

Bob reported some minor difficulty swallowing ("I used to be able to swallow a handful of pills at a time, and now I can only swallow one at a time"). He reported many years of a subtle, waxing/waning dyspnea. He said he had "always" had a "fluttering," rapid heartbeat, but he said multiple evaluations by cardiologists and multiple cardiac tests had always been unrevealing.

And there was more. Bob told me he had been having "panic attacks" roughly monthly for the prior five years; there'd never any apparent provocation, and the episodes began with acute onset of a racing pulse, dyspnea, and pallor and at least presyncope, sometimes even frank syncope. He also said he had been afflicted for many years with diarrhea alternating with constipation (which he said many of his doctors had told him was impossible). He had chronic bilateral hand and foot tingling/numbness. He also reported chronic bilateral waxing/waning tinnitus and frequent insomnia. He denied any problem with rash or sexual dysfunction.

Bob previously had been on many medications (including a trial of Allegra which he stopped after a few days because it didn't seem to help) but had been on no medications at all since being discharged by his primary physician several months earlier. He didn't think he had ever tried any of the available H_2 blockers. He said occasionally his various pains got so bad he had no choice but to borrow a narcotic analgesic of one sort or another from one or another of his relatives, many of whom also had chronic pain conditions of one sort or another, though he was certain none had ever been diagnosed with any rheumatologic conditions. He denied any known allergies except that pineapple irritated his tongue.

His only other known medical history was hypertension (remember, he was only 30!) and neonatal heart surgery to repair some sort of a pulmonic valve problem (an early tissue growth/development problem?). He had never received a blood transfusion. He was married and had two young children, both healthy. He had long smoked half a pack of cigarettes a day but has never abused alcohol. He had used several illegal drugs in the past but was adamant it had been a decade since his last such use. He had traveled very little, certainly to no places where he would be at risk for exotic infection.

Exam found, at least at rest, a trim young man appearing his stated age and in no obvious significant distress, but neither did he appear entirely comfortable, either; also, when I asked him to get up and walk, it was immediately apparent there was modest whole body discomfort, and perhaps even some modest weakness in his legs, in doing so. He was pleasant, cooperative, fully alert and oriented, and presented by himself. Key findings were his very slightly ill-appearing general countenance, a benign abdomen but for diffuse, mild tenderness to deep palpation, and a mild but clear decrease in strength in both forelegs from the knees down as well as the whole right arm and hand. Other than his report of mild tingling throughout both feet and both hands, sensation seemed intact.

My review of the limited available outside records showed, from a year earlier, a normal EKG, an unremarkable electromyogram done in both legs, a normal lumbar spine MRI, and a right shoulder MRI showing some degeneration in assorted soft tissues – certainly no findings that came anywhere close to accounting for his wide range of problems.

As I assessed at the time, there was no doubt the situation was complicated by the sequelae of multiple traumas, but overall there was a strong suggestion of a chronic systemic inflammatory syndrome of some sort as a unifying diagnosis. However, there was no rheumatologic or autoimmune syndrome I knew of that came anywhere close to fitting all or most of the findings. Rather, the whole situation had that "smell" of mast cell activation that I had learned to sense. I sent off my usual battery of blood and urine tests and asked him to try twice-daily loratadine and famotidine.

Bob returned a month later, initially reporting that although he had tolerated the antihistamines OK, he wasn't one bit better. But I had already learned not to necessarily trust such initial gestalt impressions, and that's just one of the reasons why I take such detailed reviews of systems in my patients in whom MCAS is a diagnostic consideration. Indeed, when I reviewed with him the full inventory of symptoms he had reported at the initial visit, it quickly emerged that the antihistamines in fact had yielded slight improvement in his diffuse aching, moderate improvement in severity and frequency of fevers, dramatic improvement in reflux and abdominal discomfort and dyspnea, and complete resolution of itching, eye irritation, and nasal sores. He was also tolerating a wider range of food, including reestablished tolerance for spicy foods, which he was greatly enjoying.

Nevertheless, his many other symptoms weren't one bit better. His labs from his initial visit were virtually all normal – but it was nevertheless curious that the percentage of eosinophils in his leukocyte differential was slightly elevated (as I often see in MCAS, and there certainly was no other established diagnosis in him that would account for this), and his plasma histamine level had been at the very top end of the normal range. I ordered repeats of some of the labs and asked him to cautiously try adding aspirin to his regimen.

Bob returned a couple months later, in late 2010, reporting that although he eventually had to give up the aspirin because of increasing gastric intolerance as he ramped up the dose from one children's aspirin twice a day to merely one adult aspirin twice a day, the aspirin otherwise had managed to markedly reduce his headaches, throat irritation, and sweats. Also, as I have often seen in other MCAS patients trying aspirin, his diarrhea decreased and his constipation increased (but was manageable with minimal intervention). Chronic, unimproved leg pain remained his chief complaint. His repeat labs had come back showing significant elevations in plasma histamine and prostaglandin D_2 and Factor VIII.

A trial of the leukotriene inhibitor montelukast didn't help. His insurance company wouldn't let him access the $1,000-per-year celecoxib that I prescribed for him to try, so in April 2011 we moved on to a trial – free for him due to his indigent status and the manufacturer's generous assistance program – of $100,000-a-year imatinib. (Is the American health care financing system screwed up, or what?) Interestingly, at that visit he also inquired about his six-year-old son, who he said shared many of his own symptoms including chronic fatigue and intermittent severe leg pain. He said his son's pediatrician had interpreted these symptoms as signs of ADHD and was treating it as such. Seemed odd to me, but not knowing anything more about his son, there wasn't much I could intelligently say other than suggesting he consider getting a second opinion from another pediatrician, maybe even a pediatric hematologist or allergist/immunologist if he was concerned about his son having mast cell disease.

Imatinib unfortunately quickly proved intolerable (stomach pain, nausea, fatigue, and joint pain) at the very low starting dose of just 100 mg daily. He moved on to a trial of low-dose lorazepam, which helped his anxiety but nothing else. He was still having great trouble finding any local physician to take him on.

Sequential trials over the next few months of a few other inexpensive drugs got Bob nowhere. He was beginning to notice a slowness to heal from minor wounds and traumas. Another attempt to get him a trial of celecoxib failed. By early 2012 (age 31) he was noticing his teeth were disintegrating despite a history of decent attention to oral hygiene, and his worsening joint pain and generalized muscle weakness were leading to increasingly frequent falls despite his use of a cane. A few months later, upon running out of lorazepam, he quickly discovered the drug was doing more for him than just controlling anxiety, as leg pain, sleep, malaise, migratory aching, anxiety, fevers, sweats, palpitations, and panic attacks rapidly worsened, then improved back to their prior baseline once he got back on the drug. Then, he finally found a local doctor willing to take him on, an angel who battled his insurance company and got him a trial of celecoxib, which even though it was just once a day rather than the twice-daily regimen I find usually is more helpful in MCAS, immediately decreased his fatigue, boosted his overall energy level, completely resolved his headaches, vomiting, and nasal sores, and improved his edema and eye irritation. To be sure, many problems remained and were wholly unimproved, including his leg pain, but at least he was making clear progress.

Bob next returned in late summer 2012 noting a sparse scattering of new small lipomas emerging all about his body. His insurer was still refusing to let him try celecoxib twice daily. Nearly constant, disabling pain throughout both legs was still his #1 problem. Based on some improvements in bone and soft tissue pain in response to hydroxyurea that I had seen by that point in a few other MCAS patients, plus old reports in the literature of the drug having been useful in treating symptoms in some mastocytosis patients, I started him on a trial of hydroxyurea at a standard low dose (500 mg once daily).

Bob again returned a month later with an interesting report. His pharmacist had provided him a 30-day fill of hydroxyurea consisting of roughly 15 capsules of one preparation (green/white capsules from one manufacturer) at the bottom of the bottle separated by a cotton ball from roughly 15 capsules of another preparation (blue/pink capsules from another manufacturer; this is the most commonly dispensed formulation) at the top of the bottle. For the first two weeks he was trying the hydroxyurea his leg pain was markedly improved. As he got toward the bottom of the first half of the supply, the cotton ball became twisted and he removed it, mixing the few remaining capsules from the "top" half of his supply with the full remaining "bottom" half of his supply, and he proceeded taking the drug at one capsule a day, extracting from the bottle capsules made by one manufacturer or the other at random. He said that about three days following the point where he removed the cotton ball, he noticed marked exacerbation of many of his symptoms including weakness, pallor, diaphoresis, and chest pain. He went to his local ER out of fear he was having a heart attack, but fortunately the work-up was negative. He ultimately was released after feeling somewhat better (he didn't know what, if any, treatment was given him in the ER). He had called me on his way to the ER to tell me about his symptoms (though he didn't tell me any of the particulars about the drug supply), and I instructed him to immediately cease taking the hydroxyurea. For the few days prior to his follow-up visit with me, he had been right back at his pre-hydroxyurea baseline of illness, including leg pain. His chief complaint at that visit again was his leg pain. I suspected he was reacting to the fillers and/or dyes in at least one, if not both, of the hydroxyurea formulations he had been given, and since at least initially the drug had appeared to help him, I prescribed a trial of another formulation of hydroxyurea which in my experience seemed to be better tolerated in patients who had difficulties tolerating the formulations of hydroxyurea he had already tried.

Bob returned yet another month later noting that with this third formulation of hydroxyurea (at just 200 mg once daily), his pain (including leg pain) was improved "at least 50%," falling from 10/10 to 6/10. He noted that whereas previously his activity and mobility would be limited to 5-10 minutes before he would "crash" and have to lie down for "most of the rest of the day" to "work off" the pain, now he could do the family grocery shopping and similar activities, being up for about two hours at a time, and his "crashes" were far less severe, requiring merely a few minutes seated until he was once again able to pursue activities.

Over the next few months Bob found that a dose of merely 400 mg twice daily brought his leg pain down to 3/10 at worst, 0/10 at best, and also improved all the rest of his remaining symptoms to the point

where he didn't think any other medication adjustments or trials were
needed.

I've seen similar results with low-dose hydroxyurea in several other MCAS
patients with otherwise refractory pain syndromes – and I've also observed
enough overlap between the presentation and behavior of the bone/muscle/joint
pain syndrome in MCAS patients and the presentation and behavior of the
bone/muscle/joint pain syndrome in sickle cell anemia patients (many of whom
demonstrate chronic inflammatory issues and other issues much easier to
attribute to mast cell activation than sickle cell anemia) that I have to wonder if
at least part of the reason why hydroxyurea benefits so many of the "sicker"
sickle cell anemia patients is because it's helping to control an unrecognized
MCAS in these patients. (Interestingly, another researcher at my institution (Dr.
Kalpna Gupta) and her team recently discovered that, at least in a mouse model
of sickle cell anemia, it's mast cell activation that causes the lion's share of the
pain from a classic sickle cell vaso-occlusive crisis, and mast cell stabilizers can
help decrease this pain. Another noted sickle cell researcher, Dr. Abdullah
Kutlar at Georgia Regents University, and his team recently reported that serum
tryptase levels are higher in sickle cell patients with chronic pain compared to
sickle cell patients without chronic pain. Drs. Gupta and Kutlar and now some
other sickle cell researchers, too, have proposed that clinical trials should be run
to see if mast cell activation-inhibiting drugs might be useful treatments in sickle
cell patients with frequent or chronic pain.)

There's no question that pain is the dominant musculoskeletal issue in MCAS.
Sometimes it's just pain in the bones, sometimes it's just in the muscles,
sometimes it's just in the joints (though rarely to a degree or of a pattern that a
rheumatologist will declare to be a specific arthritic diagnosis), and sometimes
it's in a combination of bones and/or muscles and/or joints. Traditional pain
medications often help little, but when they help, it's the non-steroidal anti-
inflammatory drugs (NSAIDs, like aspirin and ibuprofen and naproxen) that
more commonly actually reduce the pain, whereas narcotics simply tend to
"dull" the pain more than outright reduce it. Furthermore, both narcotics and
NSAIDs have been recognized for decades as potential triggers of mast cell
activation. For these and other reasons, I try to avoid prescribing narcotics for
MCAS whenever possible, but there is the occasional patient for whom a
narcotic clearly is the most effective analgesic, so having at least a little bit of
flexibility in one's personal prescribing policy is helpful.

Another issue with the muscles that I have repeatedly seen in a small number of
MCAS patients is an elevation in a blood marker called creatine kinase (CK).
Different types of CK are found in muscle and brain tissue, and when the CK
level in the blood is elevated beyond the normal range, it's accepted that there is
either muscle or brain tissue breakdown in progress; additional specialized
testing at that point can tell which type of CK is elevated, which can help
distinguish more specifically which type of tissue is breaking down. When I see

an elevated CK level in the blood in MCAS patients, it always appears to be the skeletal muscle type, yet the odd aspect of it is that the muscle pain or weakness one would expect in such a situation is never present. It makes me wonder whether mast cells, too, can generate CK (though that's not been reported in the medical literature), or whether aberrant mast cell mediator release of some sort can somehow induce muscle cells to release CK into the blood without necessarily going through the actual cell death process that has long been assumed to be required for a muscle cell to release CK into the blood.

I don't know whether the "bone pain" in MCAS patients is due to (likely inflammatory) mast cell mediator effects on bone tissue itself or on bone marrow – or even whether such pain might be physically due to the mild-to-moderate excess growth of blood cells in the marrow ("myeloproliferation") sometimes induced by MCAS – but I suspect such pain is usually not due to the other major processes MCAS can exert on bones: abnormal bone weakening (osteopenia or its more severe form, osteoporosis, that's totally disproportionate to any age or dietary influences) or abnormal bone solidifying (osteosclerosis). The reason I suspect the pain is not usually due to osteopenia/osteoporosis or osteosclerosis is that radiologic imaging of such painful bones usually just shows normal bones and none of the telltale signs of osteopenia/osteoporosis or osteosclerosis.

Although teeth are not bone, there's no question that teeth (and gums) often deteriorate in MCAS no matter how good one has attended to one's dental hygiene over time. I don't know whether this deterioration is due to mast cell mediator effects directly on the teeth, or the gums, or the bone tissue (the jaws) to which the teeth and gums are attached. Sometimes dental and periodontal deterioration can be due to diseases in which there is an inborn or acquired deficiency of a part of the immune system called immunoglobulin A (IgA), and I do see IgA deficiencies in many MCAS patients, but usually such deficiencies are not so severe as to be expected to enable dental/periodontal deterioration, and I've noticed no correlation between the IgA levels in my MCAS patients vs. the likelihood of a given MCAS patient developing dental/periodontal problems. Bottom line: although I can say that MCAS is associated with dental/periodontal deterioration and bone pain, I have no idea – yet! – *whether* or *how* the disease causes these problems.

The joint pain of MCAS is usually a migratory problem. Left third knuckle one day; right knee the next day, right fourth toe the next day, left shoulder the next, left great toe the next, and so on and so forth. It doesn't fit the pattern of any defined rheumatologic syndrome, and blood testing for such syndromes usually is either normal or, even more confoundingly, shows elevations in one special blood marker or another for these various syndromes – but at levels far below what would be expected in classic presentations of these syndromes. The whole situation drives rheumatologists, let alone patients, crazy – and unsurprisingly sometimes makes some rheumatologists wonder if these patients are fabricating such stories.

154

Not surprisingly, "fibromyalgia" is a diagnosis that MCAS patients have frequently acquired at some point along their diagnostic paths. Fibromyalgia, as most know, is a disease of migratory soft tissue pain of otherwise unclear cause, and it appears to be another one of the chronic inflammatory scourges of unknown cause emerging (also for unknown reasons) at epidemic levels in these modern times. Interestingly, random skin biopsies in fibromyalgia patients have been found to harbor roughly ten-fold more mast cells than random skin biopsies from healthy people. This of course doesn't come anywhere close to proving that fibromyalgia is a variant of MCAS, but it's nevertheless an interesting observation.

Another distinctive clinical syndrome notable in a subset of MCAS patients is the "Type III (hypermobility)" form of the set of connective tissue disorders collectively labeled Ehlers-Danlos Syndrome (EDS). EDS (of any type) is generally thought of as a genetic (i.e., inborn) disease in which a mutation in the gene for one connective tissue protein or another leads to production by cells of abnormal forms of such proteins that in turn lead to weakened or otherwise dysfunctional connective tissue. Each of the forms of EDS has unique and interesting features, but from the perspective of MCAS, type III is the most interesting. In type III, which also happens to be the most prevalent (by far!) type of EDS, the dominant clinical manifestation of the disease is a "looseness" (laxity) in joints that allows such patients to easily "hyperextend" their joints into configurations that healthy people find impossible to achieve. Unsurprisingly, frank joint dislocations are common in EDS Type III patients. Type III patients also demonstrate a general fragility in their connective tissue and thus suffer tears in tissues like tendons and ligaments much more easily than seen in healthy people.

But here's the really weird thing about type III EDS: it's actually not a genetic disease – at least, not as far as decades of research into connective tissue genes and proteins have been able to discover. One or more specific mutations in one or more genes for one or more specific connective tissue proteins have been found in every other type of EDS, but in type III (again, the most prevalent type of EDS by far), no clearly responsible mutation has yet been found in any gene for any known connective tissue protein. (Yes, it's true that mutations have been found in a couple of connective tissue-related genes in some EDS Type III patients, but the fact remains that for the great majority of EDS Type III patients who have been studied for mutations in connective tissue-related genes, no such mutations have been found.)

And here's where it gets even more intriguing: if you take care of, or even just talk to, enough MCAS patients, you quickly begin to realize there's a subset – small, but it's there – who either have been definitively diagnosed with EDS by an expert in such (note that without a specific mutation or other specific biological marker having been identified yet, it's purely a clinical diagnosis, i.e., the diagnostician's best estimation that the patient's findings "fit" what's described for EDS Type III better than they fit any other known disease) or are strongly suspected of having EDS Type III based on specific connective tissue problems in their history.

And thus arises the obvious etiologic question: might it be the case that, for at least some EDS Type III patients, the problem lies not in the normal assembly of allegedly mutated connective tissue proteins into connective tissue that functions abnormally but rather lies – due to aberrant mast cell mediator release –in the abnormal assembly of entirely normal connective tissue proteins into connective tissue that functions abnormally? I'm going to really stretch the bounds of how far one should analogize by saying this, but I'll say it anyway: could EDS Type III be a "connective tissue autism" in which normal connective tissue proteins are connected in abnormal ways vaguely akin to how in autism normal brain cells are connected in abnormal ways (possibly, in some patients, as a consequence of abnormal mast cell mediator release)?

Another way to think about this might be as follows: if one starts at the beginning of the assembly line for an exquisitely well designed, high-performance automobile, and one has all the (normal) parts needed to build that automobile but doesn't get the right assembly instructions at each stage of assembly, then one shouldn't expect to get a beautiful, high-performance automobile off the end of the assembly line. In fact, one should feel lucky to even get something off the end of the assembly line that's even remotely driveable.

Clearly, one "simple, small" research project that ought to be done sooner rather than later is to evaluate a small cohort of definitively diagnosed EDS Type III patients to see what proportion also harbor MCAS – and whether mutations in the genes for the assorted mast cell regulatory elements can be found in the mast cells (and thus presumably also the stem cells) of those who also harbor MCAS. If a recurring pattern of such mutations can be found, it should then be a relatively short path to track down which mediators are being aberrantly expressed as a result of such mutations and to then figure out how that particular aberrant mediator expression pattern is leading to the abnormal assembly of normal connective tissue proteins to yield the connective tissue abnormalities clinically seen in Type III EDS.

And if that sort of research is going to be pursued for Type III EDS, it ought to be pursued for fibromyalgia, too (and "chronic fatigue syndrome" (or "chronic fatigue and immune dysregulation syndrome"), "irritable bowel syndrome" (or "inflammatory bowel syndrome"), "multiple chemical sensitivity," "postural orthostatic tachycardia syndrome," refractory "GERD," and "Gulf War Illness," and the many, many other chronic (and typically inflammatory) diseases of presently unknown cause that potentially fit the profile of what could be expected from chronic aberrant mast cell mediator release).

156

To quote Dennis Miller (which is not to say I'm a fan), "*But that's just my opinion; I could be wrong.*" ☺

Chapter 18: "They Keep Telling Me It's All In My Head, But I Know It's Not": Neuropsychiatric Findings in MCAS

There are so many issues, and so many aspects of each issue, with the neuropsychiatric consequences of MCAS that I find it difficult figuring out how to even start this chapter, let alone the course it should take. Thus, I beg your pardon if this chapter seems to meander more than the others.

Basic, well-established facts are never a bad place to start, I guess. It is a fact that mast cells reside in every tissue in the body, and it also is a fact that they have a predilection for associating with (among other types of cells) nerve cells. Furthermore, we know there is extensive "cross-talk" between nerve cells and mast cells under normal circumstances. So why *wouldn't* we expect a disease of chronic, body-wide mast cell dysfunction to cause dysfunction of nerve cells potentially leading not only to disorders traditionally classified as "neurologic" but also to disorders traditionally classified as "psychiatric"?

Likely, then, neuropsychiatric symptoms are common in MCAS. Actually, it's more than just likely; it's reality, and diagnoses of assorted neurologic and/or psychiatric disorders are commonly found amongst the extensive problem lists most MCAS patients acquire as they meander through the halls of medicine in search of a sensible unifying explanation for their assorted ills.

But are such diagnoses "right"? Sure they are – sometimes. Sometimes it's just crystal clear that the MCAS patient's symptoms – or, more commonly, some portion of the MCAS patient's symptoms – precisely fit what's expected of one defined neurologic or psychiatric diagnosis or another (independent of whether there's any understanding of the actual cause of such a diagnosis). And in such cases you surely can't call such a diagnosis "wrong." (Same goes, of course, for classic presentations of diseases in other systems in an MCAS patient.)

I'll get to the "real" neuropsychiatric issues in MCAS in a little while, but I want to focus the first stretch of this chapter on what I see as the biggest problem with the neuropsychiatric aspects of MCAS: incorrect diagnosis of psychosomatism.

We doctors deplorably learn in medical school and residency – certainly not in any lecture, but from the words and actions of many of our clinical mentors (sometimes even at the bedside) – the lazy, sloppy habit of deeming "psychosomatic" or "somatiform" (classic $400 medical words commonly taken to mean "imaginary" and "not real" even though in truth they only imply central sensation without confirmable corresponding peripheral sensation) any complex of symptoms that doesn't fit any of the known entities in the pantheon of medical diagnoses, especially if objective abnormalities are not apparent or present only intermittently.

Consider the following scenarios:

Unpredictably episodic (or constant but fluctuating), often migratory abdominal pain for which all testing (that current medical standards say makes sense to perform, anyway) can't find any significant biological abnormality that could explain the pain.

Unpredictably episodic (or constant but fluctuating) shortness of breath, or coughing, for which all testing can't find any significant biological abnormality to explain it.

Unpredictably episodic (or constant but fluctuating), often migratory sensory neurologic symptoms for which all testing (if such is even available given the particular abnormality) cannot find any significant, objective, explanatory abnormalities.

And so on and so forth. You don't have to be a doctor to get the point. If somebody came to you and said, "I'm suffering this, that, and the other symptom," yet you couldn't *see* anything obviously wrong with the person (except, maybe, a vague air of "unwellness" about her), what would you think? What would you do? Would you choose the path that's easiest for *you*, call it "Option A," making the snap judgment, "It must all be in your head," and telling her "Snap out of it!" (or, more empathetically, suggesting she see a psychiatrist who can help her understand she's imagining her symptoms, and with that understanding the symptoms will go away)? Or would you choose the somewhat less lazy "Option B," thinking, and honestly telling her, "I don't know how to explain these symptoms" – and then, partly because you're already 30 minutes behind in an overfull schedule and partly because you can bill her essentially as much whether you figure out her problem or not, telling her "I'm sorry, there's nothing else I can do for you"? Or would you choose what unquestionably would be the most difficult "Option C," thinking, "I don't know how to explain these symptoms, but she doesn't have any obvious reason to make them up and she's not acting frankly psychotic, so there must be an explanation" – and then, in spite of being way behind in an overfull clinic appointment schedule, and in spite of the strong financial disincentives, telling her, "I don't know at this point what's going on, but clearly *something* is going on and I am going to keep chipping away at this until I figure it out"?

So, what would you do? It's not hard to see how Options A and B would win the vote in a landslide over Option C. A desire to help the patient is one reason why a doctor sees a patient – but it's certainly not the only reason, and doctors have way more reasons to pursue Option A or B than C.

And thus I hear, from patients found to have (or likely to have) MCAS, story after plaintive story after despondent story of "My doctors have never been able to find anything wrong and just keep telling me it's all in my head!"

Of course, once the *doctor* starts openly saying the symptoms are psychosomatic, it's often a short step to others believing and saying the same, and the patient goes from being merely a pariah amongst the medical community to being a pariah amongst society in general, even in that part of society – one's family – that's supposed to be the unshakeable bedrock of one's support.   I'm saddened to have seen it so many times; I can't imagine what it's like to live it, the loneliness, and the guilt. "What's wrong with me? Why must I be such a burden – especially with problems that are just imaginary – on my family and friends? I feel all these symptoms, but they don't exist – the doctors say so! – and I can't even begin to figure out how to just think my way out of them." (The closest I can come – and one can argue how "close" it is or isn't – is the professional isolation of dealing with a disease which 99.99% of colleagues have either never heard of or, even worse, choose to believe doesn't exist in spite of copious available data to the contrary, implicitly casting doubts about one's competency.) Humans (including both patients and doctors) are inherently social creatures; most of us *need* comfort and validation from others at least from time to time and otherwise spiral into depression and psychosis. No wonder the Internet has been a godsend for patients and doctors dealing with diseases that either truly are rare or (as for MCAS) are commonly (if erroneously) perceived as such.

Here (with some paraphrasing) are some of the sad consequences of incorrect diagnoses of psychosomatism in MCAS patients I've seen:

> Martha: "I go the ER when I have a bad flare because I never know just how bad it may get, but I bring my medicines with me when I go there and take them when nobody's looking because the doctors never believe these are the medicines that will help me and they won't give them to me no matter how much I beg."

> Bill: "My doctor started to suspect mastocytosis and gave me a prescription to have a tryptase level drawn in the ER whenever I had a flare, but every time I have a flare and go to the ER and ask for a tryptase level to be drawn and show them the prescription for it, the doctors there just ignore it."

> Cecily: "I'm so sick all the time. My doctors keep telling me it's all in my head because they can't find any other explanation, but I can't understand how something I'm imagining could cause not only so many symptoms but also so many abnormal test results that don't add up to any disease."

> Jennifer: "I keeping getting urinary tract infections, or at least what feels like urinary tract infections, all the time, except my doctors can never find any infections in my urine. They aren't even willing to give me antibiotics anymore because they're sure I'm just imagining my pain."

Heather: "I had another flare that was bad enough to go the ER, and I got admitted. The doctor said there was nothing wrong with me, that I was just making it all up. I begged for Benadryl, but he wouldn't even give me that. I had to sign this form – what do they call it? 'AMA,' against medical advice – so I could check myself out of the hospital and get home to take some Benadryl."

Amy: "My doctor told me I was having all of these problems because I wasn't praying enough." (!!!!!!)

Belinda: "My doctor brought all of his students and residents with him when he came to see me because he wanted to show them my rashes and flushing show up when obviously nothing was wrong with me – you know, how sick somebody can get just from thinking they're sick."

Marylou: "My doctor said I must be depressed because I feel so tired all the time, but I told him I'm just exhausted, I don't feel depressed, and he just said that's the way depression is sometimes."

Ginger: "My psychiatrist says my depression doesn't explain the diarrhea I'm constantly having, but my internist can't find any other reason for it and says sometimes depression can cause diarrhea, so I don't know what to think."

Julie: "I had a terrible experience following my endoscopy/colonoscopy. Actually, I never even got to the endoscopy itself because I started reacting as soon as they started to sedate me, and I wound up being hospitalized for a week with constant reactions before they finally seemed to settle down. All the doctors were basically out to prove my symptoms were psychological and gave me less than optimal treatment. It was awful. I was reacting to everything orally, which is not my normal. I would have severe muscle weakness/paralysis and hoarseness from taking a sip of Gatorade even. I reacted to the BP cuff pressure, tourniquet, heat, and many other triggers. The doctors just didn't buy into my MCAS diagnosis. They diagnosed me with vocal cord dysfunction and want me to see a speech therapist. I don't think this is needed. I only had the hoarseness with degranulation/flushing. And then the attending got angry with me for contacting you."

Bottom line: incorrect diagnosis of psychosomatism is a huge problem in MCAS and can delay diagnosis for years, decades, or even the "hypochondriac" patient's entire life. I don't walk in the psychiatrist's shoes, so I can't say that psychosomatism as the primary diagnosis for a symptom menagerie doesn't exist, but what I can say is that I haven't met the patient yet who had previously been so primarily diagnosed – and who turned out *not* to have MCAS. (Yes, I'm aware such an experience on my part is a result of "referral bias," and I'd be the last person to suggest most or all psychiatric (let alone all neuropsychiatric) illnesses likely are due to MCAS, but I *am* saying that most doctors should probably give serious consideration to the possibility of MCAS before falling back on a diagnosis of "psychosomatism.") Such situations clearly are not the fault of the patient; they are the fault of the patient's doctors and a health care delivery system that incentivizes such misdiagnosis, but all I can figure out to recommend at this time to patients who feel they are the victims of incorrect diagnosis of psychosomatism is to keep seeking additional evaluations and opinions from other doctors until you find one who is willing to pursue Option C. Worst case, such a concerned physician might still not be able to identify any diagnosis at all, but if MCAS is found, then *even if* it's thought – right or wrong – to be secondary to a primary psychiatric disorder, it nevertheless will likely be the case that co-treatment of the MCAS along with treatment of the psychiatric disorder will lead to a better outcome than would be seen with treatment just of the psychiatric disorder.

Small, more-or-less forward steps sometimes can be very helpful when the alternative is never making any progress at all.

So, setting psychosomatism aside, what are the "real" neuropsychiatric issues that can happen in MCAS?

The most common neurologic issue, unquestionably, is paresthesias – tingling and numbness to varying degrees –most commonly felt in the hands and feet, less commonly further up the arms and legs and about the head, and least commonly about the trunk. The most common psychiatric issue, if it can even be called that accurately, is generalized cognitive dysfunction – a "brain fog" that most commonly manifests as unpredictably episodic, or chronically waxing/waning, problems with memory, ability to concentrate, and/or word-finding – obviously potentially disabling symptoms (if severe enough) when one needs persistently sharp mental faculties to perform adequately at one's job.

Plenty of other neuropsychiatric issues are possible, though. *Acute* issues include flares of headaches (especially "migraine" headaches), tics, tremors, weakness (sometimes diffuse, sometimes focal but migratory), spells of "dysautonomia" (e.g., spikes or drops in blood pressure and/or pulse and/or temperature, episodic difficulty focusing vision, spells of narcolepsy (an uncontrolled sudden falling asleep), spells of cataplexy (suddenly becoming "disconnected" from, and unresponsive/unreactive to, the world around), uncontrollable spells of seizure-like movements in which no electrical seizure activity can be found in the brain on EEG recording ("pseudoseizures," though, to be sure, mast cell activation can also drive true seizures)). It's not much of a stretch to conceive of the possibility that flares of mast cell disease might underlie some cases of suicidality, homocidality, hypomania, and hallucinations. Mast cell activation disease certainly can cause a sense of anxiety, and as panic is "merely" an extreme form of anxiety, one has to wonder how many "panic spells" are "merely" flares of unrecognized MCAD (again, MCAS much more

162

so than mastocytosis due to the stark difference in prevalence between the two). Yet another research project for the future, eh? (From this one small example, extrapolating to the many other diseases that might be driven by MCAD, you can begin to better appreciate the truth of a statement I'll make and detail later about how research in MCAD could easily occupy an army of researchers for decades, if not centuries, to come.)

And what effects might *chronic* aberrant mast cell mediator release in the central or peripheral nervous system cause? Sleep dysregulations of all sorts, chronically persistent paresthesias, chronic weakness and atrophy (or spasticity) of any muscle innervated by a chronically mast-cell-affected nerve, anomalies in special senses (hearing, vision, taste, smell), depression, paranoia, anxiety, obsession-compulsion, etc. etc. etc.

What causes bipolar affective disorder (BPAD)? Decades of research and we still have no idea. Since mast cell disease can cause opposite symptoms to develop in a given organ in a given patient at different points in time (or even can cause opposite symptoms to develop at different sites in a given tissue in a given patient at the same point in time), and since the brain absolutely can be affected by mediators released by mast cells, why *couldn't* mast cell disease be the root cause of BPAD in at least some BPAD patients?

Is MCAD (again, particularly MCAS), at the root of some portion of the modern epidemic of autism? Many parents of autistic children are aware by now of the research, pioneered by mast cell expert Dr. Theoharis Theoharides at Tufts University in Boston ("Dr. Theo," as he is affectionately known to many in the mast cell community), finding that autism occurs nearly ten-fold more often in children with mastocytosis than in children without mastocytosis. Obviously, as rare as mastocytosis is, the portion of the autistic population that has mastocytosis is quite tiny, but is it possible that some portion of the autism population without mastocytosis has MCAS instead? Could chronic inappropriate mast cell mediator release (even without the inappropriate mast cell proliferation needed to diagnose "mastocytosis"), over time, cause brain development aberrations resulting in the behavior patterns we clinically label as autistic?

Is (obviously unrecognized) MCAS at the root of some cases of substance abuse? For example, might it be the case that patients with chronic pain caused by unrecognized/untreated MCAS learn that narcotics are the only drugs that even mildly dull their pain? What about marijuana? Some marijuana "abusers" report that drug as the only intervention that can ameliorate their chronic symptoms of nausea, pain, etc., so might it be the case that those symptoms in those patients are due to unrecognized MCAS and that engagement of the mast-cell-surface cannabinoid receptors by certain components of marijuana inhibits the dysfunctional mast cells' inappropriate release of assorted mediators which have been causing those symptoms? (Note that I use the term "MCAS" here –

even while aware that this scenario might apply to unrecognized cases of mastocytosis, too – only because it's far more likely that it's the prevalent disease of MCAS than the rare disease of mastocytosis that might be present in such people.)

Tobacco abuse? Many tobacco abusers report a baseline chronic anxiety ameliorated by nicotine. Is it possible that some portion of the tobacco-abusing population has unrecognized MCAS at the root of their chronic anxiety?

One could ask similar questions about alcohol abuse, too.

Given how little progress has been made, despite decades of research, in understanding the true roots of substance abuse, one can only hope these thoughts might be felt worthy of investigation by at least some future researchers.

Chapter 19: Think Puberty Is Bad? When Hormones Really Run Amok: Endocrinologic/Metabolic Findings in MCAS

Oh, man, where to start this chapter? The range of *normal* effects of the human body's endocrine system is so vast to begin with. Then there's the vaster range of what it can do when it doesn't work right. And *then* there's the even vaster range of what it can do when its malfunctions are being driven by one of the weirdest, most heterogeneous diseases ever seen.

Let's just dive into some cases:

Weirdness with gastrin and magnesium

> "Julia," a 62-year old retired receptionist, was referred to me in late 2011 by a local gastroenterologist who was beginning to become aware of MCAS. I'm not quite sure how this doctor was becoming aware of MCAS, but I suspect it was because he had had some hallway discussions with a colleague in his group practice who himself was beginning to become "MCAS-aware" due to some successes he had seen with patients he had shared with me.
>
> Julia began her first visit by telling me she had only been sick in the last three years, but it soon came out that she has been having many problems dating back much, much further than that. Actually, she said she had learned from her parents at some point that as an infant she experienced substantial difficulty with feeding and "couldn't keep anything down," but she eventually "grew out of it." The rest of her childhood and adolescence were healthy as best as she could recall, but in her 20s she started suffering attacks of presyncope and even frank syncope as well as "panic attacks," with most of these problems slowly but steadily increasing in frequency through the years. (She hadn't had a syncopal episode, though, in several years.) Around age 44 she first developed GERD, and by about age 47 it had gotten so bad that she was placed on the proton pump inhibitor (PPI) esomeprazole, which helped initially at the regular starting dose, but soon this improvement was lost. The dose was doubled, and again the problem remitted. She took this religiously for the next 15 years. Other problems diagnosed in this interval included hypertriglyceridemia, depression, and anxiety. She finally stopped esomeprazole in early 2011 when new information about potential toxicities from long-term PPI use emerged. Her GERD promptly relapsed when the esomeprazole was stopped. She was started on the histamine H_2 receptor blocker ranitidine at that point but found it completely ineffective, so she was switched by one of her doctors to omeprazole at a high dose, which again promptly remitted her GERD (though she appeared to me to be unaware that omeprazole is another PPI).

Meanwhile, about five years earlier (in 2006) Julia had begun to notice spontaneous easy bruising. Around that time she also had a breast biopsy for a mass, which fortunately was not cancer but fibrocystic breast disease. In 2008 she became newly significantly ill with sudden wakings at night with severe abdominal cramps, nausea and non-bloody vomiting, and non-bloody diarrhea. These attacks were unpredictable but overall became increasingly frequent over time. She was hospitalized for this the first time in 2009. Work-up included an EGD, which found a medium-sized hiatal hernia and a generally inflamed- (red) and thickened-appearing stomach lining. Multiple biopsies of these areas were all essentially normal, including random duodenal biopsies for celiac disease. An abdominal ultrasound was normal except for finding a fatty liver, certainly not an unusual finding, especially at her age. A gastric emptying study was unremarkable. A CT scan of her abdomen and pelvis didn't add anything new to the understanding of what was going on in her, and the same could be said for the small bowel dye study, brain MRI, capsule endoscopy, and colonoscopy (including multiple normal random biopsies) she also had done over the course of that year.

In early 2010, because of the severity of her GERD and the thickening of her stomach lining, her gastroenterologist checked her blood level of the hormone gastrin. Gastrin is made in certain specialized cells near the tail end of the stomach as well as in the duodenum and the pancreas, and it goads the stomach's production of acid. Julia's gastrin level was about 10-fold normal, but nevertheless well below the levels usually seen in a rare, specialized type of stomach cancer called a gastrinoma – and besides, there was nothing about her course or appearance, either, that suggested she had a cancer. Other blood testing was done, too, looking for evidence of pernicious anemia, celiac disease, carcinoid, and adrenal gland disease, but it was all normal. In view of the elevated gastrin level, a secretin stimulation test was done. Secretin – the first hormone to be discovered (back in 1902) – is manufactured by certain specialized cells in the duodenum which are goaded to release it into the bloodstream as the acidity of duodenal juice intensifies. Secretin both stimulates pancreatic enzyme release to help digest duodenal contents and inhibits the stomach's production of gastrin. Gastrinomas, like most cancers, don't pay much attention to the body's signals to shut down what they're doing, so if a gastrinoma were the cause of Julia's high gastrin level, secretin wouldn't be expected to reduce her gastrin level. Her gastroenterologist, though, didn't know what to make of her secretin stimulation test since not only were the post-secretin gastrin levels all normal, but so was the pre-secretin gastrin level. Clearly, no gastrinoma was present, but the cause of the earlier 10-fold-elevated gastrin level was even more a mystery at this point.

Her case was brought to the weekly gastroenterology conference at which challenging cases are reviewed, but none of her gastroenterologist's colleagues had any other ideas as to what the root of her problem was.

Thank goodness for the Internet.

Meanwhile, Julia hadn't been entirely passive about her condition. She had been plugging away on the Internet, searching for explanations of her symptoms, and around this time her explorations led to discovering there was such a thing as mast cell disease that indeed seemed to correspond with many of her symptoms, so much so that in April 2011 she just started taking loratadine on her own. This promptly helped her feel much better in general and essentially stopped her diarrheal attacks. Then, in late June of that year, she suffered – twice over two weeks – acute attacks of swelling of her tongue that fortunately didn't last very long, but these were just the precursors to "the big one" that interestingly came while at a July 4th beach outing (perhaps with sun exposure serving as a trigger?). She started feeling numb in her feet and fingers, soon feeling unwell enough in general that it was time to go home, but soon after leaving the beach she suffered a severe attack of nausea, vomiting, and diarrhea. Her fingers, too, were frozen – and she even found herself unable to speak!

Her family's immediate fear, of course, was that she was suffering a stroke, and she was immediately taken to the nearest emergency room. Fortunately, no stroke was found – but instead she was found, on the routine blood testing done for weakness, that she had a blood magnesium level of zero – absolutely undetectable. No cause was apparent (even her potassium level, usually low when magnesium is low, was OK), and she was admitted to the hospital for treatment with IV magnesium, eventually transitioning to oral magnesium supplements – lots of them – when testing showed her magnesium level quickly plummeted with lower levels of supplementation. A kidney specialist who saw her in the hospital felt the magnesium loss was more likely coming from her GI tract than her kidneys (presumably because he couldn't find any problem with her kidneys, so why not blame some other organ?). Vitamin B12, folate, and iron levels at the time were normal. She was just mildly anemic, and the rest of her CBC was normal. A serum chromogranin A was mildly elevated at 13 ng/ml (normal 0-5), but that could easily have been just a normal reaction to her PPI. Serum tryptase was checked twice and was normal both times.

Julia had continued on high doses of magnesium supplements ever since (and potassium supplementation, too, since, again, sometimes low potassium levels can cause magnesium levels to go low, even though she had never been found to have a low potassium level). At the time of her initial visit to my clinic, she clearly was (understandably!) nervous about her ability to keep her magnesium level in the proper range. Interestingly, she told me she recently had forgotten to take her magnesium supplements and quickly began again developing the same prodromal neuropathy she had felt on July 4th, so she immediately resumed her supplementation and felt the prodrome subside. She says she has not had any flares of her upper or lower GI issues since that hospitalization. However, because her diarrhea had flared at that time, she concluded the loratadine wasn't helping and had stopped it.

A rafter of chronic issues was revealed when I took a careful review of systems. Julia noted occasional acute episodes of hives across her upper abdomen (often brought on by "stress"), chronic fatigue, frequent coryza, the above-noted easy bruising, throat soreness at bedtime, intermittent mild dyspnea ("I just can't catch a deep breath") (but had not had any wheezing since quitting her 1-pack-of-cigarettes-a-day habit at age 59), occasional swallowing difficulty "when tense," an intermittent vague sense of chest discomfort, frequent palpitations, resurgent GERD as previously detailed, queasiness, nausea, vomiting, alternating diarrhea and constipation (much more so diarrhea, though), insomnia (resolved with regular use of bedtime amitriptyline), frequent episodic cognitive dysfunction, and the above-noted issues with presyncope (which had recently increased in frequency to a daily problem) and syncope (last episode a few years earlier) and "panic attacks" (improved with the benzodiazepine alprazolam taken regularly at bedtime and as needed during the daytime). Her only known medication intolerance was that codeine caused marked nausea and vomiting.

The family history was notable in that Julia's maternal grandfather had died around age 40 of the autoimmune stomach disorder called pernicious anemia, and her mother had died of complications from radiotherapy for rectal cancer at age 65. Her paternal aunt and her paternal grandfather both died of lung cancer or complications thereof, but both had long been smokers.

Julia's physical exam was completely unremarkable except that on a light scratch test on the upper back, bright dermatographism quickly emerged and was long fully sustained.

While I didn't have an explanation that day (or, frankly, since) for how MCAS might have driven her GI tract and/or kidneys to waste so much magnesium, everything else in Julia added up to MCAS being the most likely unifying explanation, and Occam would certainly argue her magnesium and gastrin problems, too, were most likely attributable to whatever one thing was likely causing all the rest of her problems, too.

I noted that although she had been on loratadine and ranitidine in the past, she had never been on both of them at the same time, so it was possible that histamine released by her mast cells was not only stimulating her H_2 receptors (on her mast cells and other cells, such as the stomach's acid-producing cells) while she was on loratadine but also stimulating her H_1 receptors (again, on her mast cells and other cells) while she was on ranitidine. I recommended restarting both an H_1 and an H_2 receptor blockade, and of course I also recommended additional testing for MCAS including not only blood and urine testing but also re-examining all of those previous GI tract biopsies for evidence of mast cell disease. I also asked her to decrease her magnesium oxide supplementation from 1500 mg daily to just 1000 mg daily.

While testing was underway, I "hit the books," as they say, to try to figure out more about the MCAS-hypomagnesemia link I was purporting. I reviewed several dozen articles I found on magnesium and mast cells and learned it was clear decades ago that hypomagnesemia is associated with mast cell activation, but it had never been clarified whether hypomagnesemia causes mast cell activation or mast cell activation (at least in some forms) causes hypomagnesemia – or both.

There also was a pretty uncommon but nevertheless well-established association between PPI use and hypomagnesemia. What made me uneasy, though, about extending this in Julia from association to causation was that although all of the reported cases showed resolution of the hypomagnesemia upon withdrawal of the PPI, the reports varied wildly (from weeks to 10+ years) in the duration of PPI therapy prior to onset of symptomatic hypomagnesemia, begging the question of how there could be a general mechanism by which PPI exposure causes hypomagnesemia. So I wondered, perhaps what's actually going on with this scenario is that something other than PPI use but which nevertheless is associated with PPI use is in turn causing the hypomagnesemia. With that thought in mind, I noted that PPIs are predominantly used for GERD, and by that point I had begun noting that PPI-refractory GERD, if fully investigated, is very frequently found attributable to MCAS, meaning that an association between PPI use and hypomagnesemia might boil down to an association between MCAS and hypomagnesemia, which is where this puzzle started, and thus I hadn't made any headway in figuring out the mechanism of this association. One possible mechanism was that since MCAS often demonstrates odd sensitivities/reactions to a huge variety of drugs, it might be possible that in some MCAS patients (depending on the particular underlying set of mutations in the regulatory elements of such patients' mast cells), exposure to a PPI leads to reaction of the aberrant mast cell with resulting aberrant mediator release which leads (somehow) to hypomagnesemia. But the question would still remain as to why there's such variability in the duration of PPI therapy prior to triggering the mast cell disease which leads to onset of symptomatic hypomagnesemia – plus there still would remain the question of the specific mechanism by which mast cell mediator release causes hypomagnesemia. Perhaps there are other acute changes in the patient's regimen or environment (i.e., novel exposures) which shortly precede the emergence of symptomatic hypomagnesemia but which simply are not being identified in the histories of these patients because mast cell disease isn't suspected and thus careful histories as to recent environmental changes aren't specifically elicited.

All of that having been said (and although cessation of her PPI with close monitoring of her hypomagnesemia (and her need for magnesium supplementation) would be an easy test to perform), I thought that, overall, hungry bone syndrome was probably the best answer. It's the only magnesium-consuming syndrome, which, as best as I could identify in the literature, could cause the particular severity and acuteness of the hypomagnesemia seen in Julia. Given the particular time course of the various symptoms in her July presentation, I didn't see that either renal magnesium wasting, GI magnesium wasting, or GI magnesium malabsorption (of whatever cause – not that any such cause, to a sufficient degree, was apparent from her history) could possibly have caused such severe hypomagnesemia so acutely. Instead, I got the sense that only an acute uptake of magnesium throughout the skeleton could cause such severe hypomagnesemia so acutely. Furthermore, it was very well established that assorted variants of mast cell disease could cause a wide variety of (potentially quite severe) disruptions of normal bone metabolism resulting in osteoporosis in some patients and osteosclerosis in other patients. (Some patients even present with mixed osteoporosis and osteosclerosis, suggesting the presence of either different clones of mast cell disease in different skeletal/periskeletal sites or the different reactions of a single MCAS clone in response to different microenvironmental conditions at different points about the skeleton.) Given that mast cell disease is well recognized to periodically shift acutely to new patterns of aberrant mediator release, and given that it's also well established that mast cell disease sometimes can result in astonishingly severe and acute floods of aberrant mediator release, I posited that what began happening in Julia in June was a shift to a new pattern of mast cell flaring (resulting in her new symptom of tongue swelling) that culminated on July 4th in a flooding release of mediators with a net impact on bone of driving bone formation – i.e., hungry bone syndrome (HBS). HBS – a phenomenon ordinarily only seen shortly after parathyroidectomy for hyperparathyroidism (i.e., a situation of acute severe deficiency of parathyroid hormone, consequentially causing an acute gross relative excess of calcitonin, which drives calcium from the blood into the bone), and which can lead to severe hypocalcemia and/or hypomagnesemia within hours – is well documented to consume magnesium as often as it consumes calcium, and there even are case reports of magnesium consumption without any apparent hypocalcemia. Thus, I thought the new pattern of aberrant mast cell mediator release which began in June resulted in a veritable flood of bone formation-driving mediators (possibly including mediators mimicking calcitonin or directly driving true calcitonin release, or mediators mimicking PTH inhibitors or directly driving release of true PTH inhibitors) which were acutely released from her aberrant mast cells on July 4th, a flood which had not since resolved (as proven by her recurring hypomagnesemia upon attempts to taper her magnesium supplementation) but rather had "merely" retreated to a steady stream/river which she had been able to manage only as long as she maintained sufficient magnesium supplementation.

Julia returned two months later. Her blood and urine testing for MCAS showed a normal tryptase level (and, interestingly, a normal chromogranin A level in spite of her ongoing PPI use, raising the question of whether the prior chromogranin A elevation actually was reflective of mast cell activation), but her plasma histamine level was mildly elevated and her plasma heparin level was 3-1/2 times greater than the upper limit of normal. An extensive set of X-rays (both a "skeletal survey" and bone densitometry) found no skeletal abnormalities at all, probably torpedoing my hypothesis about HBS as the mechanism responsible for her hypomagnesemia. She said the antihistamines had substantially reduced or eliminated her diarrhea, hives, dysphagia, chest discomfort, GERD, queasiness, nausea, vomiting, and presyncope. She wanted to try stopping her PPI, as she was now finding that both omeprazole and dexlansoprazole caused stomach discomfort. I was OK with that, but given that her magnesium level that day was still normal, I also asked her to continue tapering her oral magnesium oxide supplementation, this time down to just 500 mg daily.

At her next visit a month later, she was delighted to note further improvement. She said her fatigue had decreased and her easy bruising had essentially resolved. She remained absolutely delighted that her GERD had disappeared in spite of now being off her PPI. However, she noted her stomach continued to "grumble a lot" just like it had done when she was on the PPI and thought that drug was causing this symptom. Her coryza, however, remained unimproved, as did her episodic dyspnea and palpitations that accompanied occasional flares of "anxiety" and "panic." Given that benzodiazepines are useful not only for anxiety and panic but also in targeting the mast-cell-surface benzodiazepine receptors, I started her on a low dose of lorazepam and asked her to stop her magnesium supplementation two weeks hence. We also received her outside GI biopsies at that visit and sent them off to our pathology laboratory for re-evaluation for mast cell disease, but they were lost in transit and we never found out if they harbored hidden mast cell disease.

Six weeks later, Julia returned to report substantially decreased problems with panic and anxiety, sometimes still sensing a prodrome, which quickly spontaneously resolved, in contrast to the escalation that always had seemed to happen in the past. She noted a flare of hives on her bilateral cheeks the very morning of the visit out of nervousness about the visit, but she was intrigued that the hives had already resolved by the time of the visit. Her diarrhea was completely gone, and in fact she now was experiencing a little bit of constipation about once a week, occasionally taking some medicine for it, but overall finding it a very tolerable problem. She was proud that she had required a dose of omeprazole (a PPI) only three times since I last saw her because Tums wasn't controlling a flare of GERD at those times. She was "amazed" that she has needed omeprazole so seldom of late in view of how bad her reflux used to be. Furthermore, she had been off magnesium for a month at that point, and yet biweekly checks on her magnesium level showed it had remained just as normal after stopping magnesium as it had been while she was on magnesium. I told her it was OK to stop her potassium supplement, too, at that point.

Julia returned four months later reporting that she had run out of amitriptyline and had shortly noticed significantly worsened abdominal pain, nausea, agitation, akathisia (an inner restlessness with a compelling need to always be in motion), and nightmares bad enough to wake her from sleep with acute neck strain. She also had found that the benzodiazepine alprazolam helped her anxiety somewhat better than lorazepam and that a low dose of dye-free diphenhydramine, taken as needed, would quickly eliminate her flares of coryza. Finally, she noted that in spite of my instructions to stop her potassium supplementation, she had continued receiving fills of this from her pharmacy and thus had continued taking it. I restarted her amitriptyline and again asked her to stop her potassium supplements.

Another four months had passed when I next saw Julia in early 2013. She reported the symptoms that had relapsed upon running out of amitriptyline quickly remitted again upon resuming the drug. She had indeed stopped her potassium supplements. Since the prior visit, she had had only two "incidents," each roughly six hours long, of "stomach cramping" and marked diarrhea. She did not try any increase in antihistamines or benzodiazepines for either of these episodes. She also noted an episode of mild dysuria which, unlike prior such episodes, never "blossomed" into a full-fledged "urinary tract infection," but she saw her local physician for it anyway after it had been going on for about two weeks and (because her urine appeared cloudy) was given a 5-day course of ciprofloxacin, which she took, and the dysuria resolved at some point during that course, but she was surprised to learn later that the urinalysis obtained when the ciprofloxacin was prescribed was negative for any sign of infection. She also reported the possibly related issue that she had faced a good bit of stress related to her only grandchild about three weeks earlier, and shortly afterwards a patchy pruritic diffusely migratory erythematous rash arose about her mid-trunk, but she found diphenhydramine helped greatly with this. She also noted that her "acid reflux" started flaring about two months ago (well before the issue with her grandchild arose), and for several weeks she was "eating Tums" to little avail, so a couple of days before the visit she began a course of another PPI and was feeling significantly better within 24 hours. Her magnesium level remained normal, and in fact the mild anemia she had long had had completely resolved.

I have seen her a few more times since, and she has had no complaints at all on a regimen consisting only of twice-daily loratadine and famotidine and low-dose alprazolam, bedtime amitriptyline, and a daily morning PPI. She occasionally takes a 0.5 mg dose of alprazolam instead of her usual 0.25 mg dose when she feels an uptick in anxiety, and it quickly quashes the flare. Her magnesium, potassium, calcium, and gastrin levels have remained normal. To this day I don't know how, or, truthfully, whether, her MCAS triggered her hypomagnesemia (or her high gastrin levels), nor do I know from which organ she was losing so much magnesium. As I've said before, though, Occam certainly would have a position on that, and I've learned never to bet against Occam.

OK, so Julia didn't have weak bones, but Paul...

...had frighteningly weakened bones.

This 40-year old manufacturing supervisor was referred to me in late 2009 by his really astute endocrinologist who suspected him of having a mast cell disorder. Paul related a fascinating 38-year history – yes, since age 2 – of multisystem problems dominated by bone problems of various sorts. He fractured his left wrist in a fall at age 2, his left forearm in a fall at age 3, his left elbow in a fall at age 8, multiple ribs during martial arts exercises throughout high school, the left small toe due to trauma at age 24, the right ulna and radius due to trauma at age 25, and his left ribs due to coughing at age 34. He also had fractured numerous teeth over the years. There had never been any deformities or growth retardation. He also had been found to have a bone cyst on his right humerus at age 12, and he presently had knots of some sort on a lower left lateral rib, the right vertex, and the right zygomatic arch that might have been the same kind of problem. He had had a torn right knee meniscus and a right elbow tendinitis since 2007.

His problems weren't limited to his bones and other connective tissues, though. He had had migraine headaches frequently since childhood. He had had alternating non-bloody diarrhea (not aggravated by dairy products) and constipation ever since childhood; he didn't think his bowels had ever been regular. His eyes had been irritated since about age 20. He didn't think infections had been much of a problem; he had had a "mono"-like illness as a child and again in high school (when he underwent upper and lower endoscopy with no significant findings as best as he could remember), and he thought he got colds about three times a year on average. Around age 32 he began suffering acute-onset spells of flushing and lightheadedness. The frequency and intensity of these spells seemed to wax and wane over time. He had had chronic fatigue and migratory aches and pains diffusely about his body, including stiff joints, since about age 34. Around age 35 he had palpitations and took a beta blocker for a while for this. The problem resolved and he stopped the medication, without apparent relapse. In his early 30s he had a period of time, perhaps about a year or two, in which he would acutely develop a body-wide pruritic "chicken pox"-like rash, often in response to exposure to heat but sometimes without any apparent trigger; ultimately, this problem spontaneously resolved. He had long had occasional chest tightness but denied any frank asthmatic-type symptoms. At about age 38 he lost his appetite and about 10 lbs. of weight, but the problem resolved and he regained his weight after using megestrol acetate (a progesterone-type hormonal drug) and metoclopramide (an anti-nausea drug with modest antihistaminic activity) for several months. His past history included episodic depression and anxiety for which there had never been any obvious triggers. He denied any frank syncopal spells. He suffered a blood clot in his right foreleg around age 14 due to trauma in that area, but he had never suffered any other blood clots.

Paul had smoked one pack of cigarettes a day since age 15 and had had a waxing/waning alcohol abuse problem (at its worst, 10 beers per day), abstinent for about a month as of the time of the visit. He occasionally used marijuana and cocaine in his youth but denied any illegal substance use in more than 20 years. His father had thus far survived prostate cancer and melanoma; he also had "back trouble" and had had "stress fractures" in his feet. His mother, too, had a "bad back." His maternal uncle, a smoker and drinker, had died of throat cancer and cirrhosis. His maternal aunt had survived breast cancer. His paternal grandmother had died of melanoma. His one child, a 15-

year old daughter, has already suffered multiple fractures, all due to accidental trauma. One brother had suffered a left elbow fracture at age 5 and a hand fracture in high school, both due to accidental trauma. Another brother had suffered a femur fracture at age 9 in a motorcycle accident. There was no known family history of osteoporosis or kidney stones. His only regular medications were vitamin D and a multivitamin with calcium. He had been on risedronate (a bone-strengthening drug) but no longer took this regularly because it caused stomach upset. He had no known allergies, either drug or environmental, although a past note in his chart said he had not tolerated alendronate (another bone-strengthening drug) because it, too, caused stomach upset.

Paul had been referred by his kidney specialist in May 2009 to an endocrinologist for further evaluation of osteoporosis, which was confirmed on a bone densitometry scan in early 2006. The endocrinologist had also quickly referred Paul to a geneticist for evaluation for genetic bone diseases, but the geneticist did not feel the family history was a good fit for any such diseases. He was tested nevertheless for the two most common mutations (in procollagen genes COL1A1 and COL1A2) in osteogenesis imperfecta (OI), but both tests were negative, ruling out OI with 90-95% confidence, and no further genetic testing was felt necessary. The endocrinologist performed a variety of testing including a testosterone level, tryptase level, thyroid function tests, routine blood counts and chemistries, an erythrocyte sedimentation rate (a cheap, but not terribly sensitive or specific, screening test for inflammation), vitamins D and K, and other specialized tests looking for autoimmune inflammatory bowel diseases, adrenal gland diseases, pheochromocytomas, carcinoid, pernicious anemia, and parathyroid gland disease. Everything came back normal except for a persistently minimally elevated tryptase, mildly low vitamin B12 and folate and consequentially elevated homocysteine, and low vitamin D. The repeatedly elevated tryptase level caught the endocrinologist's eye and occasioned the referral to me. Paul was also noted to have severe hypertriglyceridemia (about 1800 mg/dl, with the normal range about 50-150) that had not responded to trials of several drugs for that condition.

My initial exam of Paul was notable for small "knots" on the right cheekbone and on the right top of the skull, plus he was mildly tender on palpation about much of his soft tissues and with movement of most of his joints. There was another small "knot" at the lateral aspect of the left 10th rib. Moderate dermatographism was promptly, easily seen on a light scratch test on his back and was long and fully sustained.

I opined in his chart that I thought his endocrinologist had hit the proverbial nail on the head with his suspicions of mast cell disease affecting the musculoskeletal, endocrinologic, cardiopulmonary, dermatologic, GI, CNS, hematologic, coagulation, and immune systems at a minimum. There simply was not another human illness that could produce the full spectrum of findings in this patient's case, and there was not a single aspect of his illnesses over the years that was inconsistent with the possible clinical expressions of mast cell disease. The barely elevated serum tryptase levels were not typical for mastocytosis, so I asked him to undergo blood and urine testing for MCAS, and we scheduled a return visit for purposes of a marrow biopsy.

Paul returned a month later (now early 2010) for the biopsy, which he tolerated well. His 24-hour urinary prostaglandin D_2 level had been found to be mildly elevated. Interestingly, he also reported that two days earlier he had spontaneously begun to intensely ache in all of the sites of prior fractures. I wondered whether this was a mild flare of mast cell disease as a result of stress from anticipating the marrow biopsy.

Paul returned another month later to review results from the marrow biopsy. The marrow was normal, including molecular-level testing (such as we could do at the time, anyway) for any traces of mast cell disease. I asked him to start loratadine and famotidine, to undergo upper and lower endoscopy with biopsies, and to return in two months.

Four months later Paul's kidney doctor contacted me to tell me Paul hadn't returned to see me because he had lost his job and his insurance and wasn't sure he could still be seen by me. Of course, I immediately got him back on my schedule and wound up seeing him five months after the prior visit. He had just suffered another fracture, while swinging a bag of ice, three weeks earlier. However, he did note that the antihistamines had improved his appetite and headaches and his presyncopal spells had essentially resolved. All the rest of his symptoms, though, persisted. He looked tired, and he hurt just about everywhere I palpated. The GI biopsies, which had been done in March, showed mildly increased mast cells in both the small and large intestines. I got our clinic's social worker involved to start helping Paul track toward temporary disability certification since he obviously couldn't work for the time being, and I also got our pharmacy specialist involved to start helping him track toward treatment with zoledronate, an IV cousin drug to risedronate and alendronate, since he so obviously needed bone-strengthening treatment so badly. I also asked him to try some aspirin.

Paul returned a month later noting that although he had quickly proven intolerant of aspirin due to stomach upset, additional time with the antihistamines had led to resolution of rash and chest tightness and improvement in fatigue, eye irritation, and itching. He mentioned his local kidney doctor had also given him a dose of IV iron, which he tolerated well, though I couldn't figure out why the treatment had been given in the first place.

What to do next? He clearly needed better control over his disease, but he was living hand-to-mouth and could afford virtually no medication that made sense to try for this disease. Ironically, his indigent status at that point led to a decision to try one of the most expensive therapies available for mast cell disease, the tyrosine kinase inhibitor imatinib, which retails for about $100,000 per year but whose manufacturer, Novartis, smartly makes the drug available at reduced prices – sometimes even free – to those who otherwise cannot afford it. I was pretty sure Paul would qualify for Novartis' patient assistance program and again got our pharmacy specialist in these sorts of affairs involved. Meanwhile, I also learned from our hospital's dentist that the dental exam required prior to initiation of zoledronate treatment (since the drug occasionally causes a potentially life-threatening bone problem called osteonecrosis of the jaw (ONJ), and people with pre-existing dental problems have a higher risk for ONJ) indeed found several teeth that needed extracting, so I had to beg upon the good graces of the hospital's chief oromaxillofacial (OMF) surgeon to perform these extractions, a few months after which Paul would finally be able to begin zoledronate.

Two and a half months later he returned, after having been on a low starting dose of imatinib for a month. He felt it was causing him 3-4 hours of nausea every morning shortly after the daily dose, and he thought it was worsening his flushing and diffuse bone aching. Interestingly, though, his triglyceride level had plummeted to a near-normal level at just 200 mg/dl, where it has stayed ever since. The disability examiners had turned down his application because they didn't see how he would be disabled for more than a year. I explained otherwise in his chart, and I asked him to try at least briefly doubling his imatinib to 200 mg once a day, a dose which, in my experience, was more likely to help control dysfunctional mast cells.

Paul returned three months later reporting that the higher dose of imatinib indeed had helped him feel much better, including complete resolution of diarrhea – until he finally got started on zoledronate, finding that the first dose almost immediately caused a marked relapse of diarrhea. I started working on trying to get him switched to pamidronate, another cousin IV drug of zoledronate, and (again in view of his financial constraints) I asked him to try a low dose of aspirin again.

Paul missed his two-month follow-up appointment, saying he couldn't afford the gas for the drive to my clinic and back, but he did return two months after that, saying many of his symptoms had relapsed. However, it also came out that due to his financial situation, he had cut back on his antihistamines to just once-daily dosing. He was tolerating a once-daily dosing of three baby aspirins (243 mg), but stomach upset precluded him taking this at 325 mg. It was also clear at this point that he wasn't going to be able to access pamidronate due to his financial situation, so I started working on getting him access to an entirely different type of IV bone-strengthening drug, denosumab, that had become available just recently. I also asked him to try to return to twice-daily antihistamine dosing.

Paul returned six weeks later reporting that returning the dosing of his antihistamines to twice-daily had immediately resolved his diarrhea, but nothing else was better. It was clear that aspirin was not going to help him, so I asked him to instead try ibuprofen, which he had tolerated much better in the past.

Another six weeks passed, and Paul returned again. He had been started by one of his other doctors on zolpidem for insomnia that he thought was caused by loratadine, and he felt the zolpidem – which is not, strictly speaking, a benzodiazepine but nevertheless works through the body's benzodiazepine receptors – had decreased his malaise. His diffuse pain seemed somewhat better with regularly dosed ibuprofen, but he otherwise was unimproved. His application for denosumab treatment was inching forward. I decided to have him try doxepin and then, if that didn't help, low-dose lorazepam.

Paul returned 2-1/2 months later reporting that he had finally gotten his first dose of denosumab two weeks earlier and had tolerated it without any apparent problems. However, he had not tolerated doxepin and had soon stopped it, and he also was finding low-dose lorazepam to be too sedating. By this point, I had managed to come across some samples of the oral cromolyn I had been wanting to try him on for a long time because of all of his GI issues, so I asked him to stop the lorazepam and try the cromolyn.

A month later Paul reported he had proved immediately intolerant of cromolyn. Many of his problems persisted. In fact, although he had tolerated the first three doses of denosumab well, after the fourth dose he soon developed a diffuse tendinitis. Despite all of his complaints, though, he actually looked pretty comfortable, the best I had seen in many months. At that visit he said his insomnia, which he still thought was coming from his bedtime dosing of loratadine, was his worst problem, so I asked him to try some alternative H_1 antihistamines. He had so many waxings and waning of various symptoms that I couldn't tell if the denosumab had caused his tendinitis, and he desperately needed bone-strengthening treatment, so I asked him to try continuing that treatment for now and to see if the tendinitis returned.

Five months later (now the summer of 2012) Paul again returned reporting he was still tolerating denosumab OK, and he had found cetirizine more tolerable than loratadine with respect to causing insomnia, but even the cetirizine was causing "weird dreams" (again, not a normal side effect of an H_1 blocker, and one has to wonder if this "side effect" was more a reaction to some filler or dye in the particular cetirizine formulation he was trying rather than a reaction to the cetirizine itself). Some of his other symptoms had worsened, too, but it turned out he had been spending quite a bit of time out in the sun during the heat wave we had that summer. I asked him to reduce or eliminate such exposures, to try reducing the nighttime cetirizine dosing and reducing the nighttime lorazepam dosing that left him too fatigued in the morning, and to try quercetin.

Paul returned three months later reporting that the lower dose of cetirizine hadn't relieved the weirdness of his dreams, but at least the lower dose of lorazepam helped him tolerate the dreams better and didn't leave him with morning fatigue. He was tolerating the quercetin well and found it regulated his bowels very well. Diffuse joint and breast pains were now the principal problems. I asked him to make some adjustments to his quercetin dosing and return in a couple of months.

He returned shortly before Christmas and said that although he had suffered yet another rib fracture from a fall while shopping, he was overall feeling the best he'd been in a long time. I made no changes.

Paul returned in March 2013 reporting that the turn of the year had brought a loss of insurance that cost him access to imatinib, denosumab, and the two medications he had been taking for his hypertriglyceridemia that had never seemed to actually help that condition. All I could do was to get our pharmacy specialist involved in trying to re-establish his access to at least his imatinib and denosumab, and in the meantime I just asked him to try increasing his quercetin.

He returned five months later reporting he had quickly gotten back on imatinib and denosumab, and he had also eventually gotten back on some cholesterol drugs, though not the ones he had been on before. Insomnia and GERD were still his biggest issues. He had finally been able to get the MRI of his neck and shoulders I had been seeking for a long time to try to help explain left back pain he had had as a particularly bad focus of pain for a long time, and it showed a torn left rotator cuff. He also had suffered a toe fracture when his 85 lb. dog bounded onto the digit. I asked him to try increasing his famotidine to thrice daily dosing and then try a PPI if necessary.

The last time (as of this writing) that I saw Paul, several months later, he was doing well on his medications, his rotator cuff had been repaired, and repeat bone densitometry showed major improvement in bone density.

Meanwhile, Jacquelyn helps us (in medicine, anyway) re-learn that not all excess ferritin is from iron overload…

Jacquelyn had sickle cell anemia, and if ever there were a disease that illustrates the old saw that the more we know, the more we know we don't know, it's sickle cell anemia (SCA). I'll tell Jacquelyn's interesting story in just a moment, but I think it would help for you to first have a bit of background in SCA.

SCA, as many know, was the first human disease to be traced (back in 1956) to a specific genetic mutation. (I won't even call it a genetic defect because the mutation actually helps people who have it survive infection, which can be lethal, by the parasite that causes malaria. The mutation, however, is nothing but bad news in people who live in places – such as the U.S. – where malaria is rare.) In people with SCA, in their DNA code (i.e., their genes) for the part of hemoglobin known as beta globin, a change (i.e., a mutation) in a single letter in the code results in a slightly different beta globin protein, and thus a slightly different hemoglobin protein into which the beta globin gets incorporated. The different hemoglobin is designated hemoglobin S (HbS), as distinguished from normal hemoglobin A (HbA). The function of hemoglobin, as many also know, is to convey oxygen from the lungs to the tissues and to convey carbon dioxide from the tissues to the lungs. HbS performs this function just as well as HbA when there's enough oxygen around, but when there's less oxygen around, the HbS protein does something that the HbA protein doesn't: it sticks to other copies of itself. When they form, these aggregates, or polymers, of HbS quickly turn the red blood cell (RBC) from its normal self as a highly flexible bag stuffed full of independent, free-floating HbS protein molecules into an inflexible bag – shaped like a sickle, actually – stuffed full of rigid aggregates of HbS protein molecules.

This change in flexibility has critical consequences because many of the smallest blood vessels – the capillaries – that RBCs need to travel through are actually smaller in diameter than the RBCs themselves, so it's only because the normal RBC is flexible and squeezable that it can get through such tight passages. RBCs full of polymerized HbS, though, aren't flexible and can't be squeezed, so they create the proverbial logjam at the point where the capillary gets too small. The medical term for this is vaso-occlusion, or occlusion of a blood vessel, and the consequences are exactly what you'd think would happen if oxygen in the RBCs, and other nutrients in the blood, can't get through to the tissues that need them: these tissues start dying. And, unsurprisingly, it hurts. This is a sickle cell vaso-occlusive crisis, or pain crisis, in action, and it can be quite severe and disabling both in the short term and, if the patient suffers crises often enough, the long term, too.

It's been more than a half-century since the discovery of the disease's ultimate cause, though, and we still can do little more to treat the acute crisis than provide the suffering patient with IV fluids (to try to help dilate the blood vessels a little bit and break up the logjams) and pain medications (such as narcotics). Even giving extra oxygen doesn't seem to help SCA patients suffering a "routine" vaso-occlusive crisis. And as far as *preventing* crises goes, we've learned a couple of tricks – a daily oral medication called hydroxyurea can help, regular (typically monthly) transfusions of normal RBCs can help – but it's the uncommon patient in whom such tricks eliminate sickle crises. There even is a small portion of the SCA population in whom we can perform a stem cell transplant that will cure the disease, but this comes at the risk of causing substantial other medical complications, not to mention a great financial cost (though that cost overall is far less than a lifetime of care for sickle cell crises).

One of the most curious aspects of SCA, though, stems from the observation that most people with SCA have relatively infrequent and less severe crises, while a relatively small minority (roughly 5-15%) have frequent and more severe crises. This is a curious distinction because if the disease is caused in every patient by exactly the same mutation, why would different patients suffer such greatly different consequences?

Clearly, there must be other factors at work in SCA patients that modulate the severity of the disease, and over time we have been learning about some of those factors. Some patients, for example, have additional mutations (either in beta globin or the other major component of hemoglobin, alpha globin) that interact with the sickle mutation. Most such additional mutations seem to have an ultimate clinical impact of lessening the severity of the disease. On the other hand, inflammation clearly worsens not only the vaso-occlusive crises themselves but also the risk for development of such crises, and it's clear that some SCA patients are chronically more inflamed than others and thus have chronically worse courses of the disease – patients I will call "the poor-phenotype sicklers." Inflammation is an awfully complex phenomenon, though, and we remain just as far from a complete understanding of why some SCA patients are chronically inflamed as we do for non-SCA patients. Regardless of why they are more inflamed, though, poor-phenotype sicklers on average clearly suffer not only more frequent and severe crises but also incur more frequently and severely the complications of SCA beyond vaso-occlusive crises, a few examples of which are strokes and other blood clots, a type of respiratory failure called acute chest syndrome, and kidney failure.

As mentioned earlier in this book, soon after I began recognizing MCAS in many of my chronically ill patients whose known diagnoses didn't account for many of their symptoms, I began seeing much the same pattern in most of the poor-phenotype sicklers already under my care. Wondering if MCAS might be one significant source of inflammation in them which might be controllable to the point of turning them into good-phenotype sicklers, I began looking for MCAS in them, and the more I looked for it, the more I found it, and the more I found it, the more I treated it, and the more I treated it, the better they got. I reported my findings in 32 such patients in an article, which the *American Journal of the Medical Sciences* was kind enough to publish in 2014.

Jacquelyn was one of those patients and certainly a "poster child" not only for the devastation that MCAS could cause in an SCA patient but also for the improvement that could be wrought upon recognition and successful treatment of her MCAS – but her case is instructive, too, with regard to one of the metabolic effects of MCAS (or, truthfully, almost any inflammatory process), namely, elevation in the serum ferritin level. We physicians are taught relatively early in medical school that the ferritin level in the blood goes up when there is too much iron in the body, and it sometimes (often, but not always) goes up when there is inflammation in the body. You can probably easily imagine, though, that when a patient has a condition requiring frequent blood transfusions – as is the case for many poor-phenotype sicklers – it becomes easy to think that most or all of the elevation in ferritin levels seen in such patients is attributable to the iron overload that inescapably accompanies such transfusions, and to forget, or at least disregard or discount, how much of the elevation might be coming from inflammation. In fact, many such patients are chronically administered chelation medications to try to leech the excess iron out of their bodies (via the urine) to avoid the substantial toxicities of long-term iron overload, and yet many of these patients never see any significant reduction in their massively elevated ferritin levels – but it's almost always the case that such elevations are blamed exclusively on iron overload, with no consideration for how much a problem of uncontrolled inflammation might be contributing.

You can also probably easily imagine that when the patient has a definitively established diagnosis of a genetically based disease, everything that happens to the patient that has ever been reported as being seen in patients with that disease – such as a flare of diffuse, migratory pain – is going to be attributed almost reflexively to that disease, with little to no consideration of alternative diagnostic possibilities. Little wonder, then, that MCAS, whose range of symptoms and morbidities overlaps a good bit with what's found in SCA, would virtually always be missed in SCA patients even if physicians were aware of MCAS and no matter how prevalent MCAS might be in the SCA population.

So with all of that as context, let's get back to Jacquelyn's story, or, as I like to summarize it, the epitome of the classic "Take two aspirin and call me in the morning" doctor's tale.

> At ages 3 and 8, Jacquelyn had suffered strokes which together had
> left her with chronic right-sided weakness (hemiparesis) and difficulty

speaking (dysarthria), and between these problems and her chronic fatigue and malaise, there was no question she was fully disabled. She also had a history of acute chest syndrome and a blood clot related to a long-term IV catheter she used to have. She was "always" in the ER or the hospital for sickle cell pain crises, which often were complicated by pneumonia and sinusitis. Interestingly, she was the daughter of a Jehovah's Witness (though not one herself), and as a result she had long refused transfusion therapy, but during a prolonged crisis hospitalization at age 31, she began accepting transfusions; however, no sustained clinical improvement was seen. There were some other oddities to her course, too. For one, she had suffered occasional periods, lasting from a few months to two years, of significantly worsened anemia attributed to a particular type of virus called parvovirus B19 which indeed can be an acute cause of severe anemia – except no evidence of this virus, not even on the most sensitive molecular testing available, was ever found in her. For another, on occasional CT scanning over more than a decade, she was found to have months-long periods of liver enlargement (hepatomegaly) that would mysteriously come on and then just as mysteriously go away all by itself. Plus, there was another remarkable oddity: although one of the supposedly inescapable consequences of SCA is destruction (and resulting gross shrinkage) of the spleen by early childhood, her CT scans found her spleen to be persistently of normal adult size. It also showed mild enlargement of a few scattered lymph nodes deep in her abdomen and pelvis, which never changed much, and the cause of this adenopathy was never apparent.

Around the time of that prolonged crisis hospitalization at age 31, new migraine headaches and frequent severe whole back pain emerged, occasioning even more frequent ER visits and hospitalizations in which these symptoms were attributed to her SCA. Jacquelyn was referred to my care at that time.

In general across multiple physical examinations, she was a thin woman appearing her stated age with right hemiparesis and a stuttering-type dysarthria from her old strokes, wearing leg braces, and frequently in moderate to severe diffuse pain. Despite her strokes, she was usually alert and oriented. Vital signs were usually unremarkable. The abdomen was usually unremarkable. She often reported pain in her extremities, chest, or along the length of her spine, but my palpation at those sites usually did not appear to provoke more pain.

I knew from the outset of her relationship with me that there was something odd about her SCA for it to be making her so much sicker than the average SCA patient, but it wasn't until a few months after she first came under my care that I finally had a chance to take a long, careful look at her record to try to begin ferreting out clues as to what might be causing her so much difficulty. Sure, there were the zillion and one pain crises and other events in her record – all attributed to her SCA, of course – but what really stood out were long-term modest abnormalities in some of her labs. (Fortunately, the electronic medical record system my institution was using at the time had lab results dating back to 1993, and it was trivial to look at the long-term trend in each lab test. I have to admit to being disappointed when the institution switched to a new system in 2012 that made it much more difficult to look at long-term trends, plus only the most recent five years' worth of data was migrated to the new system.) Her coagulation screening tests were often mildly abnormal, something you typically see only with use of anticoagulants except that most of the times at which she had abnormalities in these tests were times at which she was not using anticoagulants. Serum ferritin records dating back to age 16 showed longstanding, highly variable hyperferritinemia (898-11,424 ng/ml, normal 10-300) even before she began accepting transfusion therapy. There were also chronic mild elevations in her white blood cell count (leukocytosis) and chronic mild intermittent elevations in her platelet counts and percentages of monocytes, eosinophils, and basophils. The inflammation inherent in severely painful SCA crises might – emphasis on "might," not "necessarily did" – account for some portion of the elevations in her ferritin level, coagulation tests, white blood cell count, and monocyte percentage, but it was highly unlikely that it would account for the elevations in the eosinophil and basophil percentages. Therefore, something else – also likely an inflammatory factor of some sort – was more likely responsible for at least the eosinophil and basophil elevations, and if there indeed was another inflammatory factor present, maybe it was also responsible for at least some portions of the elevations in the ferritin levels, coagulations tests, white blood cell counts, platelet counts, and monocyte percentages.

So what might this other inflammatory factor be? None of the other things I know of that can cause elevations in both eosinophils and basophils seemed to be present, but I had learned by this point that mast cell disease could do it. And so when she returned in October 2009 with ongoing severe back pain not helped one bit by a recent significant increase in narcotics by one of her other doctors, I decided to pursue the evaluation for MCAS. I sent her off to the lab to have blood and urine taken for levels of serum tryptase and chromogranin A, serum prostaglandin D_2 (PGD_2), plasma histamine, and urinary PGD_2 and N-methylhistamine (NMH), and because pain was her major issue, I asked her to start aspirin 650 mg twice a day since it helps some patients with mast cell disease and she said she had previously tolerated it well in occasional use, so I didn't have to worry much about her being one those mast cell disease patients in whom aspirin would trigger an even greater flare of symptoms.

She returned two months later reporting reduction in average pain from 9/10 to 6/10 and modest improvement in ability to perform activities of daily living. ER visits had been virtually eliminated, and she hadn't had another hospitalization. Migraine headaches had resolved. The previously ordered blood tests were normal except for serum chromogranin A which was double the upper limit of normal; plasma histamine was at the upper limit of normal. It turned out she hadn't provided the requested 24-hour urine sample previously, but she provided it at this visit – even though the urinary PGD_2 result likely would be substantially compromised by her ongoing aspirin use. Fascinatingly, her serum ferritin, which had long been markedly elevated, including long before she started getting regular transfusions, had completely normalized. Because her pain was still at 6/10 on average, I asked her to further increase aspirin to 650 mg every eight hours (though I'll note that I no longer push aspirin dosing beyond 650 mg twice daily, as I have seen a couple of GI bleeds at higher doses, and since it's obviously my desire to make my patients better, not worse, I don't think the potential benefits at higher doses are worth the risk).

She returned six weeks later reporting her pain had reduced to an average of 0-4/10. Fatigue and malaise were much better. The frequency of her crises dramatically decreased. She previously had been bed-bound most of each day but now was fully active, participating in household chores and going on outings with friends including shopping trips and even a fishing trip! The patient and her family were very happy with her improvement. The urine sample turned in at the last visit had yielded an N-methylhistamine level of 155 ng/ml (normal 30-200), and the PGD_2 level was just barely still within the normal range at 273 pg/ml (normal 100-280), making me wonder how high it would have been if she hadn't been on aspirin while collecting the urine sample. Nevertheless, she was doing so much better, and everything was so consistent with MCAS at that point, that I didn't feel it right to ask her to stop the aspirin in order to collect another urine sample for another PGD_2 determination. Oh, and her ferritin was still normal, too.

Because of the likelihood that she would remain on aspirin for the long term, I added twice-daily loratadine and famotidine and daily omeprazole to her regimen. She eventually found she was able to sustain her improvement with just twice-daily aspirin dosing, and she also eventually learned that her "sickle crises" usually could be aborted if she temporarily increased her aspirin and antihistamines to more frequent dosing sufficiently soon after onset of symptoms.

Now 36 years old, she still requires very occasional ER visits and hospitalizations for crises. Interestingly, her serum ferritin briefly escalates to the 600-800 ng/dl range during such events – surely a sign

of an acute spike in inflammation, not iron overload – and then soon
returns to normal once the crisis is over.

Ferritin levels that don't signify what they're assumed to signify. Ridiculously weak bones at ridiculously young ages. Horrible hypertriglyceridemia controlled by imatinib. Severe magnesium deficits cured by antihistamines. These, of course, are just a few examples of the huge range of endocrinologic and metabolic abnormalities I have seen in MCAS patients. There also have been the cases of severe, "brittle" diabetes as well as cases of marked drop in blood sugar *following* each flare of symptoms. Humongous weight gain. Inexplicable, severe thyroid function abnormalities which thyroid medication could never stabilize. Otherwise inexplicable pituitary hormone abnormalities, otherwise inexplicable adrenal hormone abnormalities, otherwise inexplicable pancreatic hormone abnormalities, otherwise inexplicable sex hormone abnormalities, and so on and so forth – all with MCAS eventually identified, and all improving upon identification of MCAS-targeted therapy effective for the individual patient.

Chapter 20: How Can It Possibly Be a Blood Cell Disease When the Blood Counts are Normal? Hematologic Findings in MCAS

A book about MCAS – a disease that's fundamentally classified as a hematologic disease given that the cell at the heart of the disease is born in the bone marrow – wouldn't be complete without consideration of the hematologic abnormalities it causes.

Of course, that's one of the major confounders of the disease right there: large portions of MCAS patients exhibit no hematologic abnormalities at all. Their complete blood counts are normal, their leukocyte differentials are normal, their bone marrows are normal, and their coagulation systems are normal. No wonder hematologists are often bewildered by this disease – or even won't believe it exists.

But many MCAS patients do exhibit hematologic abnormalities. And they can be different abnormalities in different patients – and even different abnormalities in the same patient at different times.

And they can be virtually any hematologic abnormality.

Too many red cells (polycythemia). That was Shelly, in Chapter 1.

Or too few red cells (anemia, sometimes to the extreme point of pure red cell aplasia). That was Betty, in Chapter 3.

Or too many white blood cells (leukocytosis). (I'll spare you Luther's story.)

Or too few white blood cells (leukopenia, sometimes to the extreme point of agranulocytosis; I'll spare you the story of Max, which I published in *Military Medicine* in 2012).

Or too many platelets (thrombocytosis). (I'll spare you Leroy's story.)

Or too few platelets (thrombocytopenia). (I'll spare you Jolene's story.)

Or too much clotting (hypercoagulability; see Chapter 21).

Or too little clotting (that is, bleeding; again, see Chapter 21).

Or maybe any combination of the above – even a combination in which at one time there are too many of a given type of cell and at another time there are too few of those cells.

The benign polycythemia seen in some MCAS patients is usually modest[1] and, unlike the cancerous p. vera (PV), it does not progress over time. Also, in PV the kidneys should react to the excess red blood cells and shut down erythropoietin (epo) production, so the epo level in the blood should be well below the lower limit of normal. In an MCAS-driven polycythemia, though, epo is usually in the normal range and sometimes even is a little bit elevated. Clearly, there is something about the MCAS in those patients that is driving aberrant production of epo, and that excess epo is contributing to (perhaps even wholly driving) the increased red blood cells.

The anemia can be anywhere from mild to severe. In some MCAS patients with anemia, the red blood cells are normal in size (normocytic), which is what we're taught to expect in "anemia of chronic disease" (ACD). Interestingly, ACD recently has been rechristened "anemia of chronic inflammation" (ACI) – which is what we're taught to "diagnose" when the patient has a normocytic anemia and no other apparent explanation for it.

In other patients, though, the red blood cells can be increased in size (macrocytosis). Since red blood cells start out very large during their four-month life span and shrink as they mature, sometimes this macrocytic anemia reflects impaired development of the red blood cells in the bone marrow, and sometimes it just reflects premature release of normally developing red blood cells from the bone marrow. Sometimes macrocytic anemia is a result of vitamin B12 or folate deficiency or alcohol abuse, sometimes it's a result of liver disease, sometimes it's a result of hemolysis, sometimes it's due to chemotherapy, sometimes it's due to myelodysplastic syndrome (MDS), generally recognized as an assortment of pre-leukemic conditions, some of which can be shown to have mutations clearly associated with leukemia, while others of which have no (presently) detectable mutations (so-called cytogenetically normal, or normal karyotype, myelodysplastic syndromes). Given that the most common pattern of abnormality in the bone marrow in MCAS is a type of disordered blood cell development called myelodysplasia, one has to wonder whether some portion of the cases of cytogenetically normal MDS are actually cases of MCAS.

---

[1]It may not even be an absolute polycythemia. It might be a *relative* polycythemia. I teach my trainees, "normal is not always normal," and every lab test has to be interpreted in context. If the patient has a boatload of chronic inflammation, and if a boatload of chronic inflammation should cause at least a mild anemia, then if the patient doesn't have anemia, that means the patient has more hemoglobin and/or red blood cells than normal, and that's at least a *relative* polycythemia.

And in yet other patients, the red blood cells can be decreased in size (microcytosis). There are several potential causes of microcytosis, including iron deficiency and inborn thalassemia and inborn and acquired sideroblastic anemias, but sometimes there's a mild to moderate microcytosis in an MCAS patient in which no other cause can be identified, and in those cases one has to wonder whether the abnormal mediator milieu in such a patient is interfering with the iron utilization processes needed to build hemoglobin, perhaps akin to how an abnormal mast cell mediator milieu in an EDS Type III patient might interfere with assembly of otherwise normal collagen proteins, thus leading to the lax joints and other soft tissue abnormalities in such patients.

There may be leukocytosis or leukopenia, but whether the white blood cell count is high or low or normal, a significant minority of MCAS patients show (persistently or, more commonly, intermittently) increased percentages of monocytes, less commonly eosinophils and reactive lymphocytes, and sometimes also basophils.

When no other cause is apparent, MCAS patients who show increased platelets often, by default, are diagnosed (and treated) as having essential thrombocytosis even when none of the mutational abnormalities known to be associated with that low-grade hematologic malignancy can be found.

Similarly, when no other cause is apparent, MCAS patients who show decreased platelets often are diagnosed as having "autoimmune thrombocytopenic purpura" ("ITP"). It is interesting that anti-platelet antibodies can't be found in a large portion of patients diagnosed with ITP. Perhaps some of those patients actually are MCAS patients.

Chapter 21: An Invisible Hand on the Teeter-Totter: Effects of MCAS on the Coagulation System

In my 10 years of medical training, and in my 13 years of practice before beginning to recognize MCAS, nobody ever told me – and I certainly never read anywhere – that mast cell disease was a potential cause of abnormalities in the clotting system. (Given that heparin was the first mast cell mediator to be discovered, one would think the disease would at least have the potential to cause bleeding, but no, the five minutes of lecturing I got on mast cell disease in my 10 years of training never mentioned bleeding, nor did the mast-cell-disease parts of the textbooks that I read ever mention it.)

But seven years of experience with MCAS – heck, *one* year of experience with MCAS – taught me that MCAS can affect the clotting system just as much – both in severity and diversity – as it can affect any other system in the body.

You already know that different variants of MCAS in different patients – heck, different variants of MCAS at different sites within the same patient – can drive any given system in the body to polar opposite aberrancies. Red cell aplasia vs. polycythemia, osteoporosis vs. osteosclerosis, and so on.

Well, the clotting system is another perfect example. This system exists as an exquisitely finely balanced seesaw, allowing the blood to remain in liquid form to permit the circulation needed for life, yet able to clot in virtually an instant, and only where a clot is needed. It shouldn't be surprising, then, that there are a myriad of natural controls on this system, so if an anti-bleeding control is heightened, the seesaw tilts toward clotting (sometimes enough so to permit spontaneous formation of a clot without any traumatic provocation), while if an anti-clotting control is heightened, the seesaw tilts toward bleeding, most commonly manifesting an "easy bruising or bleeding" (due to merely mild trauma) that can't be attributed to any known coagulation system disorder, and sometimes manifesting as spontaneous bruising or bleeding without any apparent inciting trauma. (In women, of course, this problem can also aggravate the normal bleeding of menstruation, a condition called menorrhagia.)

You've already heard the story, in Chapter 14, of John, who had been sick with MCAS symptoms since his tween years but had never had any trouble with excessive clotting (hypercoagulability) until he had his first coronary artery stent placed (to try to address his frustrating series of heart attacks in which no coronary artery obstruction could ever be found – in retrospect, almost certainly a presentation of Kounis syndrome, or allergic angina). He had many coronary artery obstructions – clots – after that point, and every single one of them occurred not in his own coronary arteries but instead ironically within the immunosuppressive-drug-laced stents placed in his coronary arteries, strongly suggesting his dysfunctional mast cells in his coronary arteries at the sites of the stents were provoked by the drugs in those stents to release pro-coagulant mediators leading to clots at those sites.

But let me now tell you about another patient who didn't even need the provocation of immunosuppressive drugs to cause her extreme hypercoagulability.

"Ophelia" was a 41-year old married disabled nursing assistant seeking to establish a new career in social work when she was referred to me in the summer of '06 to further assess her extreme hypercoagulability that much testing by her local physicians (including a hematologist) had been unable to specifically diagnose. She dated her health problems back to early '03, when she strained her right shoulder and neck and left groin in an on-the-job accident while helping to mobilize a morbidly obese patient. (Note again here the pattern of mast cell disease escalating its baseline misbehavior in the aftermath of a significant trauma.) She had to undergo cervical disc surgery a few months later. Then, in early '05 she suffered the first of what eventually became quite a string of mini-strokes, or transient ischemic accidents (TIAs), some of which involved hospitalizations. She mentioned that she was hospitalized altogether for 29 days in '05. She also developed quite the string of bilateral upper extremity clots ("thromboses") since that first TIA, usually in association with placement of a venous device of one sort or another. She also had some hematuria and a bout of renal colic a few months before her initial visit to me; one imaging study had found a 3 mm stone, but a subsequent study found nothing. She had been on a common oral anticoagulant, the vitamin K antagonist warfarin, for roughly 7-8 months (though her international normalized ratios, or INRs (a lab test regularly monitored in warfarin users to ensure they're not being anticoagulated too much or too little), always seemed to yield widely fluctuating results despite no changes in her warfarin dosing or her diet or any other drugs that could affect warfarin metabolism. (She was never tested for the CYP2C9 or VKORC1 mutations associated with this pattern.) She only once suffered a (minor) bleeding problem on warfarin, though her INR at the time was confoundingly low (ordinarily, a high INR correlates with bleeding propensity). When she suffered another TIA while on warfarin a month before first seeing me, she was then switched to a different type of anticoagulant, the low-molecular-weight heparin-type drug called enoxaparin, and had been on 100 mg of this drug (injected under the skin, or subcutaneously, once a day) ever since. She fortunately had seemed to recover completely, or almost so, from every one of her many TIAs. She was tolerating the enoxaparin OK except for the large bruise each injection typically caused. She had had no further clots since starting the enoxaparin.

I also noted at the time (remember, this was 2-1/2 years before I made my very first MCAS diagnosis) that "interestingly, she mentions that she has been having some epigastric abdominal discomfort, early satiety, and a 10 lb. weight loss (from 139 to 128) in the last couple of months; she underwent EGD while hospitalized for her last TIA, but there were no findings of note. She is mildly fatigued by all the health problems. She has had chronic headaches since the first TIA. She also has had chronic left thigh aching ever since the job injury in '02."

Her mother had hypertension and died of an MI. Her father has survived colon and kidney cancer. Her oldest sister has survived lymphoma. There was no family history of clotting (or bleeding) problems. She had never smoked and did not use alcohol or any illegal substances.

Ophelia's past medical history was also notable for a spontaneous abortion (i.e., a miscarriage), at 3 months, of her first pregnancy at age 16, but her next three pregnancies and deliveries were unremarkable (except for extended bedrest being required during one of them, for reasons she could not remember), and her children were healthy. A fifth pregnancy was delivered at eight months, but the baby was lost after 3 days due to pulmonary complications.

She was on no medications that might be complicit in her problems. Interestingly, when a blood pressure medication in the "ACE inhibitor" class was tried, she quickly developed one of the classic side effects of that class of medications, a cough, and it resolved when the medication was stopped.

Ophelia's physical examination was unremarkable except for mild tenderness on deep epigastric palpation (the upper central part of the abdomen, about where the stomach lies) as well as numerous, minimally tender, small enoxaparin-related bruises scattered about the abdominal wall.

I'll spare you the details of her work-up for a hypercoagulable disorder and simply tell you that I ran a *very* extensive evaluation looking for a specific cause of her excessive clotting (it bothered the heck out of me that such bad clotting could evade diagnosis), but the bottom line was that she did not have any known hypercoagulable disorder, inborn or acquired, or any other disease for which hypercoagulability is a known consequence. She continued to suffer fairly frequent episodes of clotting on once-daily enoxaparin. I increased her prescription for this to twice-daily injections, and this finally decreased her clotting to just occasional episodes. I then added the immunosuppressive drug azathioprine, and she finally stopped clotting – but she didn't feel one bit better.

And then I made my first diagnosis of MCAS in late '08 and saw how much that patient had improved, as of early '09, after just a month on imatinib. When Ophelia herself returned a few weeks later, she was complaining of waxing/waning vague abdominal discomfort and diarrhea. She was having episodic difficulty focusing her vision. She reported minimal tenderness in her right anterior neck. She also reported a new tingling in her left toes with left leg heaviness; there was tingling in the right toes, too, but that is old, she said. Plus, she described episodes, usually occurring at rest, of a sudden onset of dyspneic tightening in her chest (without wheezing), which would cause her to get up quickly, only to find "the room spinning," but the episodes typically resolved in less than 5 minutes. She had not noticed any flushing with these episodes.

I "put two and two together," as they say, and performed additional testing for mast cell disease at that and later encounters. I eventually found elevated urinary prostaglandin D_2, elevated plasma norepinephrine, and markedly elevated Factor VIII in her mediator testing, mild anemia and persistent "reactive lymphocytes" in her blood counts and differentials – and I also found increased (not aggregated, as required for mastocytosis, but nevertheless increased) mast cells in the marrow biopsy I did on her as I was doing on all my MCAS patients in the early days of my experience with this (before I learned good and well, after marrow-biopsying about 60 such patients, that tryptase is not elevated in a non-proliferative mast cell activation disorder and I decided it was pointless to do a marrow biopsy unless the tryptase level was persistently above the cut-off for mastocytosis). The flow cytometry on her marrow aspirate looking for the $CD117^+CD25^+$ or $CD117^+CD2^+$ "signature" of mast cell disease was negative, and her mast cells did not harbor the KIT-D816V mutation marking for mastocytosis.

I began trying mast-cell-targeted treatments in her, eventually learning that antihistamines and cromolyn helped some of her symptoms, and a whole lot of other drugs did little to nothing for her. She continues to be chronically significantly fatigued, among many other symptoms. She remains disabled, but at least she has had no further clots. To this day I have yet to find any drug which I would consider to be "highly effective" in her. My efforts to treat her have been hampered, as is the case in many MCAS patients, by obstructionist tactics from her insurer, but there remain at least several drugs left to be tried in her and I certainly haven't given up hope yet of being able to get her feeling substantially better.

So much for clotting. What about bleeding? Can MCAS cause bleeding? Absolutely.

When "Hester" first came to me in the summer of '08 because she was consolidating all of her care in our system and needed a new hematologist to follow her decade-long problem of hypereosinophilia (i.e., increased eosinophils in the white blood cell differential), this 76 year old diabetic hypertensive atherosclerotic long-retired physician's assistant – when I asked her to take me back to the beginnings of her illness – started by telling me that she had "always" – since a tonsillectomy at age 6 – been a "bleeder." Even though "all" of her coagulation studies (she knew none of the details) had always been within normal limits, she had bled heavily with every invasive procedure (hysterectomy in the '70s, right total knee replacement in the '90s, cataract surgery, a bladder surgery in the '70s and again in the '90s for incontinence) and every delivery she had ever had, plus a long history of menorrhagia as well as two episodes of a bleeding gastric ulcer. But she had never had spontaneous bleeding, all bleeding was during her procedures (not post-op), and investigations into what might be causing such bleeding were persistently negative.

After Hester's opening remarks about the bleeding, she went on to describe how about 15 years before coming to see me, she had developed a pruritic plaque-like rash scattered about her entire body (worst on her scalp and back). Evaluations by multiple physicians including multiple dermatologists led to multiple biopsies which yielded only a diagnosis of granuloma inguinale, and when chronic eosinophilia was also recognized after having the rash for about six years, she was referred to a hematologist who she says searched intensively for a malignancy to explain the eosinophilia, but extensive bloodwork, all manners of imaging, and a marrow biopsy could not find any cause of her eosinophil percentages which typically were in the 20-40% range (normal is 0-5%). He recommended an empiric trial of hydroxyurea, and when she began it, it almost immediately resolved her rash and eosinophilia. She says her WBCs and platelets were never elevated and often were low, requiring temporary reductions or cessations of hydroxyurea. She had suffered a heart attack about four years later; treatment included placement of a coronary artery stent. In the few months before coming to see me, her hemoglobin had been dropping for no reason that could be found, so she had stopped her hydroxyurea. Her anemia was not getting better, but her itching and rash had quickly returned. Her chief complaint is dyspnea on exertion. Since stopping the hydroxyurea, the rash had begun to return, and she had had another heart attack. She said she also knew she had had a chronic magnesium deficiency since her first heart attack and reliably got leg cramps if she didn't take supplemental magnesium. At the time (i.e., before I knew about MCAS), I noted "there's nothing in the history to suggest allergic or mast cell phenomena, no wheezing or diarrhea, nor any intestinal issues to suggest a parasitosis, nor any 'aches and pains' to suggest a rheumatologic issue."

Hester's family history was rife with coronary artery disease but totally negative for eosinophilia, other blood or cancer disorders of any sort, or rheumatologic phenomena. She had never used tobacco or illegal substances and has never abused alcohol.

Her physical exam was notable only for moderate systolic hypertension (nearly 190 in spite of alleged compliance with her multiple blood pressure medications) and a few small patches of her "granuloma inguinale" rash scattered about her right forearm and right abdominal wall.

We had one lab test on file in her old chart – a CBC from 11 years earlier that was normal except for increased eosinophils at 13%. Her updated CBC now showed 32% eosinophils – within the range she had long shown at her other hematologist's office – and when I looked at her blood smear under the microscope, the "dysplasia" (abnormal development) of her eosinophils was plainly evident. Interestingly, she also had a good number – 8% – of "reactive lymphocytes," too, in her differential.

I ran a large array of tests on Hester looking for everything I knew at that time that could cause hypereosinophilia, but every test was negative. (Similarly, I again extensively tested her for bleeding disorders, but she just did not have any known bleeding disorder.) This was a classic "idiopathic hypereosinophilic syndrome" and (related? unrelated? what would Occam say?) "idiopathic bleeding syndrome." The standard treatment for this diagnosis by that point was low-dose imatinib, but, interestingly, she immediately proved intolerant of the drug.

In early '09, of course, I began to wonder if MCAS might be her root issue. It also came out that she had had a long history of poor healing. Testing eventually showed elevations in plasma histamine and 24-hour urinary prostaglandin D_2 (and normal tryptase), and she was one of only about two patients, in those first 60 or so MCAS patients I diagnosed in whom I also did a marrow biopsy, in whom I was able to find evidence of mast cell disease, just not enough to satisfy the diagnostic criteria for mastocytosis. She had a "mild increase" in mast cells in her marrow that were proven to be mast cells by CD117 and toluidine blue staining, and there was a single aggregate of spindled cells also seen in the marrow biopsy, but no proof that the spindled cells were mast cells. However, the flow cytometry on her marrow aspirate found a tiny proportion of the marrow mast cells to be "triple-positive," expressing not only KIT (CD117) on their surfaces but also CD25 and CD2 (i.e., $CD117^+CD25^+CD2^+$, which are never seen on the surfaces of normal mast cells and are accepted as a sign of abnormal mast cells. The KIT-D816V mutation, though, was not present.

I set about trying to treat her MCAS and soon found that hydroxyurea and antihistamines were all she needed to provide nearly perfect control over her many symptoms.

So why, while Hester was menstruating, did she have persistent menorrhagia, and why did she bleed – but only at the surgical sites – with every surgery?

I suspect – but have no proof – that the principal cause was release of a flood of heparin into local tissues from dysfunctional mast cells present at the surgical site and activated by the trauma of the surgery. (Wouldn't it be interesting to run a study in patients with chronic idiopathic epistaxis (nose bleeding) comparing the plasma heparin levels in the blood coming from their noses vs. their bloodstreams? Remember, heparin, like most mast cell mediators, has a very short half-life and degrades very quickly on exposure to heat, plus we're talking about *local* release of heparin usually being the problem with mast-cell-related bleeding, so one would expect the level of heparin in the (fresh) blood at the site of bleeding to be significantly higher than the level of heparin that gets absorbed into, and circulates through, the bloodstream.) However, it has also been shown that mast cell disease induces a "fibrinolytic state" in which the coagulation system proteins that break down scabs are chronically excessively released by mast cells, so the increased difficulty that mast cell patients have in maintaining healthy scabs might have contributed to her bleeding (and to her poor healing), too.

I have since seen spontaneous mysterious bleeding in many other patients eventually found to have MCAS and no other apparent explanation for their bleeding. In my experience, menorrhagia is the most common such bleeding, but nosebleeds (epistaxis) are a close second. (Given that mast cells tend to site themselves at the environmental interfaces, it shouldn't be surprising that upper airway bleeding and genitourinary tract bleeding from mast cell disease is common.) I also have seen occasional other patients presenting with bleeding limited to surgical sites in which no other known bleeding disorder could be found but in whom MCAS then was eventually found.[2] MCAS-targeted therapy of one sort or another usually eliminates (or nearly so) these sorts of excessive bleeding. However, because MCAS induces a fibrinolytic state, a "go-to" class of drugs that make sense to try when there's MCAS-induced bleeding (and not

---

[2]Interestingly, in the nearly 30 years I've now been training and practicing in hematology, the *only* times I have ever seen hemorrhage from a bone marrow biopsy was in two patients (biopsied by colleagues with much experience in doing this procedure) who had no other detectable bleeding disorder and eventually were shown to have MCAS. Even severe reductions in the platelet count, such as in autoimmune thrombocytopenia (ITP) or acute leukemia, don't seem to cause bleeding from marrow biopsies, but I can now say I've seen MCAS do it.

enough time to find MCAS-targeted therapy that's effective for the individual patient) is anti-fibrinolytic therapy, namely, tranexamic acid or aminocaproic acid. These drugs have been lifesavers at times in bleeding MCAS patients, and I wouldn't be surprised if there were unrecognized MCAS in other patients in whom these drugs have been used to quell mysterious bleeding.

So if we have at least a couple of thoughts as to what predisposes MCAS patients to excessive bleeding, do we know what predisposes MCAS patients to clotting? Unfortunately, less is known on that topic. As already discussed, MCAS can result in a wide array of immune system aberrations including incorrect production by the immune system of "autoantibodies," i.e., antibodies directed against the body's own normal tissues instead of foreign materials such as bacteria. The sorts of antibodies that such "autoimmune phenomena" can produce include, in some patients, antibodies directed against one or more of the many aspects of the clotting system. I'm oversimplifying here, but suffice to say that we generally call the autoantibodies that lead to excessive bleeding "acquired inhibitors," and we generally call the autoantibodies that lead to excessive clotting "antiphospholipid antibodies." Although I haven't yet seen acquired inhibitors in MCAS patients (it's probably just a matter of time), I have seen antiphospholipid antibodies in several, and that might be one way by which MCAS causes excessive clotting. We also know that mast cells can produce at least one of the clotting system proteins that contributes to promoting clotting, Factor VIII, and I have found two- to four-fold elevations in Factor VIII in several MCAS patients who also had proved hypercoagulable with no other identifiable cause. It may be worth noting that in the last decade, elevated levels of Factor VIII have been found in many hypercoagulable patients with no other identifiable hypercoagulable disorder, and thus I have been wondering these last few years whether MCAS – whether acting through excessive release of Factor VIII or some other mediator(s) – might underlie the hypercoagulability seen in at least some portion of "Factor VIII overexpressers."

The clotting system is so complex that I wouldn't be surprised at all if there were many other routes by which dysfunctional mast cells might significantly tilt the coagulation system's seesaw (either toward the clotting end of the spectrum or the bleeding end of the spectrum), but at present what I've related above is about the extent of what we know in this area.

Chapter 22: Infections and Hypersensitivies and Autoimmunities and Cancers, Oh My! Immunologic Findings in MCAS

As the mast cell itself is part of the immune system, it almost goes without saying that if the mast cell goes awry, the immune system is going to go awry. The alterations of immunity in MCAS may lead to overt or covert effects, but I haven't seen many MCAS patients who haven't had any problems traceable back to dysfunction in parts of the immune system other than the mast cell. And I will readily concede at this point that it's certainly possible that there might be (some? many?) clinical variants of what we presently can best demonstrate to be MCAS that might in fact be due to primary aberrancies in other parts of the immune system that lead to (reactive) dysfunction of (otherwise normal) mast cells – a so-called "secondary" MCAS. Once again you can see why readily available/affordable whole genome sequencing will prove so helpful so quickly in sorting out (by finding disease-causing new mutations) the "true" diagnosis in patients with complex multisystem disorders, but at the moment, the diagnostic criteria proposed for MCAS are the best we have, so if the patient has (1) chronic and/or recurrent symptoms consistent with chronic and/or recurrent aberrant mast cell mediator release, (2) chronically and/or recurrently elevated levels of mast cell mediators, and (3) absence of any other known disease (including mastocytosis) that can better account for the full range and chronicity of the findings in the case, then "MCAS" is the best label – the most unifying, explanatory diagnosis – we can presently assign to such patients.

The human immune system has necessarily learned not only how to defend the body against assaults by an incomprehensible number of known threats but also how to manufacture new defenses on demand against formerly unknown threats. It's not a perfect system, and that's part of why we die, but given how hostile and toxic the world about us is, it's obviously a pretty good system that keeps fending off such assaults for the several decades the average human now lives. That success, though, implies that it's a very complex system, and thus it's not surprising that when immunity goes awry, there are a great many potential consequences including:

(1) Increased risk for infections (of common and uncommon types of organisms, at common and uncommon sites about the body),
(2) Increased difficulty healing (i.e., recovering from infections and healing from wounds; there actually is a type of rat that's been genetically engineered to have no mast cells, and it's been shown that such rats cannot heal when subjected to wounding),
(3) Hypersensitivity (i.e., abnormally vigorous reactions) to potentially anything in our environment, and
(4) Increased risk for malignancy (because there are so many DNA replication events in our body every day that accidental emergence of potentially lethal mutations are virtually guaranteed to be frequent, and it

is our (normal, properly functioning) immune system that (usually) finds the cells bearing these mutations and (usually) eliminates them before they have a chance to grow into (usually eventually fatal) cancers).

There are two major arms to the immune system: the cellular arm, which obviously consists of certain types of cells (such as neutrophils, lymphocytes, and, yes, mast cells, each with a vast but unique array of roles to play in asserting immunity), and the so-called humoral arm (no, it has nothing to do with being funny), which consists of specialized proteins called antibodies (which are made by other immune cells called plasma cells), each of which is specially formed to be able to "recognize" a specific threat and "call to arms" the assorted immune system cells needed to deal with that threat.

As such, one should expect that cellular immune defects and/or humoral immune defects can be seen in MCAS patients, and that indeed proves to be the case.

I'll give you (and me) a break in this chapter from reviewing yet another (typical) patient's complicated story, but suffice to say that I have seen deficiencies of almost every type, and to varying degrees, in both cellular and humoral immunity. As a result, infections are more frequent and more chronic, especially low-grade infections that just won't go away, and stay away, no matter how much topical or systemic antibiotic treatment is thrown at them (e.g., fungal skin infections in the groin or armpits or feet, and lichen planus or halitosis (bad breath) in the mouth). Cellular immune deficiencies seen in some MCAS patients include reductions in numbers of neutrophils or lymphocytes in general, or sometimes reductions in numbers of specific types of lymphocytes (such as the so-called "CD4-positive helper T lymphocytes" or the so-called "CD8-positive suppressor T lymphocytes"). Humoral immune deficiencies seen in some MCAS patients include reductions – or, a bit less commonly, excesses – in one general class ("isotype") of antibody ("immunoglobulin") or another. Thus, the MCAS patient might demonstrate reduced or increased levels of the commonly measured immunoglobulin G (IgG), IgM, or IgA antibodies as well as the less commonly measured IgE (and least commonly measured IgD) antibodies. Or there might be *increased* levels of one or more of these isotypes. We really don't have any good way at present to identify the consequences of these abnormalities except to say in general that when deficiencies of IgG, IgM, and/or IgA antibodies become really severe, the risk for infection – and the difficulty in resolving infection – really begins to rise.

Deficiencies of IgG, IgM, and IgA are often given a diagnostic label of "common variable immunodeficiency" (CVID), another $400 "grab-bag" or "wastebasket" medical term that basically says there's an IgG, IgM, or IgA deficiency and we don't know what to expect from it except, as I said, there's a higher risk for infection if the deficiency is severe. Levels of these antibodies typically don't get checked unless the patient has suffered repeated serious infections, and since the matter hasn't been formally studied yet, it's difficult to say with any accuracy what portion of MCAS patients have CVID, but I can also say that in many MCAS patients with histories of repeated serious infections, CVID often is one of the many items on the patient's long pre-existing problem list.

When the patient has a form of CVID in which there's a severe deficiency of IgG, a very expensive treatment called intravenous immune globulin (IVIG, made by filtering IgG out of the blood of thousands of blood donors and pooling it together and purifying it) can boost up IgG levels and diminish the risk of infection and help the patient recover from infection. Interestingly, the repertoire of mast cell surface receptors includes receptors for IgG, so although there's no question that supplemental IgG can help manage infection by providing the patient with IgG antibodies that he/she is no longer capable of making on his/her own, one also has to wonder whether IVIG is helping at least some CVID patients by engaging mast cell surface IgG receptors in ways that lead the cell to make other positive contributions to immunity. I have seen several CVID/MCAS patients now who very reliably get a few days of diminished MCAS-type symptoms following each IVIG infusion. It's an unsustainably expensive way to improve symptoms in some MCAS patients, to be sure, but it's an interesting observation nonetheless.

As noted above, when the immune system goes awry (and/or when there's a heightened state of inflammation in general), the risk increases for development of malignancy of potentially any tissue (but especially those tissues with greater rates of cellular reproduction and growth such as the marrow and the intestinal tract), and we see that same risk for malignancy with MCAS, which of course is a disease that usually causes the immune system to go awry and usually creates a chronic state of inflammation.

Often, the malignancy or inflammatory disease becomes grossly evident well before the MCAS becomes evident, and it becomes the focus of attention by the patient's doctors and is used by the doctors as the scapegoat not only for the symptoms that make sense to attribute to the malignancy or inflammatory disease but also a range of other symptoms that would make more sense to attribute to MCAS than the other, more grossly apparent disease. So it's easy to understand how a co-morbid (or even underlying?) MCAS could easily be "missed in the background," outshined by the drama of the malignancy or inflammatory disease. And yet all the parts of the body interact with one another, and if there's an MCAS present alongside the malignancy or inflammatory disease, it's often the case that simultaneous treatment of the MCAS along with treatment of the other disease leads to better outcomes for both diseases.

I mentioned a moment ago that marrow (i.e., hematologic) malignancies are some of the most common malignancies seen in MCAS patients, and each such malignancy can be *any* type of hematologic malignancy. The reason I bring this up is that there are a couple of types of "early" hematologic malignancies for which a cause has not yet been identified (actually, I could say that about virtually every malignancy) and which are particularly prevalent, and I have been increasingly wondering whether MCAS might be a significant contributor to those malignancies.

One of these is monoclonal gammopathy of undetermined significance (MGUS), the precursor to the hematologic malignancy called multiple myeloma (often just called myeloma), a terrible cancer whose dominant effect is to eat away at the bones. Death from myeloma usually ensues within a few to several years after diagnosis due to complications related to weakened bones or failure of normal blood cell production in the marrow. However, it can be many, many years between when MGUS is first found and when (if ever) it evolves into myeloma. One of the principal features of MGUS and myeloma is the emergence of a set of "clonal" plasma cells that make way too much of a given antibody. Ordinarily, the body's vast assortment of plasma cells makes a vast array of antibodies. Each plasma cell makes a unique antibody targeted at a specific threat. When that threat becomes real (e.g., when a specific type of bacteria invades the body), the immune system is able to rapidly make more plasma cells that make the unique antibody that specifically targets that threat, but excessive production of that antibody is then scaled back as the threat comes under control. In MGUS and myeloma, though, the immune system permits excess production of plasma cells that produce a specific antibody, and there's never any scale-down. The whole process just keeps getting scaled up more and more. It's a slow scale-up in most MGUS patients at first – only about 1% of all MGUS patients transform into myeloma patients in any given year – but it's an inevitable scale-up that only gets interrupted if the patient dies of something else first, a distinct possibility given that it can take many decades for a given MGUS to transform into myeloma.

The cause of MGUS is unknown, but given that MCAS leads to immune system dysfunction, and given that I've seen MGUS in many MCAS patients, I wonder whether MCAS underlies MGUS in some portion of the MGUS population.

The other prevalent "early" hematologic malignancy in which I wonder whether MCAS is playing a significant role is myelodysplastic syndrome (MDS, the precursor to acute leukemia), especially the most prevalent subtype of MDS in which no chromosomal abnormality can be found.

MDS is a disease in which blood cell development in the marrow goes awry in ways that typically lead to reductions in the production of healthy red blood cells, white blood cells, and/or platelets. In an effort to compensate, the marrow often "revs up" – or, at least, tries to rev up – blood cell production, and when you examine the bone marrow biopsy from an MDS patient through a microscope, you can see not only the general efforts at increased blood cell production but also the abnormal forms of the blood cells which are then dying (often before they even make their way out of the marrow into circulation) because they're not healthy.

It's long been thought that most cases of MDS are due to mutations in chromosomes and genes that control blood cell production, but the weird thing is, in about half of all cases of MDS we can't find such mutations, at least not with presently available testing. So there's obviously a disconnect between our thinking that MDS is usually due to mutations *vs.* our inability to find such mutations half the time.

Perhaps, then, there are many more cases of MDS that are *not* due to mutations in chromosomes and genes that control blood cell production than we previously thought.

Where this potentially ties into MCAS is that in the same fashion in which many mast cell mediators can influence, in one fashion or another, growth and development of other types of cells throughout the body, these mediators also can influence growth and development of blood cells.

Furthermore, I have observed that although marrow biopsies in MCAS patients most often appear normal, the most common abnormal appearance of the marrow in MCAS patients is what is reported by hematopathologists as a non-specific myelodysplastic/myeloproliferative appearance – a phrasing that often is interpreted by hematologists as evidence of MDS. What's more, many MCAS patients have mild to moderate reductions in circulating numbers of red blood cells, white blood cells, and/or platelets, and an increase in average red blood cell size (the so-called mean corpuscular volume (MCV)) – exactly the circulating hematologic abnormalities most commonly seen in MDS.

Therefore, hopefully you'll excuse me for wondering whether some portion of normal-karyotype MDS cases are actually just unrecognized MCAS.

In summary, MCAS can cause lots of immune system-related issues, but the potential issues are so many and diverse that it's not surprising that it's usually decades, if ever, before their presence, and significance, get recognized.

Chapter 23: Diagnosing MCAS, Or, When Being Told You're Sick Is A Good Thing

Until I started figuring out that MCAS was the principal issue with some of my chronically ill patients, never had I seen patients so happy to be told there's a real illness explaining their years or decades of suffering.

I guess it shouldn't be surprising that when you've been sick in a myriad of ways for a very long time, and you've seen countless doctors who've subjected you to countless tests and given you countless diagnoses (or just "psychosomatism") that don't well account for your full range of troubles, it's a relief to finally learn there really is a biological abnormality – a disease – that can account for most or all (Occam would say usually "all") of what's been going on in you.

I can imagine what must be running through the minds of long-undiagnosed MCAS patients who, thanks largely to the Internet, have ready access to virtually as much medical knowledge as do their doctors and finally come across information about mast cell disease describing what they've been suffering. And I can imagine the fervor this must incite in them for getting their doctors to pursue the diagnostic work-up for MCAS – and the frustration this must engender when their doctors scoff at the suggestion and decline to pursue testing or even referral. And thus it is no surprise that more than once I have had a patient – who sometimes has been told by other doctors, family, and "friends" that "it's all in your head" – burst forth with tears of relief when I tell them that their testing indeed is diagnostic of a disease that can account for most or all of the long-suffered symptoms.

It might be easier if the disease were simpler and its diagnostic evaluation simpler. But they're not. The biology of the mast cell virtually guarantees multisystem complexity and, at least for the time being, a complex evaluation process. That's just the nature of our human biology and we need to accept that.

What we don't need to accept, though, is that the disease is undiagnosable. As I described in Chapter 1 about my first patient (Shelly) in whom I diagnosed MCAS, I refused to believe she had a disease that couldn't be figured out. It's important enough that I'll say it again just as I said in Chapter 1: except for the very occasional truly new infectious disease, there are no "new" diseases. There are enough patients and physicians and medical journals in the world that every way the human body can go awry has been seen and reported in the medical literature. The cause of a described illness may not be understood, its prognosis may not be understood, and we may be decades or centuries away from being able to effectively treat it, but fundamentally all illnesses have been described, and our tasks in modern medicine include not only learning the true causes of (and treatments for) all of the described illnesses but also figuring out which of the illnesses described in the literature best matches any given patient's set of symptoms and findings. And it is far more likely – again, Occam's Razor at work – that a multitude of problems in a single individual is due to a single root cause.

Therefore, "diagnosing the undiagnosable" is "simply" a matter of gathering a sufficiently comprehensive set of historical and physical exam findings and comparing that set to those reported in the literature. There has to be a match. As the complexity of the case increases, the time needed to gather the findings and peruse the literature also increases, but it doesn't change the fact that, in the end, there has to be a match. (Note I say this process is "simple" with some playfulness, since I'll be the first to admit to it being anything but simple. Gathering a "sufficiently" comprehensive set of finding and "sufficiently" scouring the literature are enormously time-consuming activities and *thinking*-centered activities, and physicians worldwide rarely have such great amounts of time available, while physicians in the U.S. also labor under a health care financing system in which they are paid to see patients and to do procedures to patients but not to truly *think* much about their patients' mysteries.

So, let's take a look at how one presently should go about diagnosing MCAS – and then at the end of this chapter I'll opine briefly on how I think we *will* go about diagnosing MCAS in the hopefully-not-too-distant future.

As I finish writing this book, it's the end of 2015, and seeing as how it's been only about eight years since publication of the first case reports of MCAS, nobody should be surprised that there still is neither consensus on diagnostic criteria for MCAS nor consensus on what the diagnostic approach, or work-up, for MCAS should be. In this chapter I will try to describe the state of the art in these areas.

To anybody who follows the literature in this area, it's no secret that there presently are two schools of similar, but nevertheless distinctive, thought on diagnostic criteria for MCAS. In early 2012 a group of experts in mast cell disease from a number of European centers and a couple of U.S. centers published a self-styled "consensus" in the *International Archives of Allergy and Immunology* (*IAAI*) in which they proposed diagnostic criteria as follows:

1. Presence of certain specific chronic/recurrent symptoms (flushing, pruritus, urticaria, angioedema, nasal congestion or pruritus, wheezing, throat swelling, headache, hypotension, and/or diarrhea) consistent with aberrant mast cell mediator release

2. Absence of any other known disorder that can better account for these symptoms

3. Increase in serum total tryptase of 20% above baseline, plus 2 ng/ml, during or within 4 hours after a symptomatic period

4.   Response of symptoms to histamine H_1 and/or H_2 receptor antagonists or other "mast-cell-targeting" agents such as cromolyn.

And, in spring 2011, I was privileged to be able to contribute to a review of MCAS principally written by the University of Bonn mast cell disease research team led by Dr. Gerhard Molderings that was published in the *Journal of Hematology and Oncology* (*JHO*). This review proposed a somewhat different set of diagnostic criteria that was structured along the lines of the World Health Organization's (WHO's) diagnostic criteria for systemic mastocytosis (SM). In our review, we proposed this alternative set of diagnostic criteria for MCAS:

Major Criteria:

1.   Multifocal mast cell aggregates as per WHO major criterion for SM
2.   Clinical history consistent with chronic/recurrent aberrant MC mediator release (symptoms as per a long table included in this article)

Minor Criteria:

1.   Abnormal mast cell morphology as per WHO SM minor criterion #1
2.   CD2 and/or CD25 expression as per WHO SM minor criterion #2
3.   Detection of known constitutively activating mutations in mast cells in blood, marrow, or extracutaneous organs
4.   Elevation in serum tryptase or chromogranin A, plasma heparin or histamine, urinary N-methylhistamine, and/or other mast-cell-specific mediators such as (but not limited to) relevant leukotrienes (B4, C4, D4, E4) or PGD_2 or its metabolite 11-β-$PGF_{2\alpha}$.

Diagnosis of MCAS is then established by the presence of either (1) both major criteria, or (2) the second major criterion plus any one of the minor criteria, or (3) any three minor criteria.

That our *JHO* review immediately became (and has since remained) the most-downloaded paper in the history of that journal caught the eye of the editor at another journal in the field, and in the summer of 2013 Dr. Molderings and I were invited to write another review for that journal, the *World Journal of Hematology* (*WJH*). Given that the #1 question we had been consistently been asked by doctors and patients following publication of our *JHO* review was detailed instructions for pursuing the diagnostic work-up, we felt that that should be the focus of our new *WJH* review.

In this new review, we analyzed the above two sets of diagnostic criteria and opined that the criteria published in *IAAI*, consensus or not, seem problematic in several respects.

First, the criteria published in *IAAI* list far fewer symptoms consistent with aberrant mast cell mediator release than listed in the other set of diagnostic criteria. Thus, for example, patients whose aberrant mast cell activation causes substantial muscle/joint/bone aching, constipation and abdominal pain, paresthesias, adenitis, and cognitive dysfunction but not the symptoms listed in the *IAAI* article would not qualify for the diagnosis.

Second, a rise in tryptase (by "20% + 2") is the only laboratory criterion proposed for diagnosis in the *IAAI* article, yet there is no published validation that this tryptase increase reliably distinguishes ordinary (i.e., normal) baseline fluctuation of tryptase from fluctuation induced by aberrant mast cell activation.

Third, there often are significant practical difficulties in providing or otherwise obtaining a specimen for tryptase within 4 hours of onset of an exacerbation of symptoms. Patients often are sufficiently disabled during a flare of symptoms and cannot easily get to a medical center, and those who do travel to an urgent care facility or emergency department often encounter doctors resistant to pursuing tests not needed for immediate care of the presenting symptoms. Such resistance often persists even when the patient presents a prescription from a mast cell disease specialist specifically requesting mast cell mediator testing at times of such flares.

Fourth, the "20% + 2" formula means that for many MCAS patients, a tryptase in the normal range (for example, increased from baseline 2.0 to an acutely symptomatic 4.2 (but not 4.1)) would be acceptable for diagnosis, and yet I know of no other disease in which a lab result in the normal range is accepted as the sole laboratory criterion for diagnosis of that disease. (I know, I know: soon after this book is published, some smart person somewhere is going to school me on this, but all I can say now is what I know now.)

Finally, these criteria require treating the patient for the disease (before the disease has been diagnosed) and observing at least some improvement. Not only is this a "Catch-22" that's at odds with the general principle of diagnosing before treating, but it's also at odds with the observed marked heterogeneity of the clinical behavior of MCAS (which, as you know by now, I strongly suspect is due to underlying marked mutational heterogeneity), in which some patients benefit little from the first few or several MC-targeting therapies tried. It would seem that if the patient demonstrates clinical and laboratory evidence of mast cell activation and has no other identifiable illness that can better account for the full range of findings in the case, it would be premature to reject the diagnosis if the patient fails to respond to merely a few lines of therapy. (To be sure, as the patient fails to respond to each successive line of MCAS-directed therapy, it is

206

imperative that the doctor reconsider what other diagnostic possibilities might be appropriate in the patient, a process that may involve yet more hours of history-taking or literature-searching, but if the sum total of symptoms and findings continue to argue more strongly for mast cell disease than other disease, then additional trials of MCAS-directed therapy may well be warranted given the possibility that that patient might "simply" have a variant of MCAS that's resistant to the types of medications commonly tried early on in treating MCAS.)

In my opinion, the criteria published in *JHO* seem more accommodating of the clinical heterogeneity of MCAS, allowing a wider spectrum of symptoms and laboratory indications of mast cell activation without requiring demonstration of response to treatment and without needing to interpret mediator test results in their normal ranges as indicative of disease. However, the criteria published in *JHO* neglected to explicitly state that other diseases better accounting for the full range of findings in the patient needed to be excluded. One could say that such a criterion is implicit, but it would have been better to be explicit about it.

The *WJH* review discussed in detail the diagnostic approach to both systemic mastocytosis and MCAS.

Step 1 is simply to establish suspicion of the disease. Are there classic *signs* of mast cell activation (e.g., unprovoked flushing or anaphylaxis)? Are there *symptoms* of mast cell activation? (A long table of such was included in the review.) Are there more symptoms or signs than can be explained by the patient's existing, definitively established diagnoses? Are there "odd," "strange," "weird," "bizarre," "unusual," "mysterious" symptoms and findings? (Sometimes this is as relatively easy to find as simply reading the patient's records, as many patients with unrecognized MCAS have long had chart entries incorporating exactly these words.)

Step 2 is initial testing. If there are skin lesions suggestive of the cutaneous forms of mastocytosis, they should be biopsied to look for that disease. Also, the serum tryptase level remains a good "fork in the road." If it's persistently above the 20 ng/ml cut-off defined as one of the WHO criteria for systemic mastocytosis (SM), then further evaluation should be directed toward SM (principally, bone marrow examination including appropriate molecular testing). If not, then further evaluation should be directed toward…

…Step 3 in which additional mast cell mediator testing is performed.

The *WJH* review goes on to discuss the details and nuances of properly performing all of this testing, and it's freely publicly available at http://www.wjgnet.com/2218-6204/journal/v3/i1/index.htm. More recently, I've discussed some other aspects of mast cell mediator testing in an American

Society of Hematology 2015 abstract freely publicly available at http://www.bloodjournal.org/content/126/23/5174.

Two final notes to diagnostic testing in MCAS: (1) I want to emphasize the importance, as noted in the second diagnostic criterion in the *IAAI* article, of ruling out potential alternative diagnoses (which for patients suspected of having MCAS often include other uncommon and rare disorders that manifest unusual symptoms and behaviors, e.g., inborn autoinflammatory syndromes, porphyrias, amyloidosis, etc. etc. etc.). Such "rule-outs" of course require fairly good awareness of the pantheon of disease, which is why self-diagnosis by those without formal medical training is often risky. There's no sense going to effort and expense to rule out diseases which don't behave as the patient's illness has behaved, but one wouldn't want to risk failing to assess for a diagnosis other than MCAS that does behave as the patient's illness has behaved. (2) Although it's beginning to appear that most MCAS patients bear mutations in key regulatory elements in their mast cells, there is the additional possibility (which is not mutually exclusive with the mutational hypothesis) that, at least in some MCAS patients, autoantibodies directed against various elements at the surface of the mast cell might trigger activation. Although some of these diseases might manifest as the so-called autoimmune urticarias, it might well be possible for such autoimmune disorders to manifest other, non-urticarial forms of mast cell activation, too. There aren't many such mast-cell-activating autoantibodies for which testing is presently clinically available, but particularly in patients with remarkably severe or persistent mast cell activation, checking for antibodies against immunoglobulin E (a.k.a. "anti-IgE IgG") and antibodies against the IgE receptor (both now available at some clinical reference laboratories) might be worthwhile because if such autoantibodies are present in a given patient, there would be more justification for considering trials in that patient of the kinds of immunosuppressive therapies typically used to treat autoimmune diseases.

So that's how MCAS is diagnosed presently. But what does the future hold?

It really all rides (see Chapter 27, Research Needs in MCAS) on whether we are able to confirm the preliminary findings reported twice now by Dr. Molderings' group that mutations are commonly present in the mast cell regulatory elements of MCAS patients and that such mutations are the principal drivers of the aberrant mast cell activation in such patients. (Note these observations are very similar to observations subsequently by multiple other groups that almost every mastocytosis patient bears multiple mutations in multiple mast cell regulatory elements.) If such a model of mutational heterogeneity can be proven (by independent confirmation of the results from Dr. Molderings' group) as the operative model for most MCAS patients, then it is my hope that within the next 10-20 years, it will become economically sensible, upon coming to suspect MCAS in a patient, to basically do routinely in the clinical laboratory what Dr. Molderings' team has now repeatedly done in their research laboratory: extract mast cells from the patient's blood, determine the entire DNA sequence in these cells, and identify whether there are mutations present which are known to drive aberrant activation of the mast cell. If such mutations are found, *voilà*, diagnosis made, without any need to go hunting for ephemerally elevated levels of assorted mast cell mediators with ridiculously short half-lives and chilling requirements.

Time will tell. For what it's worth, in July 2015 I launched a study attempting to confirm the key findings of Dr. Molderings' group – again, that mast cell KIT is significantly mutated in a wide variety of ways across most subjects in an MCAS patient population (and, importantly, not significantly mutated in healthy control subjects). My study will be looking in the study subjects' blood samples for mutations in a wide array of other mast cell regulatory genes, too. Results hopefully will be published by late 2016.

Chapter 24: What We Know About the Genetics of Mast Cell Disease (Short Answer: Not Much – Yet)

We've been hearing for several years now that the era of genomically personalized medicine is almost upon us, a time when at a cost of perhaps a few hundred dollars we will be able to determine anybody's complete genetic code which – and here's where we wave our hands in a magic gesture – will tell us all that's wrong with us now and all that's likely to go wrong with us.

Yeah, right.

If only.

I don't have a problem with the first part of that supposition. There's really no question at all that "any time now" we will be able to determine anybody's complete genetic code for a few hundred dollars, or less. That's the pace at which the technology is advancing. After all, it cost a few billion dollars to determine the first complete human genetic code (finished in 2003), and today the cost for doing the same is already down to a few thousand dollars, so it's inconceivable that it won't "soon" (a few years? a few months?) be down to a few hundred dollars – and once it gets down to a hundred bucks or less, I wouldn't be surprised if complete genomic determinations start getting bundled in as a standard maternity service. Leave the hospital with not only your newborn but also the genetic map that will determine some portion of your newborn's health for the next several decades.

No, I don't have any problem with the notion of how soon complete genome sequencing will be here at so cheap a price that it would be silly not to integrate it into "routine testing" for a zillion different conditions.

Rather, the problem I have is the notion as to how soon we'll know the *patient* any better just by knowing his or her *genome*.

Here's an analogy for you: the *data* as to the macrostructure of that part of our universe that's visible to our naked eye – the ground under our feet, the lights in the night sky that are the planets and stars, and that foggy band across the night sky that is our Milky Way galaxy – have always been all about us, before our eyes night and day, for the duration of our species' existence, but only in the last few hundred years have we been able to *make sense* of these data, these observations, to understand their true significance. We used to think the various constellations were gods; it was the most sensible interpretation of those lights in the sky that we could conjure at the time. Our modern interpretations, of course, are substantially different.

Shortly now, patients and doctors will be inundated with genomic data. We're just now seeing the leading edge of this, in services that for a hundred bucks or so analyze a dollop of your saliva and determine a million or so excerpts from your genome that may ("may," not "will"!) be significant for identifying present disease or risk for future disease. You pay your hundred bucks, send off your saliva to one of these service providers, and 2-4 weeks later you get an e-mail containing a link to your personalized web page at the service provider's website. You logon, and voilà, pages and pages and pages and pages reporting all the analyses that have been done. You have Mutation Code A, which puts your risk for Disease B at Level C. You have Mutation Code D, which puts your risk for Disease E at Level F. And so on. And it's so much data that it's mind-numbingly overwhelming at best – "I don't know what *any* of this means!" – and downright scary at worst: "Aaaauuuggggghhhhh!! I've got a 25% chance of developing prostate cancer by the time I'm 60? I'm 58 right now! Maybe I've already got it!"

And so you forward the link to your page to your doctor with an e-mail subject line of "HELP!" to which your doctor responds by saying, "This is way too complicated to discuss in e-mail, so come on in the office." And you print your whole report, maybe circle the worst parts of it (as best as you can tell, anyway), and dutifully march in to your doctor's office (maybe forking over another co-pay and certainly incurring another cost burden for your insurer, who will see a diminishing profit margin the current year and start thinking about the need to raise premiums for next year), at which point the doctor spends maybe 10-30 seconds glancing through the thick sheaf of paper before handing it back to you (or, if he feels a need to pretend that he takes any of this seriously, he hands it to an assistant to have it added to your chart), and he says, "Well, there's a lot of stuff here, and the truth is, we really don't yet know what 99.99% of this stuff truly means, and there's really nothing to be done about it at this point."

And he's exactly right.

And this situation is only going to get a lot worse before it gets better, because right now these services are providing analyses of only a million or so *excerpts* of your genetic code (with different services looking at different excerpts, yielding wildly varying estimates of risk for a given disease), while in the near future such services will upgrade to reporting your *entire* genetic code. Diseases are complex systems, each with many, many interlocking/interacting phenomena, and to think one can understand the entire system by knowing merely a few tiny parts of it is the height of naïveté. If we already don't understand how to accurately interpret the million or so excerpts currently being examined by these services, what are the odds that we will understand – anytime soon – how to interpret the full code that's roughly a hundred times larger?

Even if one assumes that your genetic code that's being delivered to you or your doctor is accurate – and in a "game" where a single incorrect code letter at just the right place can have *huge* implications for current and future health, accuracy is *crucial* – we simply won't know what most of the code *means*, let alone what the implications might be of aberrations in the code.

The reason I've taken a couple of pages or so for the above diatribe is to preclude any (grossly incorrect) presumptions that even if we don't presently know most of the genetic issues in mast cell disease, we'll likely have most of it figured out soon.

Wrong. Completely wrong.

That said, let's now move on to what we do know – and suspect, but don't in truth yet know – about the genetic issues in mast cell disease.

We know that many mutations have been found in the genes and proteins that regulate mast cell behavior across various patients with mast cell diseases of various types. And we know that many of these mutations result in mast cell misbehavior in one fashion or another. Sometimes this misbehavior is a reduction in a specific process, but it more commonly seems to be the case – at least with the mast cell mutations studied thus far – that the mutationally driven misbehaviors result in increases in specific processes, particularly processes that lead to production and release of mediators.

Thus, most of the mast cell mutations found thus far result in the cell – which ordinarily is supposed to be quiet unless something happens in the environment that requires the cell to react – *always* acting as if it's reacting. (It's this "always on" state that we technically refer to as "constitutive activation.") It's clear, too, that in some patients with mast cell disease, their dysfunctional mast cells also react to many environmental provocations not in normal fashions but actually in hyperactive fashions.

The mast cell gene (and corresponding protein) that's been studied the most to date is called "KIT." To the best of our knowledge, KIT is the most important controller (certainly not the only controller, but indeed the most important controller) of the mast cell's activities. Among other functions, KIT regulates the mast cell's ability to survive, move, grow – and activate.

KIT is not a gene that's unique to mast cells. Actually, there are no genes that are unique to mast cells – or any other cells, for that matter. All the genes found in any one cell in the body are also found in all the other cells in the body, but any given gene functions at different degrees (sometimes even not at all) in different cells. The KIT gene, in fact, is an important gene in many blood cells and other types of cells because of what its corresponding protein does. The KIT protein is in a class of proteins called tyrosine kinases that regulate, among other processes, growth and differentiation of cells. (Differentiation is the process by which a stem cell can mature into many different types of cells depending on various influences.) KIT is a "transmembrane" tyrosine kinase, meaning it's a protein that's anchored in the cell membrane, with part of the protein waving around up above the cell surface and part of it waving around down below the cell surface (i.e., inside the cell). The extracellular portion of KIT (the part waving around outside the cell) is a receptor, sort of like a lock, and when the matching key – in this case another protein called stem cell factor (SCF) – floats by the mast cell and inserts properly into KIT's extracellular "lock" and thereby "activates" KIT, the interaction between key and lock causes the intracellular portion of KIT to instantly change shape, which might seem a modest consequence, but it turns out that this one little change in shape in one little protein molecule is like the lead domino whose toppling results in the triggering of many other domino falls which proceed, in parallel, in rapid chain reactions throughout the cell.

And that's what happens *normally*, once KIT is activated by the "binding" of the SCF "key," or "ligand," to the extracellular, "receptor" portion of KIT. Many of the mutations in KIT discovered thus far, though, result in (permanent) shape changes in KIT. Some of these shape changes diminish KIT's activity, but many of these shape changes result in KIT being in a permanently activated shape even when SCF is not around. Again, we call this constitutive activation of KIT. It's abnormal activation because it doesn't require SCF, but it's also abnormal because the KIT proteins the cell makes based on the mutated KIT gene are not normally shaped, and thus the domino reactions that result are not normal reactions.

The KIT mutation that's been studied the most is the one that's found most commonly in mastocytosis. It's called the D816V mutation – you'll find it written in the scientific literature as either KIT-D816V or KIT^{D816V} – and it's what happens when a one-letter mutation in the KIT gene causes the cell's protein-making machinery to make KIT proteins in which the 816th amino acid in the unique chain of amino acids that makes up the KIT protein is erroneously switched from the normal "aspartic acid" amino acid (amino acid code "D") to an incorrect "valine" amino acid (amino acid code "V").

The KIT-D816V mutation is found in the mast cells in about 90% of patients with mastocytosis. We know KIT-D816V can't cause mastocytosis by itself – it's even found in some people who, as best as we can tell, are completely healthy – but given that it's the most common mutation we've found yet in mastocytosis, it's almost certain that the KIT-D816V mutation works together with other mutations (whose identities we are just beginning to discover) to cause the mast cell misbehavior that we clinically recognize as mastocytosis. Among other consequences, the KIT-D816V mutation in mastocytosis has been associated with the mast cell's overproduction of tryptase, a change in the mast cell's shape to an abnormal "spindled" appearance, and appearance on the mast cell surface of the CD25 protein which is never seen on the surface of the normal mast cell.

In the same way in which we now know that patients with mastocytosis have mast cells that have gone awry as a consequence of a bunch of mutations, we also are beginning to learn that the mast cells in many MCAS patients have (usually multiple) mutations, too. Interestingly, the KIT-D816V mutation that's so common in mastocytosis seems to be quite rare in MCAS.

Now, some mast cell disease experts think that MCAS is rare and that it's almost always a phenomenon in which the mast cells are normal but are reacting to provocations that haven't been identified yet. I respectfully disagree – I think that from what we've learned to date about mast cell biology, myeloproliferative neoplasms, and the genetics of mastocytosis, it makes a whole lot more sense that MCAS is mutationally rooted in most cases – but I acknowledge we haven't yet acquired much scientifically rigorous evidence to support either position.

Of course, if most cases of MCAS are secondary/reactive, the big question is, what are they reacting to? And if most cases of MCAS are primary/mutational, the big question is, how and why are such mutations developing?

I'll take authorial license and not dwell on the question of what mysterious provocation(s) might be present in secondary MCAS, since I think that theory is wrong, but I'll touch a little bit on the questions surrounding mutation development since I suspect that theory is right.

The fundamental conundrum of the scenario of mutationally rooted MCAS is not how MCAS can clinically present in so many different fashions. That's easy. Different sets of mutations lead the cell to misbehave in different ways, producing different aberrant patterns of mediator production and release, and each mediator has such diverse functions that it's easy to see how different aberrant patterns of mediator production and release could easily lead to very different patterns of clinical presentation. Rather, the mystery is how so many different sets of mutations could develop, as the studies of Dr. Molderings and his team at the University of Bonn have repeatedly suggested is the reality of MCAS. And we also have to account for how the risk of MCAS in the relatives of an MCAS patient is roughly triple the risk in the general population, and yet when you look at the mast cell mutations in related patients, you find completely different sets of mutations from one relative to the next. So on the one hand, it would seem that "something" must be getting inherited, while on the other hand it would seem that nothing is getting inherited. How can these diametrically opposed scenarios be reconciled with one another? Furthermore, even within the individual patient, there clearly is the curious behavior of MCAS that the disease often "steps up" its baseline level of misbehavior soon after the patient is exposed to a stressor of one sort or another – almost as if at least some of the patient's dysfunctional mast cells are acquiring, as a result of a stressor, yet another mutation (or two or three…) that then causes even more aberrancy in the cell's pattern of inappropriate mediator production and release, inescapably leading to new symptoms.

The (hypothetical! – nothing proven yet) scenario that would seem to best explain all of these intrapatient and interpatient observations would be the presence of one or more inheritable "genetic fragility factors" which interact with different stressors (e.g., different infections, different traumas, etc.) to cause *additional* (non-inheritable) mutations, either different specific mutations depending on the particular stressor and the particular genetic fragility factor(s)) in the individual patient, or perhaps – even more confounding – mutations virtually at random. Perhaps some – heck, perhaps even most – such mutations result in non-viable cells, but you know the old saying: "that which doesn't kill us, makes us stronger." Thus, mutations that don't result in non-viable cells will either have no effect on the cells (i.e., silent mutations) or result in cellular misbehavior which then results in clinical misbehavior. (I guess it's possible, too, for mutations to develop that cause *beneficial* misbehavior. After all, that's how evolution works – but it seems much more likely that a mutation would have no effect or ill effect.)

What might such a genetic fragility factor be like? Might it be a mutated gene itself, leading to cellular production of a dysfunctional regulatory protein? Might it be a mutated epigene? Epigenes are patterns of addition of methyl groups to the DNA strands comprising genes. An epigene controls aspects of how functional a gene is within a cell. The same gene may function in very different ways (e.g., different transcription rates, different splicing patterns, etc.) in different cells as a result of bearing different methylation patterns, or epigenes, in the different cells. Epigenetic mutations, then, might also conceivably predispose a given gene, or set of genes, to becoming mutated themselves, with such mutations perhaps being more likely in provocative circumstances such as exposure to stressors of one sort or another.

And there might well be other forms the hypothetical genetic fragility factor could take, forms such as silent genes, microRNAs, hidden viruses, and so on and so forth.

It's all just hypothesis for now that there *is* such a thing as a genetic fragility factor underlying the personal and familial development of MCAS, let alone the hypotheses as to what form(s) such factor(s) might take – but at the moment, variable interactions of inheritable genetic fragility factors with variable stressors leading to variable mutations provides the best accounting for what's been observed clinically.

I can only conclude this chapter as I concluded the last one: time (and a whole lot of research) will tell, eh?

Chapter 25: No, It's Not Just "Take Two Aspirin…": Treatment of MCAS (Warning: Long Chapter)

I'm hesitant to write too much in this chapter because I suspect there's more "information" in this chapter that will soon be obsolesced, or proven flatly wrong, than in any other chapter in this book.

At the same time, though, I don't want to skimp on this chapter because I'm well aware that both doctors and patients want as many treatment ideas as possible, and doctors in particular feel uncomfortable about treating mast cell disease because just about the only thing they're taught to do for mast cell disease (no matter the form) during their decade or so of training is to give antihistamines. Allergists (I'm guessing) are taught to use antihistamines and other allergy medications. Oncologists (I know) are taught that chemotherapy doesn't help much, interferon maybe helps some (but often is a tough drug to tolerate), and there are too few cases of stem cell transplantation (which theoretically is the only therapy with curative potential) for mastocytosis to really know the true potential of that therapy, though most of the mastocytosis/transplant cases published to date have been anything but cures.

I should probably focus first on some general principles of treating MCAS rather than specific treatments.

Principle #1: Based on what I've seen these last seven years in more than 1,000 MCAS patients, the odds of getting better are good, by which I mean most patients are eventually able to identify some regimen that helps them feel significantly better than their pre-treatment baseline the majority of the time. This is the "therapeutic goal" that I explain to my patients. Importantly (i.e., so that the patient doesn't have unreasonable expectations), that doesn't mean feeling perfect, and it doesn't mean feeling significantly better *all* the time. It means what it says, and, I'm sorry to say, the average MCAS patient should not expect to ever again feel "perfect" or, once improved, to never again deteriorate. (That's of course not even normal for life in general.) Furthermore, given the complexity of the disease, the degree of improvement varies significantly amongst patients, but the basic principle remains as I've stated. It is easy to become frustrated/disappointed/sad/depressed/despondent when intervention after intervention fails to help, but that doesn't change the principle, and thus by definition the MCAS patient who achieves the therapeutic goal must find some way internally to get past the disappointments of treatment failures. The key difference in the newly diagnosed MCAS patient's future life vs. past life is that the patient now has a diagnosis, which can rationally guide therapeutic decision-making. I have had plenty of patients who have finally found "the right drug" on their 5th or 10th or 15th medication trial. There are *lots* of medications that have been found helpful in various patients with mast cell disease (bespeaking the enormous assortment of mutations I suspect underlies the disease), and the biggest frustration at this point is not being able to predict which of these medications is most likely to be helpful in the individual patient. But not knowing ahead of time which drug is most likely to be helpful is a whole lot less frustrating than not even knowing what's wrong to begin with (i.e., not having a diagnosis). The doctor's job is to know which medications are reasonable to try for any given diagnosis in his field and to provide guidance as to how to dose them and how to sequence the medication trials. The patient's job is to follow the doctor's instructions and "hang in there" (see principle #2 below). Most newly diagnosed MCAS patients have been ill from the disease for *decades*. It hasn't killed them yet, and it's not likely to kill them anytime soon. If they had the patience and wherewithal to survive a few decades with it, they can survive the next few weeks, months, or even years that it might take to identify an effective regimen. It should be kept in mind, too, that as the general medical community and the pharmaceutical industry become more aware of how prevalent MCAS is (i.e., how much of the mysterious chronic multisystem polymorbidity of a generally inflammatory theme that's out there is actually MCAS), there will be increasing attention toward developing new therapies. As just one example, there's a new class of medications – the "JAK inhibitors" – just now emerging for various hard-to-treat inflammatory diseases as well as a previously very-difficult-to-treat, rare hematologic malignancy called myelofibrosis, and there are excellent reasons why the drugs in this new class might be very helpful in treating MCAS. (In fact, a few pharmaceutical companies have begun patenting their medications for MCAS even though they haven't yet begun testing them in MCAS.) All that has to be done is to convince the makers of these new drugs that MCAS is a significant enough problem that it's worth testing them against MCAS, which might constitute a vastly larger market for them than the diseases they're currently studying. (Believe me, I've been trying to convince them, but they're as handcuffed by the traditional understanding (i.e., the alleged rarity) of mast cell disease as most physicians are, so I haven't been successful yet, but I'm a long way from giving up on this quest.)

Principle #2: Identification of the optimal regimen for the individual MCAS patient requires patience and persistence (on the part of the patient, the patient's support system, and the patient's health care providers, most especially the one who is primarily coordinating the treatment trials) and a methodical approach.

Persistence and patience, of course, go hand-in-hand. I guess it's possible to persist at something without being patient about it, but impatience in this endeavor will not get you to the end result one bit sooner and it likely will make you appear to be the dreaded "difficult" patient that no doctor wants to work with. And if you don't have a doctor to work with on this, it likely will take you an awful lot longer to get to the end result, whatever that may be, good or not. So, please, try to be patient. Yes, you don't feel well, it's been going on a long time, and it's *really* dragging on you. You know all this, your family and acquaintances know all this, and your doctor, too, knows all of this. But the fact of everybody knowing the depth and duration of your suffering is still not going to get you to the end result one bit sooner. So, be (politely and reasonably) patient…

…but *persist*. The person whose actions – actions! – are most likely to get you a successful result is you. When it seems to you that you might have MCAS but your present doctor doesn't "believe" it, you need to *act* and take up the matter with another doctor. And, if necessary, another, and another – at least until your doctor has either given you a satisfactory explanation why it's highly unlikely for you to have MCAS or until you have had it ruled out by proper testing (which, as you've learned by now, involves a good bit more than just having a tryptase level checked). And when it comes to therapy, don't give up in the hunt for effective therapy until your doctor has told you there's nothing left to be tried – and even then you should persist in the hunt by getting at least one second opinion, preferably from a mast cell disease expert.

I didn't say it was going to be easy. Your parents, too, never promised you a rose garden when they conceived you. Your life to this point, good or bad, is what it's been and can't be changed, but that certainly doesn't mean your future can't be better than your past. Maybe your future won't be better than your past, but the only way to make *sure* your future won't be better than your past is to not try to make it better. You must *persist* – but, please, remember to be polite and patient about it. Somebody with as complex a disease as MCAS needs more friends a whole lot more than he or she needs more enemies.

And let's not forget the criticality of a methodical approach. As I've said before, someday we'll get to the point where dealing with this disease will be as straightforward as sending off a blood sample for mast cell genome sequencing in the patient suspected of having the disease, identifying the mutations present in the mast cells (and thus establishing the diagnosis), and, finally, consulting a "library" of MCAS treatment studies to tell us that the mast cell misbehavior that stems from such-and-such a combination of mutations is best controlled by such-and-such a combination of therapies.

But until we get to that far more efficient future method, we'll still be better off for dealing with this via some *method* rather than just random therapeutic efforts. And what method should that be? I have a few suggestions, espoused in Principles 3 through 5 below.

Principle #3: Whenever possible, try to change only one thing in the MCAS patient's regimen at a time. Maybe that's trying a new medication, or trying a new dose, schedule or formulation of an old medication. Maybe it's trying a new food or soap or detergent. Maybe it's trying new clothes (which may be pretreated with some modern miracle textile chemical which might provoke a mast cell reaction). Sure, it's often difficult or impossible to limit changes to just one at a time – when you visit a new place, for example, it almost goes

218

without saying that you'll be exposing yourself in one fell swoop to multiple new foods and chemicals – but, *whenever possible*, try to limit changes in the MCAS patient's regimen to just one at a time – and allow suitable time to judge the impact of the change. At the time the change is made, set a date on which to judge the impact of the change (consulting with your doctor regarding the pharmacologic behavior of the drug being added, increased, decreased or stopped can help guide your decision how long to wait to judge the impact of the change), and then try to stick to that appointment (with yourself or with your doctor) for reassessment so that a definitive decision can be made and you can move on to the next change to be tried.

Any change in an MCAS patient's exposures has the potential to yield positive and/or negative effects. If you make more than one change around the same time and you get either better or worse, you'll have no idea which change led to the observed result and it becomes somewhat messier to try to sort it out. You want to reverse and avoid changes that have resulted in negative effects, but even when the effects of multiple changes are positive, you won't know whether the positive effects might be attributable to just one of the changes, and surely you don't want to be persisting with a useless change. For example, who in his right mind would want to keep taking a medication that wasn't bringing about some benefit?

Principle #4: Since at present we do not have readily, economically available testing (full sequencing of the genes for the mast cell regulatory proteins) or knowledge (which mutations cause elevations of which mediators causing which symptoms) to predict which medications are most likely to help which MCAS patients, the most sensible approach, in my opinion, is to start with the cheapest medications and escalate in expense only as necessary.

At least with regard to MCAS, it is a mistake to assume that the likelihood of a therapy helping is proportional to the cost of the therapy. I have seen plenty of patients get substantially better just with antihistamines and aspirin, costing merely a few bucks per year, and I have seen plenty of patients not get substantially better until they wound up trying $100,000-per-year tyrosine kinase inhibitors such as imatinib. (Caveat: imatinib is already much cheaper (as low as $300 per year!) in many other parts of the world, and its patent in the United States is presently expected to expire in February 2016, meaning that much cheaper generic formulations of the drug are likely to become available soon in the U.S., too. This change, of course, may have implications for how early this drug will be tried in some MCAS patients, and may even have implications for the drug's availability in different excipient packages and its availability for compounding. As always, time will tell. Meanwhile, it will be at least several more years yet before other tyrosine kinase inhibitors lose their patent protection in the U.S. and become more affordable.) I understand there is a *natural* human expectation that more expensive therapies are more likely to be helpful, but I am telling you that, at least with regard to MCAS, it is an *irrational* expectation.

You would serve yourself (and your bank account) well to fight this expectation and instead persist through therapeutic trials in order of cost until we have better scientific tools to better biologically characterize the individual patient's disease and thereby rationally identify the therapies which – irrespective of cost – are most likely to control the patient's misbehaving mast cells.

Principle #5: Whenever a stabilized MCAS patient destabilizes, the first thing to do – and the second, third, fourth, and fifth things to do – is *carefully* review the events of the few days to few weeks prior to the destabilization to try to identify *what changed*. It has been my experience in these last seven years of learning about this disease that it is virtually always the case that when a previously stabilized MCAS patient acutely or subacutely destabilizes, there has been a change of some sort which can be identified with a sufficiently careful review of the history. (For example, sometimes it's as simple as a medication refill in which the pharmacist, as directed by the insurer, substituted a less expensive little round white pill for a more expensive little round white pill containing the same active ingredient but very different binders. Sometimes a change in medication formulation is obvious from a change in pill shape, size, color, taste, or smell, but sometimes you have to call the pharmacist to figure out that there was a substitution in medication formulation.) Careful review of the history is very important, as some changes (e.g., new medications, new environmental exposures) can be reversed, and even if an offending change can't be reversed, at least it can be identified as a trigger so that steps perhaps can be taken to avoid similar changes in the future. There will be more about this principle later on.

Principle #6: *No* medication consists solely of the active ingredient, and although any active ingredient might be a trigger in some MCAS patients, it's also the case that *any* allegedly inactive ingredient (e.g., a "filler," "binder," or dye in an oral medication, an adhesive in a patch medication, a carrier fluid in an intravenous medications, etc.) has potential for triggering a flare of mast cell activation in some MCAS patients.

Principle #7: "The simpler the better." Many MCAS patients wind up on zillions of prescription medications, over-the-counter medications, and "supplements." The reasons their regimens become so complex are obvious. They visit a zillion doctors for their zillion symptoms and acquire a zillion diagnoses to explain those zillion symptoms, and each doctor prescribes one or more therapies and interventions (medications, environmental adjustments, exercises, and even surgeries) to address those symptoms. And with most such interventions, specific goals – at least with respect to reversible, non-surgical therapies – are rarely laid out in advance. Rarely does the doctor say to the patient, or the patient say to herself, "If this treatment doesn't reduce my Symptom X by Y% in Z weeks, then it's not worth it and I'll drop it." So because MCAS patients often have felt so awful in so many different ways for such a long time, *any* improvement (even when minimal) from a new

220

intervention is seen as justification for continuing it regardless of what its long-term financial cost might be or what its potential for causing other harmful effects might be.

Each and every intervention has potential to cause trouble. (Even a "simple" multivitamin or multi-supplement can cause trouble. Yes, some MCAS patients have significant dietary intolerances, and some have nutrient absorption problems, but most MCAS patients don't have these problems, and most MCAS patients who eat a relatively normal diet do not need *any* nutritional supplements.) Troubles from assorted interventions might be due to allegedly inactive ingredients (see Principle #6), might be due to *drug-drug interaction* effects (potential for which multiplies as more therapies are added to the regimen), might be due to poor tolerance of environmental or activity adjustments, might be due to poor healing from surgery, etc.).

To limit potential for medical troubles and unnecessary financial expenditures, MCAS patients should eliminate from their regimens all interventions that have not *clearly* resulted in *significant, sustained* improvements. Furthermore, when a new intervention is tried which yields major benefits, the possibility should be considered that other interventions that have long been part of the patient's regimen might no longer be necessary. But, if you are going to try to stop old treatments that used to provide significant benefit, beware Principle #3 and try to make just one change at a time.

Principle #8: Just because you failed to improve upon trying one drug of a given class does not necessarily mean you will fail to improve with all drugs of that class.

First of all, when a given drug that's expected to yield improvement or, at worst, no change at all, actually winds up causing trouble, the question of toxic fillers/binders/dyes has to be raised, and it may well be worth trying the same active ingredient again, though in a different formulation with different fillers and dyes, or perhaps even in a simpler formulation that can be custom-prepared by a compounding pharmacist. Some of my patients have even found that both commercial and custom-compounded formulations of a given medication are intolerable – but that it sometimes (with some patients and some medications) is the case that when the custom-compounded capsule is opened and the active ingredient therein is taken all by itself, it works well.

Secondly, even though there may be molecular features of different medications which lead to them having similar properties in "normal" patients, each different medication is fundamentally a different molecule that has the potential to interact with mast cells differently. For example, I have seen patients who reacted adversely to lorazepam but then benefited greatly from lorazepam's sister drug clonazepam. And vice versa!

221

So if a given medication is tried from a class the patient hasn't tried before, and it proves unhelpful, consideration needs to be given to trying not only at least another one or two alternative formulations of the same medication but also to trying at least another one or two drugs from the same class before necessarily concluding it's unlikely that class will be of help for the particular variant of MCAS harbored in this patient.

Principle #9: Triggers are bad. Duh. Therefore, you can take this as "Step 1" in the therapeutic plan for any MCAS patient is identification and avoidance of triggers, such as is possible. Also, if possible, desensitization therapy (if available for identifiable but unavoidable triggers) is a reasonable intervention to consider.

Principle #10: An ounce of prevention is worth a pound of, well, treatment. I won't say "cure" since MCAD, for all practical purposes, can't be cured. But preventive measures are smart. Handwashing. Mammograms and colonoscopies for those ages 50-80. Stop smoking and other (primary and secondary) tobacco exposure. (Smoke is a well-recognized trigger of mast cell activation in many patients. Alcohol, too, often is a trigger.) Vaccinations for those who aren't triggered by them into bad flares. Bone density screenings with appropriate treatment if osteoporosis is found. And so on and so forth.

Principle #11: Eat as normal/balanced/healthy a diet as you can tolerate. I'm often asked, "Might Diet X help control my MCAS?" My answer is always the same: "I don't know." Not only is it difficult with many diets to find agreement on what actually is allowable and disallowable, but also I've yet to see any consistent results (good or bad) with any specific diet. This is not to say that a specific dietary alteration can't help some MCAS patients. I'm fine with MCAS patients trying (reasonable) dietary adjustments, but a dietary adjustment is an intervention and only one intervention at a time should be pursued whenever possible (Principle #3).

Now, on to treatment, but let me very explicitly state the critical caveat that treatment of MCAS often is complex and involves drugs with significant potential toxicities, and thus all efforts to treat MCAS should be performed under a doctor's supervision.

Symptoms and other clinical consequences (e.g., blood count abnormalities) in MCAD result virtually exclusively from the consequences (direct or indirect) of aberrant mediator release. It should be remembered, too, that because of potential circulation of released mediators, and because of potential interaction of released mediators with elements of the nervous and hormonal systems, the dysfunctional mast cells that release the mediators that cause a particular clinical consequence at a particular clinical site, or in a particular system, may not be located near the affected site or system. Thus, therapies for MCAS and non-aggressive mastocytosis primarily aim to (1) reduce mast cell production and

222

release of mediators, (2) interfere with released mediators, and (3) counter unavoidable effects of released mediators.

The doctor who tries to identify effective therapy in an MCAS patient must keep in mind how differently the disease behaves in different patients, both in its clinical presentations and its responses to any given therapy. With the exception of classic histamine-related symptoms, at present it is virtually impossible to predict effective therapy for the individual MCAS patient based on the presenting symptoms and findings.

Thus, in each patient being treated, each medication tried should be dosed appropriately for the disease and should be given an appropriate period to demonstrate effectiveness. Ineffectiveness of one medication of a given class does not necessarily condemn all other medications of that class to ineffectiveness, and it is not at all unreasonable to try at least one or two other medications of a class if the initial medication tried of that class proves ineffective or intolerable. Medications that have clearly demonstrated efficacy and tolerability by the end of a suitable trial period should be continued; medications not achieving such criteria should be stopped (or, if necessary (such as with high doses of glucocorticoids), weaned). Once the effectiveness of a tolerable therapy has been identified, consideration should be given to trying to identify the lowest effective dose and frequency of the therapy.

Given the rarity of systemic mastocytosis, together with how recently MCAS has come to be recognized, there are no large controlled studies of any intervention for mast cell disease. The absence of such data, together with the suspected great underlying mutational heterogeneity of MCAD in general, means that at present the clinician treating MCAS has no way to know in advance which medications are most likely to benefit the patient. Most clinical and laboratory consequences of the disease can arise via multiple mechanisms. As such, there presently are no symptoms or laboratory findings which can reliably foretell effectiveness of any given therapy, and absent such foreknowledge of effective therapy, an economics-based strategy for determining the order in which to try assorted therapies is a reasonable approach, starting with the most inexpensive therapies and escalating in cost as necessary (Principle #4). Such an approach is often appreciated by patients who, due to chronic disability from the disease, are underemployed or unemployed and may face difficulties affording health care. Fortunately, in many patients MCAS is easily controlled with one or two inexpensive therapies – but there also are many patients who require moderately and even stratospherically expensive medications. Doctors treating MCAS often are asked by their patients to write letters supporting application for disability qualification. (The disability certification process is complex. Patients pursuing disability certifications should carefully document (i.e., keep a detailed diary!) the consequences of their disease and, if affordable, engage lawyers familiar with the disability certification process.) Dialogues with senior-level personnel at insurance companies, especially chief medical officers, may be necessary, too, to address denials of coverage due to the insurer's insufficient understanding of MCAS. MCAS patients also sometimes require their doctors' assistance in enrolling in drug manufacturer assistance programs to access expensive therapies at reduced or free rates.

Largely due to how recently awareness of MCAS has dawned on the medical community, clinical trials (of both diagnostic approaches and therapeutics) in MCAS presently are non-existent. However, in light of the increasingly apparent prevalence of the disease, trials – particularly of newer, better targeted (and often more expensive) therapies – are greatly needed, and both patients and doctors should seek to participate in them when they become available.

The glucocorticoid class of steroid medication (including drugs like prednisone) can be helpful in controlling MCAS chronically and emergently, and most drugs in this class are pretty inexpensive, but the rafter of well-known toxicities from their chronic use makes them less preferable for chronic use.

The most inexpensive sustainable therapies for MCAS (and non-aggressive mastocytosis) generally include histamine H_1 and H_2 receptor blockers (which engage H_1 and H_2 receptors on surfaces of many types of cells including mast cells), benzodiazepines (which engage benzodiazepine receptors on many types of cells including mast cells), and non-steroidal anti-inflammatory drugs (NSAIDs, including aspirin).

Antihistamines typically are first-line therapies for chronic control of MCAS and often are highly useful in the emergency management of the disease, too. To minimize histamine-mediated mast cell activation, most MCAS patients should try a histamine H_1 receptor blocker in combination with an H_2 receptor blocker.

Diphenhydramine (also commonly known by the trade name Benadryl) is the prototypical histamine H_1 receptor blocker and is highly effective in many MCAS patients suffering flares of symptoms, but its principal side effect of sedation is undesirable in patients who work or operate heavy machinery and in patients whose disease causes chronic fatigue. In the United States, approved non-sedating histamine H_1 receptor blockers include loratadine, fexofenadine, cetirizine, and levocetirizine, but unlike diphenhydramine, none of these drugs is commercially available for intravenous administration, making diphenhydramine the histamine H_1 receptor blocker of choice in the emergency management of MCAS. Loratadine may have fewer drug-drug interactions than the other products. Loratadine may be effective at the recommended over-the-counter dosing of 10 mg daily, but many patients respond to it better when it is taken every 12 hours. Some patients even can identify further improvement when dosing is increased from every 12 hours to every 8 hours. Higher individual doses of 20 or even 30 mg sometimes provide more benefit, too. However, some MCAS patients on multiple daily doses of loratadine complain of excessive dryness (of eyes, sinuses, or mouth, and possibly also constipation and difficulty urinating), and in such patients it may be more beneficial (with respect to sustaining control over the dysfunctional mast cells) to try decreasing the individual dose (e.g., 5 mg, still taken 2-3 times daily) rather than the frequency (e.g., 10 mg taken daily).

Dosing strategies for fexofenadine, cetirizine, and levocetirizine are similar to those used with loratadine. Initial dosing for fexofenadine typically is 180 mg every 12 hours; for cetirizine, 10 mg every 12 hours; and for levocetirizine, 5 mg every 12 hours. Outside of the United States (where it is not yet available), the histamine H_1 receptor blocker rupatadine (dosing typically 5-10 mg every 8-12 hours) has been shown to help control mast cell activation.

Less desirable, of course, but still sometimes useful are the relatively sedating histamine H_1 receptor blockers. Diphenhydramine was already mentioned above. Others in this class include hydroxyzine, doxepin, and cyproheptadine, all typically dosed 2-4 times daily. Also, diphenhydramine has even been used recently with some success as a continuous intravenous infusion in some particularly severely afflicted (i.e., virtually continuously anaphylactoid) MCAS patients. (I published my early experience with this (in 10 patients) as a peer-reviewed American Society of Hematology 2015 abstract, freely publicly available at http://www.bloodjournal.org/content/126/23/5194, and have gone on to see similar results in the great majority of another three dozen or so such patients, but readers should be cautioned that these latter results are not yet published and thus overall it has to be said that this is essentially anecdotal experience and not the results of a rigorous study. Also of note is that no such patient has yet found another, even more effective drug that has permitted successful weaning off the infusion.)

Although cimetidine and ranitidine are effective histamine H_2 receptor blockers, famotidine and nizatidine have fewer drug-drug interactions. Unlike the non-sedating histamine H_1 receptor blockers, most of the H_2 blockers are commercially available for intravenous administration if necessary. As with the H_1 blockers, the H_2 blockers sometimes are optimally effective in providing what control they can over mast cell activation when taken just once daily. However, many patients respond better to twice-daily use of H_2 blockers. Famotidine often is begun at 20-40 mg every 12 hours, while ranitidine is begun at 75-150 mg every 12 hours. Nizatidine can be used at 150-300 mg every 12 hours. Cimetidine is uncommonly used because of its rafter of drug-drug interactions but, when necessary, can be tried starting at 400 mg every 12 hours.

Given recent recognition of the involvement of inflammation in the development and evolution of a wide range of psychiatric morbidities, it is an open question as to whether benzodiazepine-driven inhibition of mast cell activation causes (directly or indirectly) a significant portion of the anxiety-relieving effect seen with these drugs in diseases such as panic and anxiety disorders.

Benzodiazepines (such as lorazepam or Ativan, clonazepam or Klonopin, alprazolam or Xanax, and the longer-acting diazepam or Valium) also are helpful in some patients with inflammatory bowel disease, again raising the question of whether it is benzodiazepine receptors on gut cells or on mast cells that result in greater benefit from these drugs. Benzodiazepine therapy certainly can result in a wide range of other improvements, too, in MCAS patients, likely underscoring what can be accomplished solely from blocking mast cell benzodiazepine receptors.

Other inexpensive antihistamine drugs can be helpful in controlling MCAS, too. The anti-depressant doxepin, the anti-inflammatory ketotifen, the whole class of tricyclic antidepressants, the whole class of phenothiazine anti-nausea drugs, and the antipsychotic drug quetiapine all have histamine H_1 receptor blocking effects. Dosing starts low and escalates, as tolerated, to maximal benefit. Ketotifen is not presently available in the United States in a commercial oral preparation (though some are working to fix that), but it can be obtained by pharmacists for compounding into oral forms.

Some MCAS patients have long suffered symptoms of major depression and are already taking one drug or another from the class of selective serotonin reuptake inhibitors (SSRIs) that are the front-line drugs for treating depression at present. Addition of antihistamines to SSRIs increases the risk for the life-threatening "serotonin syndrome," for which the clinician must remain alert; should such develop, cessation of the offending drugs and immediate institution of aggressive benzodiazepine therapy (such as lorazepam, initially dosed at 2-3 mg 3-4 times daily) should be the emergency response.

Like antihistamines, benzodiazepines often are useful not only in chronic management of MCAS but also in emergency management of the disease. Although benzodiazepines with longer half-lives such as diazepam can be helpful, most MCAS patients who benefit from benzodiazepines use shorter half-life drugs such as lorazepam, clonazepam, or alprazolam, typically dosed every 8-12 hours. Although dose-finding experiments initially should use the same dose given at regular intervals, many patients report eventually discovering optimal benefit from benzodiazepines upon using slightly different doses at different times of the day possibly involving slightly irregular intervals; the shorter half-life benzodiazepines obviously are more amenable than the longer half-life benzodiazepines to such personalization of therapy. Flunitrazepam is another benzodiazepine reported to be useful in mast cell disease but has a longer half-life; dosing typically is daily, more convenient for some patients but allowing less of the intraday variability in dosing and response appreciated by other patients.

Imidazopyridines such as zolpidem (Ambien) also target the benzodiazepine receptor and sometimes are useful in treating MCAS. In my experience, the likelihood for benefit from imidazopyridines seems independent of whether

226

benzodiazepines are already being used and whether they are proving beneficial. Imidazopyridines seem to help somewhat with the insomnia frequently seen in MCAS, but unlike benzodiazepines, beneficial impacts on other MCAS symptoms are not often seen with these drugs. Also unlike benzodiazepines, currently available imidazopyridines do not seem to have any role in the emergency management of MCAS.

Non-steroidal anti-inflammatory drugs (NSAIDs) can be very helpful in some MCAS patients, but the physician needs to be aware that these drugs (and many narcotic analgesics, too) can trigger flares of mast cell activation, even to the point of anaphylaxis, and even at seemingly trivial doses. Aspirin, of course, is the least expensive NSAID. Patients who report prior intolerance of aspirin sometimes can gain tolerance by being started on very low doses (e.g., 1-10 mg, which may require the services of a compounding pharmacist) and doubling as often as every 6 hours as tolerated, with full precautions in place for managing anaphylaxis – meaning that such efforts usually should be conducted under a doctor's supervision. Patients who report prior tolerance of aspirin typically can be started at 325 mg twice daily. It is unclear whether there is any advantage (or disadvantage) to "enteric coating" of aspirin in MCAS as different studies have reached opposite conclusions. Patients who are unaware of any prior exposure to aspirin (somewhat unusual given the wide range of products into which aspirin is integrated) may be best served by starting with a dose of 40-80 mg and doubling as often as every 6 hours as tolerated. Once tolerance of lower doses (e.g., 325 mg twice daily) is demonstrated, dosing can be escalated as often as daily until target dosing is reached. Some patients respond quite well to just 325 mg twice daily and do not require higher doses, but many patients do not clearly respond until dosing reaches 650-1300 mg twice daily. The need to dose aspirin as high as 1300 mg four times daily (felt to be sustainable with maximal ulcer prophylaxis in place) in order to achieve a desired therapeutic salicylate level of 20-30 mg/dl has been reported in the literature, but I have seen enough trouble (typically in the form of GI bleeding), and not enough benefit, at doses higher than 650 mg twice daily that I'm not willing to advise going higher these days. Patients should be counseled regarding potential toxicities. Patients who benefit from aspirin at total daily doses of 650 mg or higher need to consider methods to improve their ability to tolerate chronic use of the drug. Concurrent use of histamine H_1 and H_2 receptor blockers is helpful and probably should be the first therapy to be considered for ulcer prophylaxis; consideration can also be given to addition of a proton pump inhibitor to the regimen, though the doctor should recognize that excessive acid suppression can interfere with iron absorption.

If aspirin is intolerable or ineffective, other NSAIDs can be tried. Particularly (but not necessarily) if kidney disease or a low platelet count is present, use of a "COX2-selective" NSAID such as celecoxib (typically 100-400 mg twice daily) can be considered. Chronic use of some NSAIDs may increase risk for a heart attack.

Leukotrienes are another class of inflammation-driving mediators that are synthesized and released by mast cells (and, to be sure, other types of cells, too) and clearly drive a wide variety of events categorized as inflammatory in nature. As such, it is not surprising that leukotriene receptor blockers such as montelukast (Singulair) and zafirlukast (Accolate) are clearly helpful in some forms of MCAS, but they have to be used with particular caution in patients with pre-existing liver disease.

Cromolyn has long been recognized for its mast-cell-stabilizing activity in some patients, though its specific mechanism of action remains unclear; in fact, it's been argued that its principal effects aren't even against mast cells but rather against nerve cells. It is an expensive drug, each dose has only a short period of activity in the body, and it is absorbed so poorly that it essentially has no ability to affect mast cells beyond the ones it directly comes in contact with as it passes through the body. It is not available yet for intravenous administration (though some are working to develop such a formulation). It is available as a nasal spray, an eye drop, for inhalation, and for oral ingestion typically in commercial liquid form but also compoundable into capsules. It can be compounded as a cream, too, for topical use, usually on wounds that are healing poorly due to local mast cell effects. Due to an initial flare of mediator release, some patients experience a flare of symptoms in the first few days of exposure to cromolyn before seeing symptoms reduce to well below their prior baseline.

Pentosan is another mast cell stabilizer whose mechanism of action remains unknown. Its activity seems far greater against mast cells in the urinary tract than elsewhere. It has been used for many years to treat interstitial cystitis, which has increasingly come to be recognized as a form of MCAS.

Quercetin is a natural component of many foods in a normal diet (e.g., apples, onions, berries, red grapes, citrus, broccoli, and tea). It is poorly absorbed but has a range of properties potentially useful in MCAD. It seems to result in reduced production of inflammatory mediators (e.g., leukotrienes and histamine). It may also serve as an inhibitor of tyrosine kinases and other regulatory proteins of interest in activated mast cells. Quercetin seems to provide general anti-inflammatory effects and seems to impede prostaglandin D_2-driven flushing. A more recently developed form, quercetin chalcone, is water soluble, which might make it more absorbable and permit lower dosages.

Pancreatic enzyme supplements are helpful in some MCAS patients whose symptom complexes include features of (painful or painless) chronic pancreatitis such as chronic diarrhea, weight loss, and certain micronutrient malabsorption syndromes.

Allergen-driven cross-linking of multiple IgE molecules bound to mast cell-surface IgE receptors is a major route of mast cell activation. Omalizumab (Xolair) is a "monoclonal antibody" that blocks IgE from binding with its mast cell-surface receptor. As with all monoclonal antibody therapies, omalizumab presently is very expensive. Omalizumab has been reported in a small number of patients to be effective in controlling MCAS, and I've seen such benefits in several of my own patients, but in contrast to the 2-8 weeks it typically requires to identify effectiveness for most of the drugs patients try in attempting to control their MCAS, a trial of omalizumab should be pursued for at least 3-4 months before making a conclusive assessment of its efficacy. One other note: although the usual uses of omalizumab tie the drug's dosing to the patient's IgE level, responsiveness of MCAS to omalizumab so far has appeared to be independent of IgE levels, so a normal IgE level should not dissuade a doctor from trying it for an MCAS patient who hasn't responded to several less expensive therapies. I also sometimes use omalizumab "sooner rather than later" in MCAS patients who are having "more reactions than usual" from foods and odors.

As demonstrated by Dr. Molderings and his team at the University of Bonn, most MCAS patients harbor one or more mutations in mast cell KIT, and most of these mutations lead to constitutive activation of the KIT protein. Activation of KIT in turn leads to activation of the Janus kinases (JAK1, JAK2, JAK3, Tyk2), which in turn lead to activation of the assorted Signal Transducer and Activator of Transcription (STAT) proteins, which then migrate to the cell nucleus, where they bind to the DNA in our genes and promote transcription of genes responsive to STAT. It is well demonstrated that activation of STAT proteins leads to increased production and release of a number of inflammatory mediators. In view of these biological insights, the tyrosine kinase inhibitors (TKIs) of KIT such as imatinib (Gleevec), dasatinib (Sprycel), nilotinib (Tasigna), and sunitinib (Sutent) can be predicted to be useful, and have been seen to be useful, in some forms of mast cell disease. Imatinib is less useful in systemic mastocytosis (SM), as most cases of SM harbor mutations in the region of KIT codon 816 which render KIT resistant to imatinib binding. However, imatinib can also inhibit constitutive activation of KIT caused by mutations at certain other sites in KIT (such as the region of the protein near the cell membrane). Also, via mechanisms not yet clear, even some SM patients with the KIT-D816V mutation can respond to imatinib. Underscoring the "mutational overlap" between SM and MCAS, responses to imatinib have been reported in MCAS. (I've written some of those reports.) In contrast to the dosing of imatinib typically used in chronic myelogenous leukemia (CML, the disease for which imatinib was designed to control), lower dosing has appeared sufficient thus far in MCAS patients who respond to tyrosine kinase inhibitors. As compared to imatinib, dasatinib targets a wider spectrum of tyrosine kinases, has additional immunosuppressive/anti-inflammatory effects, and may be the better initial choice in patients with renal insufficiency, but it may have a greater propensity for clinically significant pulmonary complications; a few responses have been reported in systemic mastocytosis patients thus far. There have been no reports in the peer-reviewed literature thus far of the use of this drug in MCAS patients – but that's as much my fault as anyone else's because I haven't gotten around yet to writing such reports on any of the few MCAS patients I've had who have responded very nicely to dasatinib. (To be clear, though, I've also had several patients I tried on the drug who didn't respond at all.) Nilotinib has a somewhat different toxicity spectrum than imatinib and dasatinib and requires somewhat closer monitoring; a few responses have been reported in systemic mastocytosis patients thus far, but there are no reports yet of use of this drug in MCAS patients. (I've tried it in a couple, with no improvements seen.) Finally, with regard to sunitinib (Sutent), I'm aware of one MCAS patient who has benefited spectacularly from it, but there aren't yet any published case reports about the use of this drug in any form of mast cell disease. Bosutinib, too – a TKI approved relatively recently for CML – might be predicted to be useful in some forms of mast cell disease and indeed has been seen to control mast cell activation in the laboratory but hasn't yet been reported to help any patients with mast cell disease. No generic versions of the tyrosine kinase inhibitors are yet available, and all of these drugs are very expensive. Retail prices are roughly $100,000 a year or more. "Cheaper" generic versions will start emerging in the next few years, but nobody will be surprised if they still cost many thousands of dollars per year (at least in the U.S.).

Tumor necrosis factor (TNF) alpha is a well-established mast cell mediator, and TNF-alpha antagonists such as etanercept, adalimumab, and infliximab are approved for use in a variety of systemic inflammatory diseases increasingly suspected to involve mast cell dysfunction (such as rheumatoid arthritis, psoriatic arthritis, and inflammatory bowel disease). Thus, there is reason to suspect such drugs would be useful in reducing TNF-alpha-derived symptoms in some patients with MCAS, but no data regarding the use of any of these drugs in MCAS have been published and there are no reports of such trials in progress or development.

There is another entire class of inflammatory mediators called the interleukins, and there is hardly an interleukin known which is not produced and released by the mast cell. Thus, there is reason to suspect that interleukin-1 antagonists (e.g., anakinra or Kineret) and interleukin-1-beta antagonists (e.g., canakinumab or Ilaris) may be helpful in some forms of MCAS, but, again, no data regarding the use of any of these drugs in MCAS have been published and there are no reports of such trials in progress or development.

Along with calcium and vitamin D supplementation, the class of drugs known as the bisphosphonates has proven helpful for weak bone conditions such as osteopenia and osteoporosis. A small case series demonstrated that concurrent use of interferon alpha and the bisphosphonate drug pamidronate (Aredia) in patients with SM led to significantly bone strengthening which was subsequently maintained with pamidronate alone. However, no controlled trials have been performed, and interferon can be substantially toxic. A new class of bone-strengthening therapy called anti-RANKL monoclonal antibody therapy has recently emerged, and the first drug in that class, denosumab (Xgeva or Prolia), has demonstrated effectiveness in certain osteopenic/osteoporotic situations equal to or better than bisphosphonate therapy. In theory, such antibody therapy should be useful in reducing the osteopenia/osteoporosis of MCAS. No controlled clinical trials regarding the use of any of these bone-protecting therapies in MCAS have been performed, but use of any therapy approved or generally recommended for osteoporosis/osteoporosis seems reasonable in MCAS patients also found to have osteopenia/osteoporosis. Osteonecrosis of the jaw (ONJ) is a topic that must be considered when contemplating use of the bisphosphonates or denosumab. ONJ is a rare but serious complication of such therapies. It is known to be more prevalent in cancer patients than osteoporosis patients, and it has not been reported in mast cell disease patients receiving these therapies. Nevertheless, it seems prudent to practice with mast cell disease patients the preventive measures advised for other populations receiving these drugs including pre-treatment dental evaluation, good dental hygiene, and suspension of therapy in the period surrounding invasive dental therapy.

Interferon-alpha is a well-recognized modulator of the chronic myeloproliferative neoplasms including SM. Its activity in MCAS has not been specifically investigated, but it seems reasonable at present to presume it would have similar activity (as in SM) in reducing aberrant mediator production and release. However, interferon alpha therapy is expensive and associated with many toxicities, which not infrequently lead to patients choosing to stop therapy. The most common such problem is a flu-like syndrome. Use of the "pegylated" form of interferon appears to decrease toxicity, and pegylated interferon treatment of chronic myeloproliferative diseases in general appears to require lower doses than needed with non-pegylated interferon. A case of SM with secondary osteoporosis successfully treated with pegylated interferon has been reported, but use of the pegylated product has not been specifically investigated in any form of mast cell disease.

Tryptase inhibitors remain in the early stages of clinical development (generally, pre-clinical development and Phase 1 clinical trials). Histamine H_3 receptor antagonists, too, are in development (primarily for neurologic diseases).

Ivabradine, a relatively new drug used in Europe for the last decade for angina, has been found by some MCAS patients to help control the palpitations and tachycardia caused by the disease. It's presently available only in Europe, but a major U.S. drug company is working to make it available in the U.S. (for congestive heart failure, to start with – but once it's available here for *any* purpose, it may become easier to access it anyway for mast cell disease).

Hydroxyurea is an oral RNA synthetase (a.k.a. ribonucleotide reductase) inhibitor useful chronically and acutely in a wide range of hematologic malignancies. It also has been recommended for essentially lifelong use in sickle cell anemia patients. A modest degree of efficacy has been reported with hydroxyurea in SM. I have seen some MCAS patients improve with hydroxyurea, but initiation of this therapy in MCAS patients should be monitored cautiously, as in this population the drug sometimes causes more rapid and severe drops in blood counts than seen in other populations. Such reactions may be due to the fillers or dyes in one hydroxyurea preparation or another, as I have seen some such patients turn around and benefit greatly from hydroxyurea when subsequently re-tried in an alternative formulation (for example, switching from the Hydrea 500 mg hydroxyurea capsule to the Droxia 200 mg hydroxyurea capsule).

Cyclophosphamide, a chemotherapy drug, seems to have little activity in human mast cell disease but nevertheless can be helpful sometimes in management of steroid-refractory cases of the autoimmune diseases which can emerge from mast cell disease. The drug can be given as a daily oral dose or as an intravenous dosing every few weeks. Although such regimens tend to be tolerated well in the short run, chemotherapy treatment of this sort inevitably conveys some increased risk for secondary malignancy.

Other single- and multi-agent chemotherapy drug regimens have been used in SM. Though durable responses are rare, cladribine may be the best performer to date. The rationale for use of chemotherapy (i.e., mast-cell-killing) drugs in relatively non-proliferative MCAS seems weak, and there are no reports of the use of such drugs in MCAS patients.

Similarly, there are scarce reports of other immunosuppressive drugs (e.g., cyclosporine, azathioprine, methotrexate, alemtuzumab, daclizumab, etc.) being used with widely varying degrees of success in SM, but no reports of the use of these drugs in MCAS have been published yet.

Stem cell transplant therapy in theory might be curative but has been used in SM only rarely to date. This approach seems to be used most in the setting of associated refractory blood cancers such as leukemia (sometimes with the mast cell disease being recognized only in post-transplant retrospect) and generally (but not always) failing to eradicate the mast cell disease component, providing little reason a priori to consider using this approach for MCAS patients without associated refractory blood cancers.

Secondary issues in MCAS – e.g., inflammation, infection, autoimmunity, malignancy, coagulopathy, osteopathy, etc. – not uncommonly come to clinical attention first, but whether such issues present prior or subsequent to diagnosis of mast cell disease, they warrant standard therapy and may fare better when the mast cell disease is recognized and concomitantly specifically addressed.

Many patients with mast cell activation disease suffer pain. Sometimes the pain is diffuse, while sometimes it is focal but diffusely migratory. It often is described as a deep-seated muscular, bony, or marrow-based "aching" rather than a distinct "pain." Narcotic and non-narcotic analgesics help some patients, but often are ineffective. (In fact, in a fashion similar to how NSAIDs can trigger flares of mast cell disease, so, too, can narcotics.) Sometimes other classes of mast-cell-targeted agents not expected to have analgesic effect are nonetheless effective at achieving such (e.g., antihistamines relieve chronic migraine headaches in some MCAS patients). I have reported, too, that hydroxyurea is helpful in relieving pain in some MCAS patients.

Patients with mast cell activation disease often suffer presyncopal events. (Frank syncope seems somewhat less common but certainly is not "rare.") When hypotension can be demonstrated during such events, and when the trigger appears to typically be postural change, medications such as fludrocortisone, midodrine, and pyridostigmine can be helpful. Ivabradine has helped some MCAS patients with this symptom, too.

Emergency and perioperative management of severe flares of mast cell disease has been amply discussed in the medical literature and is available publicly (e.g., at the website of The Mastocytosis Society, http://www.tmsforacure.org). In general, histamine H_1 and H_2 receptor antagonists, glucocorticoids, and benzodiazepines form the core of the therapeutic attack at such a problem, and of course epinephrine is the #1 go-to drug for anaphylaxis. Patients susceptible to anaphylaxis should be prescribed epinephrine autoinjectors (unless, of course, they have demonstrated anaphylaxis to the metabisulfites typically used as preservatives in epinephrine preparations) and should be counseled to fully recline before using the device to prevent trauma from falls should dysrhythmias or other complications develop to further weaken a patient likely already weakened from the flare.

Some MCAS patients are highly reactive to a wide assortment of foods. Elimination diets such as described for the eosinophilic esophagitis population may be helpful, but efforts to identify and control the underlying mast cell disease probably are the best approach in the long run.

In spite of the substantial fatigue and malaise many MCAS patients experience, and in spite of their many physical sensitivities (e.g., heat, cold, ultraviolet radiation, exertion, etc.) and antigenic sensitivities (e.g., pollen, perfumes, etc.), MCAS patients should be strongly encouraged to regularly exercise – but only to the usual individual limit of tolerance each patient likely has learned from experience, as, again, exertion clearly can trigger a flare of mast cell activation in some patients. At the same time, although the mechanism likely is complex and remains quite unclear, exercise can help many patients with chronic inflammatory diseases improve both subjectively and objectively, acutely and chronically. Brief (15-30 minute) periods of exercise of mild-to-moderate intensity may be more helpful, at least subjectively, than longer periods and high intensity of exercise. Also, some workers in the field have observed that activities causing frequent sharp abdominal motion (e.g., jogging, tennis, soccer, etc.) may be more prone to provoke flares of mast cell activation than less abdominally provocative activities (e.g., bicycling); a potential mechanism for this difference may be aberrantly heightened response of constitutively activated gastrointestinal tract mast cells to physical force.

Overall, in my opinion, the single most important aspect to successful management of mast cell disease is identification of a local physician/partner who will help the patient not only access local health care resources as needed for tactical management of acute issues from the disease but also access remote resources which may be able to help determine strategic management of chronic issues. Absent an effective local physician/partner (which can be challenging to identify for many reasons), the MCAS patient often faces great difficulty gaining initial control over the disease even after consulting remote expertise which for many reasons cannot provide care for acute issues with the disease.

Chapter 26: Why Diagnosis of MCAS Likely Won't Get Much Easier Anytime Soon

Perhaps MCAS will turn out to be the "invisible elephant in the room" – the root cause for a significant portion of the modern epidemic of chronic inflammatory diseases – that I have come to suspect. (I'll have more to say in the next chapter about what I think needs to be done in the MCAS research arena.) But even if I'm wrong, I regret to report I suspect MCAS will remain an elusive diagnosis for most patients suffering with it for a long time to come. Thus, perhaps millions will suffer without diagnosis, let alone treatment, longer than might be necessary, but even if "only" thousands so suffer, I think it's important to understand the problem of diagnosing MCAS. Call me a product of my training: only by dissecting a problem can we learn its component issues, what makes them behave in the manners they do, and devise rational approaches to overcoming the issues.

To be sure, there usually isn't any one culprit in the failure to make other diagnoses, and that's no less a truth in MCAS. Here are my thoughts on the issues in MCAS:

Reason #1: Insufficient training and insufficient existing literature.

For roughly a century now, the medical profession has consistently taught its successive generations that mast cell disease occurs, for all intents and purposes, in only a couple of forms – allergy (common, and certainly recognized since the dawn of our species) and mastocytosis (rare, and not first recognized until the latter part of the 19th century) – and both forms, despite the wide disparity in their frequencies of occurrence, are relatively easy to recognize.

Respiratory and/or gastrointestinal reactivity is generally regarded as an allergy to elements of the environment, foods, or medication. If you repeatedly sneeze, or get nauseous or produce diarrhea, upon exposure to the same trigger, then you are allergic to that trigger. Even young children often are capable of quickly figuring out what they are allergic to and wisely practice avoidance; one has never needed a formal medical education to recognize allergy.

Mastocytosis, though rare, is relatively easy to suspect: your physician probably only got 5 minutes of exposure to the disease – all book-learning, as such patients are sufficiently rare that the average doctor will never see one – but the symptoms are so flagrant and almost unique (unprovoked flushing and anaphylaxis) that even the average physician will soon come to consider mastocytosis in the differential diagnosis for such a patient.

MCAS, though, is the ultimate chameleon, and this is just Reason #1 why it will long be difficult to diagnose.

Reason #2: Experience counts.

It's no surprise that the more cases of a given type a physician has to deal with, the better he (usually) becomes at dealing with them. Well, what's the experience base with mast cell disease? Extremely few physicians worldwide presently have experience with bona fide mast cell disease (i.e., not just allergy and asthma), and the great majority of those few physicians know mastocytosis fairly well but are still "coming to terms" with MCAS.

Reason #3: Subspecialization.

MCAS is the prototypical multisystem disease, but we live in an era in which most physicians focus in single systems, either by dint of training (as for subspecialists) or dint of time constraints (as for generalists, who only have time to focus on one or two problems in the typical 5 minutes visit). As a multisystem disease, though, MCAS is just too complicated to reveal itself to the physician who focuses on a single system or the physician who only has a few minutes for each patient.

Reason #4: Sorry to break this news to you, but doctors don't get paid to think…

…nearly as much as they get paid to do other things. The health care financing system in the U.S. has long incentivized only two things: performance of procedures and seeing as many patients as possible. Also, U.S. physicians have been paid based on what they've done, not based on the outcomes of what they've done. This isn't the physicians' fault, nor is it the insurers' fault – and it certainly isn't the patients' fault. It's nobody's fault. It's just that physicians have to be paid based on some factor(s), and it's far easier to account simply for the number of procedures performed, or the number of patients seen, than to account for outcomes. Think about it. In any given physician-patient encounter, the physician will have one sense of the value he provided the patient, the patient will have a different sense of how valuable the encounter was – and the insurer likely will have its own sense of the encounter's value. How does one fairly reconcile these three perspectives – and do it in a way that can be replicated, in automated fashion, across millions of encounters every day?

Perhaps there is some reason for encouragement. The health care financing system in the U.S. is beginning to be reformed. Outcomes-based incentives are beginning to be introduced into the system – and it is only with such incentives that physicians will begin taking the far greater amounts of time needed to successfully manage patients with mast cell disease and other complex diseases – but procedures and patient volume likely will continue to be the primary drivers of physician payment for a long time to come.

Reason #5: Establishing a definitive diagnosis of MCAD is not a trivial process…

236

…even if the patient is so lucky as to find a physician who can take the time needed to get to a point where he suspects mast cell disease, establishing a definitive diagnosis is not a trivial process. Many of the tests that need to be ordered are not tests the average physician is familiar with, and there are substantial logistical challenges in getting the tests done correctly. No NSAIDs for the last several days. No PPIs for the last several days. Most of the tests require – in order to determine results that are as accurate as possible – that specimens be drawn into chilled containers, which then must be carefully kept continuously chilled. The physician needs to be educated about this, the patient needs to be educated about this, and the lab staff need to be educated about this. MCAS patients are challenging to laboratory technicians. A typical non-MCAS patient may consume 5 minutes of a lab technician's time; the MCAS patient may easily consume 30-60 minutes. Shortcuts which may invalidate results become tempting when technicians, too, are graded based on the patient volume they handle.

Reason #6: The self-fulfilling prophecy of never finding it if you don't look for it.

Fairly early in these first seven years of learning about MCAS, I lost count of the number of patients I diagnosed with the disease in whom I had asked the pathologist to re-visit old biopsies with a new eye toward the possibility of mast cell disease, and voilà, it turned out the disease had been sitting in the pathology warehouse for years just waiting to be discovered.

It's not that pathologists don't know how to evaluate biopsies for mast cell disease. Rather, this part of the problem in diagnosing MCAS is two-fold.

First, when "routine" stains are applied to tissue sections, mast cells rarely look like physicians are taught they look like. Instead, just as the disease itself is so chameleon-like at a clinical level, the cells themselves are chameleons, easily masquerading as lymphocytes, plasma cells, histiocytes, macrophages, or spindle cells.

Second, doctors have been taught for a century that mast cell disease is rare, so why on earth would a pathologist ever suspect that some of the lymphocytes, plasma cells, histiocytes, macrophages, and spindle cells he's seeing under the microscope might actually be mast cells?

No, the pathologist needs to be given a reason to do the special staining required to reveal the mast cells for what they are – and the only person who's going to give him that reason is the clinician who's obtaining the biopsy in the first place. But given that that clinician, too, was taught (and, as far as he knows, has experienced) that mast cell disease is rare and is just that one disease, mastocytosis, that shows up with flushing and anaphylaxis, why would he ever suspect mast cell disease and ask the pathologist to look for it?

Don't despair. All of these hurdles will eventually be overcome. But it will take time. Until then, it will continue to be the case – thanks largely to the Internet – that many patients will figure out they might have MCAS long before their physicians will figure it out, and it will simply require patients to persist in their search for physicians who are willing to listen and take the time and make the effort needed to help their patients get to a diagnosis and then effective therapy.

Chapter 27: The Rumsfeldian Research Needs in MCAS: The Known Knowns, Known Unknowns, and Unknown Unknowns

Oh, man, how does one start this sort of a chapter? The research needs in this area are enough to occupy an army of researchers for centuries.

To start with, we need to identify "improved" techniques for diagnosis. If the ultimate objective is to improve the lot of the patients who have this, they'll need to be treated, but you can't (sensibly) treat what you haven't (accurately) diagnosed, so improving diagnosis is paramount.

But, "improved" in what ways? Well, we (as in, the entire medical profession) need to somehow make it easier to both suspect the presence of the disease and to prove its presence.

Clearly, the primary means to improving the ability to suspect the disease is to train doctors (and nurses and other health care providers who diagnose) to recognize it. There need to be lectures and treatises about how the disease behaves – what it clinically looks like – that health care professionals and trainees need to see and read. I have had medical students work with me for only a single half-day clinic in which I've taught them the basics of how the disease operates, and then the students rotate elsewhere, recognize it in other patients, and refer those patient to me – and they've almost always been dead-on right. We'll need to improve training at all levels: medical (and nursing and nurse-practitioner and physician-assistant and dental) schools, residencies, and fellowships – plus continuing medical and nursing and dental education for those already practicing. But this is really more along the lines of the educational needs in MCAS, so I'll save more comments on this matter for Chapter 28, which specifically addresses that topic.

How else can we make it easier to spark that initial suspicion of the disease? There exists at least one validated questionnaire that patients can fill out to help identify those who likely have symptoms of mast cell activation, but there are a couple of problems. First, I've seen the questionnaire, and although it covers many of the clinical behaviors of mast cell disease, there are many such behaviors it doesn't cover. Second, it's a chicken-and-egg problem: no health care professional will provide such a questionnaire to the patient unless the professional already has come to initially suspect the patient of having the disease. Perhaps, though, this questionnaire, or improved versions that could be developed and subjected to equally rigorous validation, could be made publicly available so that *patients* who come to suspect they might have the disease could fill it out, and if they meet the questionnaire's threshold for likely identifying abnormal mast cell mediator release, they would have a validated research tool they could present to their doctors rather than what they're limited to doing now, i.e., telling their doctors, "Even though I have no medical training or experience,

I have an idea what I may have, and it's something about which, in spite of all your medical training and experience, you might not know anything at all." You can imagine that line, or any variation thereupon, doesn't get received well by most doctors (regardless of what that may say about the average physician's ego).

In the end, perhaps the most productive way to spark initial suspicion of such a complex, heterogeneous disease might be to program our electronic medical record (EMR) systems to recognize it (or what likely is it) in its many forms. This would be a sizable medical informatics research project, but I contend a properly programmed computer is far more able to recognize complex patterns in a sea of data than a human being whose cognitive capacity is so limited that Ma Bell (i.e., the Bell Telephone System, the precursor to the modern corporate telecommunications behemoth AT&T), after rigorous research into human mental abilities, limited phone numbers to just seven digits.

In every one of the patients I've diagnosed with MCAS, the signs of the disease – symptoms, exam findings, and laboratory abnormalities – were present for years to decades prior to diagnosis. Even if physicians had been aware of MCAS years earlier, *putting together* all of these scattered clues to construct a coherent jigsaw puzzle is, and will always be, a very difficult task, especially when it's a different set of clues from one patient to the next and when physicians are heavily incentivized to look only at the problem of the moment rather than at the big picture. While there always will be physicians who will indeed put together the big picture, I believe most physicians will need – and eventually come to welcome – automated assistance to recognize complex diseases. Such assistance will wind up benefiting not only the patient but also the doctor. Not only will the doctor gain recognition from the payer for getting to the root of why the patient has had so many problems and been so expensive to take care of, but he also will gain recognition from the patient and from the patient's other physicians (and whatever referral traffic such recognition might engender) for getting to the root of the problem. And the doctor won't even have to reveal that his diagnostic insight was EMR-aided, now, will he?

Beyond improving the initial ability to suspect the disease, though, there must be improvement in the ability to prove the presence of the disease. Although there are ways in the research laboratory to test for any of the 200+ mediators the mast cell is presently known to produce, at present we can test in the clinic for only a small handful of these mediators, and even those tests are difficult to perform accurately. At present most of them are run by only a small handful of laboratories around the world, so specimens – which have to be maintained at chilled temperatures – have to be transported great distances to get to these labs. Not only is time an enemy when trying to measure mediators that disappear within minutes in unchilled environments, but there also is a small army of technicians and transport workers who have to handle these specimens and their containers. It's sort of like the old game of "telephone" or "grapevine": the

240

more links in the chain of handling (especially when the individual links are not familiar with the sensitivity of the specimens), the greater the likelihood of the specimen getting corrupted.

We can look forward to a day when it will be possible to affordably test – in the local clinical laboratory, rather than at distant reference clinical laboratories – for a far greater array of mast cell mediators, but it will take much research and business effort to develop and market/distribute such tests. And it will still require much education of laboratory personnel to get this testing done right, but, again, that strays into Chapter 28's domain.

Probably the single most important research question that's got to be answered about this disease is whether the mast cell misbehavior seen in these patients is a result of fundamentally *normal* mast cells *reacting normally* to known and/or unknown provocations, or a result of fundamentally *abnormal* (i.e., mutated) mast cells *reacting abnormally* in response to provocations and/or *acting abnormally* in response to no provocation at all. As I've mentioned repeatedly in prior chapters, the data from repeated experiments performed by Dr. Gerhard Molderings' team at the University of Bonn strongly suggests the latter scenario is the reality here, but a fundamental tenet of scientific truth is its reproducibility, and to date the Bonn experiments haven't been reproduced by anyone else. It's not that others have tried and failed to reproduce them; it's that nobody has yet even tried to reproduce them. (Update as this book nears press: as I mentioned in an earlier chapter, in July 2015 I launched a study to try to reproduce these findings. Results hopefully will be published by late 2016.)

Especially given that we now know that there's a bevy of mutations in the mast cells of each mastocytosis patient, it makes far more sense that there should be a bevy of mutations in the mast cells of each MCAS patient (as the Bonn data suggest), and nailing down the truth or falseness of this contention is crucial to directing the large body of mast cell disease research down the road. If the Bonn team is wrong and the mast cells in most MCAS patients are normal mast cells, then research efforts to understand what's truly at the root of MCAS must turn (at least somewhat) away from the mast cell and toward other cells and environmental factors that may be serving as signals to cause the mast cell activation that's so obvious in the symptoms and exam and laboratory findings in MCAS patients. Because the range of such cells and factors is virtually infinite, such research will necessarily be very, very difficult.

But if the Bonn team is right, then clearly the right direction for further research becomes identifying the full range of mutations in the disease, what each mutation does on its own, what each mutation does in combination with any other given set of mutations, and how best to combat each unique mutation set. Such research, while not necessarily easy in an absolute sense, would nevertheless be relatively a whole lot easier and more straightforward than the previously mentioned alternative scenario.

Furthermore, if the Bonn team is proven right, then clearly the whole diagnostic process for MCAS needs to change – and get a lot easier. Presently, the way to *prove* somebody has MCAS is to find laboratory evidence of increased mast cell mediators (in conjunction with symptoms attributable to abnormally increased mast cell mediators), but it's a difficult task because mast cell mediators typically have short half-lives, their elevations often are evanescent, and different mediators are elevated at different times in different patients. In other words, there's nothing *constant* about the presently testable laboratory manifestations of the disease. But if the Bonn team is right, then the way to go about diagnosing MCAS is to sift mast cells out of a blood sample (or other tissue sample) and look for the mutations which if present are, of course, constantly present.

At least one such specific genetic/mutational variant of MCAS has already been defined, the inborn autoinflammatory syndrome called cryopyrin-associated periodic syndrome (CAPS), in which a mutated, non-functional form of the NLRP3 gene in the mast cell leads to overproduction of interleukin-1-beta, in turn driving excessive inflammation all throughout the body virtually from birth.

A decade ago, figuring out the sequence of a cell's DNA cost tens of millions of dollars, which itself was down from a billion dollars or so in the prior decade. Today, that cost is down to somewhere in the range of a thousand dollars, and by a decade from now, if not sooner, it should be down to $100. Compared to the cost of treating for decades a bevy of recurring symptoms whose origins are unknown, it becomes nonsensical *not* to run a mast cell genomic sequencing in a patient whose symptoms are consistent with a mast cell activation disorder.

We can imagine the research progressing to the point where once a given patient's set of mast cell mutations have been identified, that set is compared against a library of such sets. The library will in turn provide information correlating each mutation set with not only the mediators that are produced abnormally as a result of that mutation set but also the resulting clinical consequences – and the medications (existing and hypothetical) that are, or ought to be, most likely to be effective in controlling that particular variant of MCAS.

But the research challenges for MCAS go well beyond determining, and then leveraging, the disease's clonality. We also need to understand the epidemiology of the disease – is MCAS the true root of some portion of chronic fatigue syndrome? fibromyalgia? irritable bowel syndrome? refractory gastroesophageal reflux disease? asthma? obesity? hypertension? diabetes? Gulf War Illness? etc. etc. etc. – and we need to understand what causes the disease.

MCAS is too heterogeneous a disease for us to understand its prevalence in the general population (not anytime soon, anyway). I doubt anybody is going to design, much less fund, a study in which a random sample of the population is investigated for MCAS. Instead, what I predict will happen is a "divide and conquer" approach in which cohorts of patients with different diseases of unknown cause will be assessed for MCAS. We then will come to know what percentage of patients with, say, fibromyalgia, have MCAS, and we will come to know which mast cell mutation sets are more commonly associated with fibromyalgia than other diseases caused by MCAS – and I believe it is the knowledge of the mutation sets that will lead to the best ideas for treatment.

What causes the disease? That question alone will require decades of effort by an army of researchers. Given that there is a familial predilection for mast cell disease but that different affected members in a given family almost always bear different mutation sets in their mast cells, clearly the mutations causing the mast cell activation in any given patient are not inherited. And yet, if there is a familial predilection for the disease, *something* involved in the development of the disease must be getting inherited. As I hypothesized earlier, perhaps there is some sort of a "genetic fragility factor" that is inherited and which, upon interaction with one stressor (e.g., infection) or another, causes in the marrow stem cell the mutations that eventually "filter down" to the mast cell. If so, perhaps certain mutations result from interactions of certain stressors with the fragility factor, or perhaps the mutations that result occur at random. Or perhaps there are multiple such fragility factors, further increasing the potential complexity of interactions between them and various stressors. Or perhaps this entire line of reasoning is cockamamie and there's some other theory that can explain at least as plausibly both the disease's observed familial predilection and its observed intra-family mutational heterogeneity. What do you think?

Chapter 28: When Ignorance Is More Blissful for the Doctor than the Patient: Education Needs in MCAS

There's an old joke in which the dean of the medical school is giving his welcome address to the matriculating freshmen medical students and tells them, "Half of everything we're going to teach you is wrong. We just don't know which half is the wrong half."

The best jokes are the best jokes, of course, because of their essential truth, and boy is there an awful lot of raw truth in this joke. Indeed, mast cell disease is the perfect demonstration of that truth, since so much of what all medical professionals have been taught for the last century about mast cell disease, and are still being taught today, is now so clearly in the "wrong" half.

Mast cells were first associated with disease – the proliferative cutaneous mast cell disease called urticaria pigmentosa – in 1887, and then another six decades passed before these cells were first associated with proliferative systemic disease in finding that systemic mastocytosis had killed, via wasting, a 1-year-old.

The many other case reports and treatises on various forms of mastocytosis and its biology that ensued formed the basis of the medical profession's tenets of "knowledge" of mast cell disease for the last 130 years, to wit:

(1) "Mast cell disease" is, for all intents and purposes, one (rare) cancer-like disease of too many mast cells, namely, mastocytosis, typically a skin-only disease in childhood but a (ten times less common) systemic disease in adulthood.

(2) Tryptase is a sensitive and specific marker for mast cell disease. If you don't have a significantly elevated (more than double the upper limit of normal) tryptase level, then you don't have mastocytosis, which is to say you don't have a mast cell disease.

The papers on MCAS that have entered the literature since 2007, though, have completely upended this "understanding" of mast cell disease. While it certainly remains true that mastocytosis, in its cutaneous and systemic forms and other, even rarer forms, is a rare disease, it's now crystal clear that mastocytosis is merely the tip of the proverbial iceberg that's now termed in whole "mast cell activation disease," with the body of the iceberg (below a "waterline" of easy clinical recognizability) being the collection of variants of MCAS. Although the overseers of mast cell disease terminology continue, for the time being, to officially recognize a few other mast cell activation diseases (e.g., "idiopathic anaphylaxis") in distinction from MCAS, it seems to me to be quite likely that each of them is actually just another variant of MCAS.

Preliminary research by Dr. Molderings at the University of Bonn, and his colleagues, on the prevalence of MCAS, at least in the German population, shows that roughly one in six adults have a clinical history compatible with MCAS, a figure that's not at all surprising in view of the equivalent prevalence figures for the modern epidemics of chronic inflammatory diseases which increasingly are being found to manifest inappropriate mast cell activation (though causative roles for mast cells in such diseases remains unproven).

Thus, while the medical profession (and the obviously closely related pharmaceutical and health insurance industries) continues to "know" that "mast cell disease = mastocytosis" and "mastocytosis is rare" and thus "mast cell disease is rare," the few physicians world-wide specializing in mast cell disease, and a rapidly enlarging body of Internet-enabled savvy patients, know well that, except for "mastocytosis is rare," these century-old truisms are wrong.

This dichotomy necessarily creates tensions and problems between the joint body of mast cell disease-specializing physicians and MCAS-aware patients vs. (1) the 99.9% of the medical profession that still thinks mast cell disease is rare and is only mastocytosis, (2) the 99.9% of the pharmaceutical industry that still thinks mast cell disease is rare and is only mastocytosis, and (3) the 100% of the health insurance industry that still thinks the same.

As famed astrophysicist and science popularizer Dr. Neil deGrasse Tyson famously quipped, "The great thing about science is that it's true whether you believe it or not." That is, the scientific process/method, when uncorrupted, ensures the truth of a matter will eventually be revealed. Thus, it's inevitable that the medical profession and the pharmaceutical and health insurance industries – the three horsemen of mast cell science, if you will – will come to fully appreciate the true size and character of the iceberg of mast cell activation disease. The path from here to there, though, likely will be long and winding, with a specific route and a transit time that are anything but clear.

(In truth, the (non-pharmaceutical) biomedical research funding "industry" is a fourth "horseman" that can have a substantial impact on advancing mast cell science, though it's my sense of the matter that their present understanding of MCAS is largely in line with the health insurance industry's 0% understanding. I'll leave the biomedical research funders out of further discussion for the time being since I expect their contribution to advancement in this area will be dwarfed by the pharmaceutical industry's contribution once the pharmaceutical industry figures out how prevalent MCAS is.)

Along the way, the horsemen will need to be educated. Let's discuss how to proceed with each of them in turn, but I'm going to save the toughest nut to crack – the medical profession – for last.

I actually don't think it will be all that difficult to educate the pharmaceutical industry or the health insurance industry because there's only one thing that motivates each of them: making money. Make no mistake about it: both of these industries say they're here to help the patient, but the utterly unavoidable fundamental truth of the matter is that they are *businesses*, and aside from the occasional non-profit business (constituting an insignificant fraction of these two industries), businesses exist first and foremost (by a wide lead over any other mission) to make as much money as possible (and preferably in as short a time as possible). In fact, both the pharmaceutical industry and the health insurance industry have the ability – all the more impressive given what behemoths they are – to adjust their operations with almost lightning speed once they sense an opportunity to make more money and/or make it faster. This fact of life has been seen over and over again, but when was the last time (if ever) that anyone ever saw a pharmaceutical firm or a health insurance firm make an adjustment to their operations (e.g., develop a new product) to improve the health of their customers if they didn't think they could make (a lot of) money at it?

The pharmaceutical industry ("Pharma") has one principal way to make money: develop and sell drugs shown to be safe and effective. Pharma has largely ignored mast cell disease because, again, Pharma still has the traditional understanding of the disease, i.e., that it is rare, and given how difficult (not impossible, but difficult) it is to make a lot of money selling drugs to a tiny patient population, Pharma has presumed it would be very difficult to make a lot of money from mast cell disease. But show Pharma that mast cell disease is present in a sixth of the general population, and Pharma will shift its attention to this "new" area so fast it will give you whiplash if you try to watch it.

The health insurance industry is better off than Pharma because it has *two* principal ways to make money: increase what it charges you for insurance, and decrease what it spends on your care. There's nothing about a newfound understanding of mast cell disease by this industry that will reduce the premiums you pay. However, this industry knows very well the vast sums it pays to care for its clients with chronic inflammatory diseases of unknown etiology, so as soon as it becomes aware that mast cell disease underlies many of these diseases, it will muster resources to foster improved diagnosis and treatment of the disease.

So it won't be too hard – maybe just a couple of decades – to educate Pharma and the health insurance industry. But educating the medical profession? That's a whole different ball game, as they say, and to needlessly invoke another metaphor, the medical profession will be the toughest nut to crack because, unlike Pharma and the health insurance industry, there are *two* things that motivate physicians: making money *and* helping patients. As with Pharma and the health insurance industry, making money comes first for the simple reason that, absent the making of money, nothing else is possible. (As they like to say even at academic medical centers with missions that include research and

246

teaching, "No margin, no mission.") But once a reasonable degree of economic security is achieved, most physicians still really do go to work every day for the reason they entered the profession in the first place: they want to help patients. But with mast cell disease perceived (correctly) as a complex disease (and that's just with awareness of mastocytosis, let alone MCAS), physicians know that they generally can't make money taking care of mast cell disease patients – at least, not within the structures of most of the health care financing systems on earth today. Although the Affordable Care Act ("Obamacare") is a step toward reformation, the vast majority of the current U.S. health care financing system still compensates physicians for only two things: seeing patients (regardless of whether such encounters actually help the patients) and performing procedures on patients (regardless of whether such procedures actually help the patients). Mast cell disease patients tend to need few procedures, yet they are so complex and require so much time that they necessarily reduce the number of patients a physician can see in a given unit of time. The physician enters the exam room to see a mast cell disease patient knowing he probably will lose money either in a relative sense (compared to what he could make seeing a greater number of less complex patients in the same amount of time that the one mast cell disease patient will require) or in an absolute sense (where the payment received for seeing the mast cell disease patient literally fails to equal or exceed the costs incurred in seeing the patient). Thus, the absence of any ability for the physician to make money seeing mast cell disease patients is the proverbial Strike One against such patients trying to find physicians to tend to their needs.

Strike Two comes from the fact that the vast majority of physicians have essentially no training in how to manage mast cell disease. If you were an auto mechanic good at managing an internal combustion engine and suddenly somebody asked you, with no training on your part, to manage a nuclear reactor, how would you feel? And what if you were also told, oh, and by the way, if you do agree to try to manage the nuclear reactor out of a good samaritan desire to help those who depend on the reactor, you nevertheless will bear the same legal responsibility for safe, effective management of the reactor as you bear for safe, effective management of internal combustion engines? So what would you do? Almost certainly, you would refuse to take care of the reactor. And in the same fashion, most physicians understandably, and not unreasonably, refuse to take care of mast cell disease patients.

And Strike Three comes from most physicians' naturally conservative behavior. For all the press about how quickly medical *science* is advancing, and in spite of modern requirements for continuing medical education and board re-certification of more recently trained physicians, the fact remains that most physicians, young or old, are very set in their ways and very resistant to change. This can be a good thing – most of the time you want there to be a substantial body of evidence supporting the decisions your doctor makes on your behalf, and there's no getting around the fact that it takes a long time to develop a substantial body of evidence – but it also can be a bad thing in the situations when traditional medical understanding isn't helping and you need your doctor to "think outside the box." Good thing or bad thing, though, the fact is that most physicians are very set in their ways, so when they come out of medical training "knowing" that mast cell disease is rare, and when they see patients with an established diagnosis of mast cell disease only very rarely, they will continue to think the disease is rare and thus warrants far less attention than common diseases (even if the truth of the matter, as they will eventually learn, is that mast cell disease underlies many of the common (if idiopathic) diseases they routinely manage).

Need a Strike Four? The very heterogeneity of mast cell disease certainly qualifies. Diagnosis is an exercise in pattern recognition. How can a physician recognize a disease that can present with virtually any complaints, a vast array of physical exam findings, and requires esoteric lab testing for confirmation of diagnosis?

Thus, most of the time the mast cell disease patient strikes out in trying to find effective local medical care. That's not to say it's impossible to find such care. I'm just openly acknowledging all the "dirty little secrets" about why it's so difficult to find such a doctor.

What needs to be done to fix this? Simply put, a modern understanding of mast cell disease must be infused into medical training at all stages. The fundamental biological concepts of mast cell activation disease need to be taught beginning in the early years of medical school and continuing throughout the rest of the young doctor's clinical training. An appreciation of the clinical heterogeneity of MCAD needs to be taught in the later years of medical school, and basic approaches to diagnosis and management of MCAD need to be taught in residency. Advanced (subspecialty fellowship) training should be upgraded to further reinforce the understanding that new generations of subspecialists will possess as to the myriad different ways that MCAD can present, and subspecialists also must be trained in advanced methods of controlling the disease as it affects the systems of the body they are trained to manage. Continuing medical education programs must be developed for generalists, specialists, and subspecialists to help the existing base of physicians understand the diversity of MCAD presentations and at least the basics of how to manage it.

None of this will come easily, especially given that this fundamentally new concept of the widespread prevalence of mast cell disease, and its heterogeneity of presentation, is 180 degrees opposite from what the profession has been teaching its successive generations for the last 130 years. Thus, all of these training program enhancements will take many years, if not a few decades, to develop. In the end, though, because the profession values adherence to science above all, the truth will eventually come out.

Chapter 29: A Final Case for Thought: Just When You Think You've Seen It All..., or, Smoking Is Bad For You In Ways You Couldn't Possibly Have Imagined

My appreciation for the heterogeneity of the disease has been fueled by the fact that, while there certainly are some symptoms (such as fatigue, rash, aching, and itching) which are more common across the MCAS patient population and many other symptoms which are less common, the full range of problems in each patient is unique to that patient. As I've noted many times in this book thus far, each MCAS patient I've seen has taught me more about the wide range of symptoms and problems the disease can cause, from the polycythemia, burning mouth, and severe anemia (pure red cell aplasia) in the first three patients I diagnosed with MCAS, to the many other patients I described in later chapters with assorted constitutional, gastrointestinal, cardiovascular, pulmonary, neurologic, genitourinary, hematologic, musculoskeletal, endocrinologic, and other troubles. As I've seen more MCAS patients, the range of issues I've seen which seem to be attributable to the disease has steadily expanded.

But in February 2011 I first encountered a patient whose key presentation feature was an abnormality so spectacular that case reports of this phenomenon have been excluded from the peer-reviewed medical literature and presented only in the forensic literature and popular media, strongly suggesting that the treating physicians or medical journal editors (likely both) have been reluctant to jeopardize their credibility by writing and publishing such cases. Indeed, before he would reveal his signature problem to me, the patient – who told me that some of his prior physicians, upon hearing this complaint, had threatened to commit him to a psychiatric hospital – made me swear that I would not do the same. But let me first give you some more background about this patient before I get to the heart of the matter.

> "Mark" was a routine referral to my clinic for recommendations for managing a previously diagnosed "lupus anticoagulant," a type of anti-phospholipid antibody (see Chapter 21) which, despite its name, usually tilts the clotting system away from the bleeding end of the spectrum and toward the clotting end of the spectrum. At the outset of the evaluation, at age 47 Mark, who had already retired from his second career as a corrections officer due to chronic illness, had ostensibly already suffered several heart attacks and strokes (fortunately, and somewhat curiously, without any apparent neurologic sequelae) since about age 37. Two potential clotting system issues – his lupus anticoagulant and a compound heterozygous MTHFR mutation (C677T and A1298C) – had been found by another physician only about four years after his first heart attack.
>
> Thus, before I even started speaking with him, the oddness of the situation – multiple heart attacks and strokes since his 30s? no

neurologic sequelae? *two* clotting system abnormalities? – my "MCAS radar" was already on high alert, and the oddities continued rapidly accumulating as I perused his chart. He had first come into our system around age 42, for evaluation similar to what I was now being asked to perform. My colleagues at that earlier time had noted he had been "in good health" until age 41 when chest pain developed and he was found to have significant coronary artery disease. Two coronary artery stents were placed. Because the prematurity of his vascular disease was recognized, a hematologist was consulted, and she soon found the lupus anticoagulant and the compound heterozygous MTHFR mutation. (The initial consulting hematologists in my system properly noted, however, that his plasma homocysteine level was normal, meaning the MTHFR mutations likely were clinically insignificant.) No other cause for hypercoagulability was found on a fairly thorough search. Chronic anticoagulation was begun, and Mark appeared to be compliant. However, seven months later chest pain recurred, a heart attack was diagnosed, and another two coronary artery stents were placed. During that hospitalization he also developed a left arm clot thought to be catheter-related, but he also developed clots in both legs. Anticoagulation was continued, and the symptoms of these clots soon dissipated.

The initial consulting hematologists in my system also noted his complaints of memory loss for about six months as well as unprovoked syncopal attacks and that he was "very frustrated with his current situation," as one could well imagine. His only other past medical history noted at the time was elevated triglycerides and an old rotator cuff repair. Medications included baby aspirin, clopidogrel, a modest dose of warfarin, ezetimibe and carvedilol, atorvastatin, paroxetine, and alprazolam. Understandably not recognized at the time for the red flag that it was, he reported that diphenhydramine caused confusion. The only family history of note was that his father had died of an aggressive lymphoma in his early 60s, his grandmother had died of stomach cancer, an uncle had died of prostate cancer, and another aunt and uncle had both died from leukemias of some sort. He previously had been a very healthy Marine (discharged at age 34) who used to run (15-20 miles a day!). He had never used tobacco products or illegal substances.

He was recommended by the initial hematology consultants in our system to continue his platelet-inhibiting drugs but to stop his warfarin given that his venous clots had occurred more than six months previously; he also was advised to continue with an evaluation for the syncope that the patient said a neurologist had recently initiated. The lupus anticoagulant test was repeated and was now mysteriously found to be negative.

Almost a year later, at age 43, he suffered his first "seizure," but two EEGs were reportedly unremarkable. He was started on a low dose of an anti-epileptic, but he continued having "seizures" once every 3-6 months. Nearly a year after that, he presented with an automobile accident-related re-injury of the right shoulder rotator cuff tear that originally had been repaired at age 35. He was noted at the time as denying "syncope, paresthesia, or paralysis" but endorsing a history of seizure activity ("of unknown etiology – EEG negative") requiring daily use of a low dose of an anti-epileptic drug, phenytoin. He was noted to have shortness of breath on exertion, and he said he slept with his head elevated on "several" pillows because of this shortness of breath. He reportedly had a low cardiac ejection fraction (30%), presumably from his prior heart attacks. He also complained of intermittent diarrhea (certainly difficult to attribute to any of his other established diagnoses). The diarrhea was ignored (no easy way to fit it into the overall picture, I guess), his cholesterol medication was increased, and he was referred to a psychiatrist for his anxiety and to a neurologist for another evaluation of his seizures.

The neurology consultant interestingly reported learning "...[The seizure] episodes may last up to 20-30 minutes but marked by periods of time where patient will seem to be coming out of it. Occasionally, he'll have bladder incontinence and tends to be very emotionally labile for hours to days after an episode. He does not exhibit automatisms prior to his events nor does he report feelings of aura. He does have a history of syncope but states before his syncopal events he'll feel exhausted, his equilibrium is off, and he sees 'fireflies' in front of his eyes and then he'll pass out. Of note, 2 days ago he had an event at home where he woke up in the hallway and had discovered hours of time had elapsed. He did not have urinary incontinence during this time nor bite his tongue but was very confused afterwards. Patient states that all of his current problems started happening after patient had his heart attacks and stents placed in 2007. He complains of worsening memory problems and worsening anxiety because he never knows when he is going to have another event. He does not work and has lost all interest in his hobbies and activities. He states he used to be a pro golfer and artist as well as very enthusiastic about proper diet and exercise but has lost interest in these things...Of note, patient states he has had major head injury as a child after being beaten and has had 2 episodes when he 'died' – when he was told he had no pulse due to his heart attack in 2007 and when he had an anaphylactic reaction related to Benadryl." The consulting neurologist also recorded that Mark had had a clotting abnormality found at the time of his first heart attack, but he incorrectly identified it as an abnormality in clotting Factor V called the Factor V Leiden mutation – even though the records from that post-heart-attack clotting evaluation clearly stated the Factor V Leiden mutation analysis had yielded a negative, or normal, result and that the actual abnormalities had been the lupus anticoagulant and the MTHFR mutations.

The neurologist was unclear whether Mark was truly having seizures. She ordered a brain MRI and an inpatient video EEG. Mark obtained neither. However, a brain MRI done a year earlier, a few months after the first seizure, had shown only "mild microangiopathic changes" and "increased signal on the FLAIR in the hippocampi which may represent mesial temporal sclerosis" (fibrosis in the brain? how unusual!) but was otherwise normal.

A few months later he was noted to be feeling "frustrated, angry, losing [my] mind, agitation persists, reports amotivation (gives example of not wanting to work on art despite having a gallery interested in his work, reports it is because of frustrated mood). Relations with spouse reportedly difficult; he conveys that immediate family informs him he accuses spouse of being stupid, and his extended family is hostile toward his spouse and stepdaughter, thus creating hostile communication between him and spouse. Reports anhedonia, anergia, difficulty concentrating and making decisions. Denies sense of worthlessness, denies excessive guilt. Reports appetite as stable without weight gain or loss. Denies thoughts of death, suicidal ideation, homicidal ideation or auditory/visual hallucinations. Last played golf 2 weeks ago, shot a 75, reports had not played for 6 months prior. Reports having problems at times if there is new staff that do not recognize him as a golf pro and being charged for a bucket of balls, reports difficulty in resolving such situations in a calm manner."

A few months later (January 2010) he again suffered chest pain and went to his local hospital, where another heart attack was diagnosed. An angiogram found "complete thrombotic occlusion of the mid left anterior descending coronary artery" and another stent was placed. He was seen in follow-up by a cardiologist in our system a month later (one year before I first saw him). The errant history of a Factor V Leiden mutation was carried forward (and without any mention of the true clotting system abnormalities). Mark reported to the cardiologist that "since his recent [heart attack], he is extremely tired and weak, gets short of breath with minimal exertion and goes back to bed. No chest pain… Unclear if he has severe atherosclerotic coronary artery disease or it is all related with thrombus formation secondary to his Factor V Leiden mutation… Given his increasing fatigue, we will plan to obtain an echocardiogram… Since his most recent [heart attack] was on clopidogrel and aspirin, we will start him on prasugrel."

The echocardiogram was done in March 2010; there was diminished movement of several aspects of the heart, but overall it was still pumping a normal amount of blood (well improved from the earlier 30% figure) and showed no other abnormalities.

At the end of 2010 his primary physician joined the parade of errant notations of the patient's Factor V Leiden mutation status (and also failed to note the true coagulation system abnormalities). He reported the patient had been doing well following his most recent heart attack "until the past few months when he started with multiple syncopal episodes. He has been to the ER a few times for these emergencies. He complains of being overheated, and most seriously he has become extremely fearful and anxious he is going to have another heart attack. He is depressed in spite of citalopram and alprazolam... Generally feels miserable, anxious depressed fearful, has weight loss, and anorexia, chest pain, shortness of breath, palpitations, erectile dysfunction, urinary frequency, and low back pain and other joint pain."

He was referred to my clinic for further evaluation of his clotting problem, and that's what led to my initially seeing him in February 2011. As I previously said, the oddity of his situation already had my "MCAS radar" on alert. As I wrote in his chart at the time, "This 47-year old white male is kindly referred in consultation regarding further evaluation and management of hypercoagulability from compound heterozygous MTHFR mutations and lupus anticoagulant – and though these hypercoagulability issues may have played some role in his MIs in '05, '06, and '10 as well as his seizures which have been attributed to thrombotic stroke-like events these past few years, the hypercoagulability clearly is just one more aspect of a much broader syndrome of illness he has been suffering for at least a dozen years. This formerly healthy, formerly very physically active man provides a fascinating history of chronic multisystem polymorbidity beginning with onset about a dozen years ago – shortly after a relocation from California to Louisiana – of relatively frequent syncopal episodes which have continued ever since and which have always been attributed to heat stroke/exhaustion even though most of the episodes clearly have not been associated with major heat exposure or physical activity anywhere near extreme enough to cause heat stroke. He also endorses frequent migraine headaches, fevers, chills, feeling cold all the time, diffusely migratory pruritus, frequent soaking sweats, mild irritation of both eyes, minimal nasal irritation, absent oral/pharyngeal/laryngeal irritation, absent dysphagia, chronic waxing/waning dyspnea, frequent anginal-type and non-anginal-type chest pain, treatment-refractory GERD, frequent nausea, frequent post-prandial diarrhea and abdominal pain/discomfort, absent constipation, diffusely migratory rashes, migratory edema, migratory sensory (tingling/numbness) neuropathies, and frequent spells of cognitive dysfunction. He reports many additional odd events including severely pruritic, instant reaction to Benadryl (same to

Vistaril), and an episode a year or so ago when large welts spontaneously developed across his back. Note he relocated from Louisiana to South Carolina around 2001. He's presently retired. Review of systems otherwise negative. The family history is rife with cancer and leukemia but not hypercoagulability."

In medical school physicians are trained to prize "open-ended" questions over "closed-ended" questions. At the end of the history, I asked him if he had anything else he wanted to tell me, and this open-ended question ultimately yielded the most fascinating piece of history I have ever gotten from any patient (MCAS or otherwise). First, though, Mark appeared to carefully contemplate my question. It was obvious he was weighing whether to reveal something else that was on his mind. Eventually he acknowledged there was something else going on, but he wanted me to first promise him that I would not commit him to a psychiatric hospitalization if he told me about this other problem. I asked why he would want me to promise him this, and he said that more than one of his doctors in the past had threatened to "put me away" after he revealed this mystery problem, so he understandably had become quite wary about discussing this with anybody who might have the power to "put him away."

Of course, I promised him I would do no such thing and again asked him what else was on his mind. As I noted in his chart, he then told me about "…an episode some months back when, while engaged in a basketball game, he began 'smoking' (smoke-like mist began emanating from all about his body and was visible to passing motorists 50-100 feet away) and 'it looked like I was going to spontaneously combust.'" I also noted he was "under the care of a psychiatrist, as it has been implied he has been hallucinating or otherwise imagining much of the bizarreness that has been happening to him these past dozen years."

The exam was notable for its complete normality – except that "a light scratch test on the upper back resulted in mild-moderate dermatographism quickly arising, sustained for at least 15 minutes."

My goodness. What to do with all of this? Clearly he had a hypercoagulable state – and clearly that state was none of the hypercoagulable states we're trained to look for. But, just as clearly, there was no way that any hypercoagulable state could possibly cause anywhere close to the full range of problems he had had and was continuing to have. The range of issues here was such that only MCAS could be the root issue here, and I could readily imagine how the episode of spontaneous arising of bruise-like welts all about his body (such that the ER physician had separated him from his wife and asked him whether he was the victim of spousal abuse!) might be the result of an MCAS flare dominantly featuring heparin release, but that still left the extreme mystery of how MCAS might cause him to literally smoke, i.e., how MCAS might cause the temperature of the human body to rise so high as to cause spontaneous combustion of human tissue. I mean, it was still possible that he was hallucinating such an event, but at the next visit, when his wife accompanied him, she made it clear that if it was a hallucination, it was a mass hallucination that had been shared by dozens of people who had all seen what really looked to be smoke emanating from all about the extremely hot body of the acutely greatly weakened and confused Mark. Teammates and other onlookers had applied various methods to help cool him down (pouring cold water on him, fanning air at him, etc.), and the smoking had stopped after perhaps about 5-10 minutes. He finally rallied enough strength and clarity of thought about an hour later to return home.

I guessed it was also theoretically possible that some issue other than MCAS was causing this "smoking" while MCAS was causing all of the other problems, but obviously it made a whole lot more sense – Occam's Razor! – if MCAS were causing all of the problems including the "smoking."

Clearly, Mark needed to be tested for MCAS, but it was also once again – as I have had to do so many times since starting to figure out Patient #1 – time to hit the books.

Actually, I had heard previously of the alleged phenomenon of spontaneous human combustion, and, like every other normal person, I hadn't thought much of it, imagining it to be hallucination or hoax of some sort – but here I had in front of me a real, live patient who had had a real, live, multiply witnessed episode of spontaneous human combustion (actually, by the time of the second visit it was now two such episodes), and there simply was no way it was mass hallucination, nor was there the slightest reason for the patient or anybody else to be perpetrating any hoax, let alone a hoax as bizarre as this. No, this was not imaginary. He really had started smoking, and therefore spontaneous human combustion must be possible. Furthermore, it was most likely that MCAS was the root of all of his problems, so it was now "simply" a matter of figuring out at least one mechanism by which MCAS might theoretically drive spontaneous combustion.

In the pre-Internet (indeed, the pre-Yahoo/Google) era, reviewing the literature on something like this would have been very challenging. There simply was no medical literature on the subject (not that I could readily find, anyway). But lack of medical literature didn't mean the phenomenon didn't exist. Clearly, the phenomenon, while rare, did exist, so I would have to turn to other literature.

And, as Google and Google Scholar quickly revealed, it was the forensic literature that bore what I was looking for.

It turned out that about 100 cases of spontaneous human combustion have been reported in the forensic literature and popular media over the last century. The great majority of the cases were deaths, and the pattern was essentially always the same: the victim had had no known prior medical problems and was later found, alone and dead, with all of the body fat and bones reduced to ash, with all of the rest of the tissues remaining relatively intact (perhaps with a bit of charring). If the incident had happened indoors, there almost always was a pink grease stain on the ceiling, presumably the residue of combusting human fat. And no matter how much combustible material (paper, wood, fabric, etc.) was in contact with, or in immediate proximity to, the body, such material was never found burnt. Autopsies had never yielded any medical explanation, and these cases all remained total mysteries. There also were a few cases of survivors who had only produced smoke for a few minutes, never flames, but no other details of their ordeals, let alone their medical histories, were available.

First: why just the fat and bones? Actually, the issue with the bones was immediately obvious to this hematologist: bone marrow typically contains great quantities of fat. If all the rest of the fat in the body is burnt by some metabolic catastrophe, one would expect at least the marrow in the bones, and perhaps also the adjacent bones themselves, to also burn. So, for all intents and purposes, we could eliminate one variable and simply say that it was all the fat that burned.

But why just the fat? What is it about human fat that would make it so much more (reliably!) susceptible to combustion? Another quick answer from a bit of Googling: fat actually has a lower ignition point than any other human tissue, actually less than the boiling point of water, about 90 degrees Celsius.

So what on earth could cause human fat tissue, ordinarily at 37 degrees Celsius (i.e., normal body temperature), to suddenly ramp up its temperature by a phenomenal 53 degrees Celsius?

More Googling, and reading of a number of papers on certain aspects of basic human biochemistry, led to a possible answer.

As it turns out, human fat tissue is perfectly primed to be an engine of hyperthermia because it already is the principal source of heat in the human body (in addition to being one of the principal sources of energy in general). Like all cells, fat cells ("adipocytes") contain little energy/heat-generating power plants called mitochondria, and mitochondria contain a regulatory protein called UCP-1 (uncoupling protein 1). Ordinarily, mitochondria convert fatty acids (via oxidation, for you biochemists out there) contained within the adipocyte into the principal form of energy that's used throughout the human body, a molecule called adenosine triphosphate (ATP). UCP-1, though, is a "switch" which, when turned on, causes the energy coming from oxidation of fatty acids to be released as heat rather than being channeled into production of ATP.

Obviously, under normal circumstances, the "decision" as to how much of the energy in the fatty acids is to be converted to ATP vs. how much is to be released as heat is a very carefully regulated process. And even when one has an infection and a fever is produced, obviously the balance between ATP production vs. heat production is set off from normal by only a slight amount.

But what if – *what if?* – a hugely greater number of the UCP-1 switches in the adipocyte mitochondria than normal were suddenly flipped on? How much heat could be produced?

Time for a bit more Googling and a little bit of math…

It turned out that various research teams had already done most of the work. It had long been known that the average human adipocyte has about 1000-2000 mitochondria. And it also turns out that the average human has about 50 billion adipocytes (more like 70 billion in the average weightier American). And, finally, it turned out that the average adipocyte could generate around 5 nanowatts of heat.

A little bit of multiplication (50 billion times 5 billionths) and…oh, my goodness, it turns out that if most of the UCP-1 in our adipocyte mitochondria were to suddenly get switched on, the fat alone in our bodies could suddenly generate 250 watts of heat. A little more math…and now we see that, yes, indeed, sudden severe dysregulation of UCP-1 could easily escalate the temperature of at least some portion of our fat tissue to the ignition point – all the while the rest of our cells keep working (albeit less and less as the ambient temperature in the body keeps rising) so that blood keeps pumping and the fat cells survive just long enough to finally hit that ignition point. And once some portion of the fat ignites, the combustion process should become self-sustaining, since obviously fat itself is an excellent fuel. And all of the fat in the body will just keep combusting – at a low enough temperature that the rest of the tissues don't ignite – until all of the fuel (the fat) is gone.

All of which leaves one critical question: how on earth could mast cell dysfunction cause UCP-1 to switch on?

Again, a bit of Googling and reading some basic human biochemistry papers leads us to a possible answer.

As it turns out, there are many proteins that regulate the "position" of the UCP-1 "switch" – and one of them is norepinephrine, which is a known mediator product of the mast cell.

And as it also turns out, adipose tissue is a known mast cell reservoir.

Therefore, what if "just the right" (or, more appropriately, "just the wrong") variant of MCAS were to yield a reservoir in adipose tissue of mast cells dysfunctional in a manner such that, in response to a sudden great stressor, these cells were to suddenly release a flood of norepinephrine (or some other UCP-1 activator) – much as Mark's mast cells obviously were occasionally releasing floods of heparin – which would then cause enough acute adipocyte heat release to ignite at least one field of adipose tissue, after which it's inevitable that all the rest of the adipose tissue will eventually burn, too. Meanwhile, of course, once the ambient temperature in the other tissues rises much above 42 Celsius (about 108 Fahrenheit), death quickly ensues (be it cardiac or neurologic in origin likely matters not), but meanwhile the fire has already started, and it will continue until the fuel is gone, regardless of whether the victim is still alive or dead. (Mark, fortunately, was surrounded by friends and family who saw the process beginning and cooled him down so he never fully ignited.)

(Parenthetically, I feel inclined to note at this point that there has long been recognized a rare catastrophic acute illness called neuroleptic malignant syndrome (NMS). NMS can be seen with use of any neuroleptic agent and manifests with mental status changes, muscular rigidity, hyperthermia, and autonomic instability. Is it possible that malignant hyperthermia is a less spectacular form of drug-exposure-triggered MCAS-driven hyperthermic catastrophe than spontaneous combustion?)

Ironically, only two months after I first met Mark, I heard of yet another case of spontaneous human combustion covered by the popular media. A man in a porn shop in San Francisco reportedly had suddenly erupted in flames and had run out of the shop into the street before collapsing. He was taken to the burn unit of a local hospital. Police investigation found no source of combustion. Given my hypothesis by that point that spontaneous human combustion might be the consequence of an acute stress causing enough release of norepinephrine by adipose tissue mast cells to raise the temperature of such tissue to the ignition point, I wondered whether it might have been the stress of sexual excitement that could have caused the event in this victim. Through news reports and Google, I tracked down the San Francisco medical examiner and the chief of the burn unit at the hospital to which the patient had been taken. I e-mailed them regarding my theory and suggested that a work-up for MCAS would not be unreasonable, but, unsurprisingly (☺), I never heard anything from either of them.

> Meanwhile, what happened with Mark? Indeed, his urinary prostaglandin D_2 level was significantly elevated (500 pg/ml, normal 100-280). With H_1 and H_2 antihistamines alone, he stopped having his episodes of smoking and bruise-like welting, and when benzodiazepines were added in, anxiety significantly improved. Clearly, he met all of the current proposed consensus diagnostic criteria for MCAS. Unfortunately, soon after starting benzodiazepines, he relocated a significant distance away for family-related reasons, and I've never received any follow-up.

I am convinced spontaneous human combustion is real, though it obviously will be difficult to prove my hypothesis as to its etiology. To this day, though, I haven't come across any evidence proving my hypothesis can't hold water.

One final comment about this case: remember how the wife of a very bruised Mark was taken aside in one ER visit and questioned about whether she had been beating her spouse? She's certainly not the only spouse/partner of an MCAS patient who I've heard so accused. And it's not necessarily just accusations of beating vis-à-vis bruises. One husband of a patient told me that during *several* of his chronically mysteriously markedly ill (and often confused) wife's presentations to the ER, he was taken aside by the ER doctors and accused of "somehow" poisoning his wife, and the ER doctors were forever suspicious but couldn't do anything about it because all of the extensive toxicology testing (metal exposures, legal and illegal drugs, etc.) they performed trying to find the poison all kept yielding negative results. How inclined would you be to keep seeking emergency care for your acutely-on-top-of-chronically markedly ill spouse if you *knew* the ER doctors almost certainly weren't going to find the cause and, even worse, were going to threaten you once again with criminal accusations that you knew were nonsensical?

Chapter 30: "What's Next?"

I really enjoy Aaron Sorkin's dramas, and though I haven't had a chance to watch the productions of all this remarkably prolific man has written, I managed to catch almost every episode of *The West Wing*, whose lead character, U.S. President Jed Bartlet, had a catchphrase I appreciated: "What's next?" Even at the worst of times (such as when post-op from a nearly successful assassination attempt), his strength was evident from his utterance (a whispering, really, at that particular point) of that merely two-word phrase – and I think it's an apt title for this last chapter, which is intended to suggest direction.

You now know what MCAS is. The question for *you* now is, "What's next?" Where do *you* go with this knowledge?

Left to its own ends, modern medicine will figure this out – eventually. For all of its faults, medicine nevertheless remains grounded in science, and, again, the great thing about science is that it eventually speaks the truth of what is studied. There may be great delays in getting around to studying a particular subject, and there may be all sorts of biases and other reasons why initial and intermediate determinations about a particular subject are errant in one direction or another, to one degree or another – but in the end, science really does speak the truth of what is studied. It must, for describing the truth of the natural world is the very essence of science. Anything else isn't science, and since medicine is grounded in science, medicine, too, must – eventually – see and speak the truth of the natural world of human biology and disease.

So the issue really isn't *whether* MCAS will be recognized more widely as a "real disease" or *whether* we will ever understand its molecular roots. There's already copious data proving it's a real disease (regardless of whether one "believes" it's a primary disease of mutational origin or a secondary disease reacting to some mysterious provocation). It's beginning to get discussed at some professional society meetings and in some medical school classrooms and some teaching clinics, and it's beginning to be studied more, such that it's just a matter of time until it's widely accepted as a real disease and it's routinely taught and diagnosed and treated and studied.

It's just a matter of time.

And *that* is the real issue: how much time?

Again, left to its own ends, modern medicine will figure all of this out – eventually.

But do you want to wait for modern medicine to figure it all out at modern medicine's own (typically very slow) pace? Or do you want to see it get figured out sooner?

If you want to see it get figured out sooner, *you* need to do something about it.

Perhaps you are, or someday will be, in a position in which you can do *a lot* about it (e.g., help connect a potential major funder to a doctor leading to diagnosis and successful treatment of MCAS). More likely, though, you're in a position in which you can do *at least something* about it. I seriously doubt you are in a position to do *absolutely nothing* about it. But *your* doing even a little bit about it, together with many other folks also doing little bits about it in their own ways will quickly add up to a whole lot being done about it.

First, and perhaps most importantly, if you have MCAS or think you might have MCAS, you need a local physician (or nurse practitioner or physician assistant) to be your "primary partner" for dealing with it. Here and now in the 20-teens, that physician – who might be a primary care physician or might be a specialist/subspecialist – likely won't know much about MCAS (at least, not to start with), but he can still be your "first contact" for problems you're having from the disease and your conduit to other expertise (whether in the MCAS area or other areas) for dealing with the acute and chronic problems the disease causes. Fundamentally, though, everybody with MCAS – indeed, everybody with *any* disease as complex as MCAS – needs a *local* primary professional partner to be the *first* resource to consult for assistance (except, obviously, in cases of emergency, in which case an emergency resource such as 911 or an emergency room should be the first resource to visit or consult). Expertise may be available at a distance, but the distance itself makes distant expertise a decidedly *secondary* resource.

Therefore, if you have MCAS or think you might have MCAS, and if you don't have such a "primary partner" among your present assortment of local health care resources – especially if none of your present physicians "believes" that MCAS exists or is willing to serve as your primary partner for dealing with it – then you need to begin a search for such a partner and *keep searching* until you find one. I understand that many patients live in smaller communities with limited physician resources, and I understand it's possible (in both smaller and larger communities) to search all *presently available* local physician resources for an "effective partner" and come up empty – but that doesn't mean it will always be that way in your community, and when your first search comes up empty, you simply need to keep (politely) urging the available physicians in your community to consider exploring MCAS as a potentially better diagnosis for you than "I don't know," and you need to remain alert for new physicians coming into the area, especially younger physicians whose more up-to-date education might have inculcated in them a very different attitude of "Of course MCAS exists."

You can join mast cell disease support organizations, national and regional, and participate in their activities. Patient privacy interests are paramount, but if you have a diagnostic or therapeutic success story that you're willing to share, then share it! Post your story on-line. Submit your story to your local newspaper and ask if they'd be willing to publish it – or if they'd even be willing to have one of their journalists write a story about you and/or the disease. (Direct the simple stories to video and radio outlets; save the complicated stories for newspapers and on-line forums. For lots of obvious reasons, video and radio are far less effective than print at conveying complex stories.)

If you have an effective local physician partner, try to leverage his connection network and ask him/her how you can advocate for MCAS awareness within the local community of health care professionals. Perhaps there is a hematologist, or allergist, or rheumatologist, or internist who would be interested in giving, at a local professional society meeting, a talk on the subject that would be enlivened by a patient's (i.e., your) personal presentation. Even if you don't have an effective local partner, you can still write to relevant local and regional professional societies and ask if they'd be willing to have a patient contribute a story for their proceedings or journal or speak at one of their meetings; perhaps the leaders of some societies, intrigued by such an opportunity, might then solicit for a society member to provide a professional presentation to accompany your patient's-perspective presentation.

Contact potential research funders (e.g., the National Institutes of Health, major pharmaceutical firms) and those who influence those funders (e.g., legislators, major investors), asking if they're aware of MCAS and how it might be connected with the diagnoses you've been given (e.g., fibromyalgia). Include, or point them to, a review article – any review article – from the peer-reviewed medical literature. They may have no interest in reading it, but the mere appearance of a subject being discussed in the peer-reviewed medical literature conveys influential *gravitas*. In your letters and contacts, encourage research into potential connections between MCAS and other chronic inflammatory diseases of yet unknown cause. It may be impossible at present to get research funding for "MCAS," but it might be a lot easier to get research funding for, say, "fibromyalgia." You may well never get any response to any of your letters and contacts, but it is your very planting of an idea sure to be novel to the recipient that will be your greatest contribution. As Christopher Nolan penned for his 2010 film *Inception*, "Once an idea has taken hold of the brain, it's almost impossible to eradicate." Your letter may be dismissed by a recipient today, but a year from now, when the recipient becomes aware of an acquaintance or family member suffering a wide range of inflammatory problems with no evident unifying diagnosis, the idea of MCAS may resurface, to possibly significant ends on both small and large scales.

Finally, whenever possible, try to coordinate with others in your efforts so as to demonstrate strength in numbers (larger wheels are squeakier than smaller wheels, and squeakier wheels get more grease) while minimizing wastage of the recipient's time in managing redundant supplications. No sense irritating those who are best positioned to help.

Thank you for buying this book, thank you for your attention these last 200 pages or so, and best of luck in whatever your dealings with MCAS may be.

"What's next?"

Do Something.

I'm doing something. Will you?

Appendix 1: Medical Terms Used in This Book: How to Pronounce Them and What They Mean

5

5-HIAA

See 5-hydroxyindoleacetic acid.

5-hydroxyindoleacetic acid

"fĭv hy-drox´-ee-in-dohl´-ee-uh-seet´-ik ass´-id." Quite a mouthful, which is why it's always abbreviated (in writing and in speech), as simply "5-HIAA." 5-HIAA is a natural chemical product in the human body whose level in the urine is expected to substantially elevate when the patient has a type of neuroendocrine cancer called "carcinoid" which can produce some symptoms (e.g., flushing, diarrhea, wheezing) which can mimic mast cell disease. Although carcinoid is rare, traditionally it has been taught that it is more common than the ultra-rare mastocytosis (which, again, has long been, and still is, the only mast cell disease taught in most medical training programs), so it's common for patients with mast cell disease of any form – particularly if their symptoms include otherwise mysterious flushing, diarrhea, or wheezing – to have been previously suspected of possibly having carcinoid and thus to have been previously tested for urinary 5-HIAA levels. In a mast cell disease patient, the 5-HIAA level (usually tested on a 24-hour urine collection rather than a small, random (or "spot") urine collection) will be normal or perhaps slightly elevated, far below the substantially elevated levels (many times above the upper limit of normal) seen in most carcinoid patients. A special type of radiology procedure, too – an octreotide scan (or "Octreoscan"), performed in the radiology department's nuclear medicine section – is sometimes used to detect the location of a carcinoid tumor (a starkly elevated 5-HIAA level merely says a carcinoid is likely present but doesn't say where; the scan then can help pin down the location in case it's localized enough where surgical removal might be helpful), and thus some patients ultimately diagnosed with mast cell disease have previously undergone not only a urinary 5-HIAA test but also an octreotide scan to try to detect the carcinoid that the doctors think surely must be present to explain the patient's otherwise unexplainable flushing, diarrhea, or wheezing.

A

Abscess

"Ab´-sess." A collection of infecting microorganisms, usually together with a range of white blood cells responding to the infection at that spot. These infection-attacking blood cells are naturally white in color and create the whiteness of the pus that one sometimes drains from an abscess, which is how they came to be called "white" blood cells, or leukocytes, in the first place. Since mast cell disease often impedes the functioning of the immune system, leading to increased susceptibility to infection among other effects, it is not uncommon to find abscesses (though fortunately usually small, such as in acne-like "folliculitis" in the skin) from time to time in patients with mast cell disease.

Accolate

See Zafirlukast.

Acetaminophen

"Uh-seet´-uh-min´-oh-fen." Also known around the world (i.e., outside the U.S. and Japan) as paracetamol (pronounced "par´-uh-seet´-uh-mol") or APAP (pronounced "ay´-pap"), this commonly used, inexpensive oral drug reduces pain and fever but has too little anti-inflammatory activity to be classified among the non-steroid anti-inflammatory drugs (NSAIDs). Although its mechanism of action is not entirely understood, acetaminophen seems to work in at least two principal ways, one by blocking some of the cyclo-oxygenases such as COX2 and COX3 (the cyclo-oxygenases are enzymes which help produce mediators that result in a sensation of pain; note that it's the COX1 cyclo-oxygenase, blocked little by acetaminophen but much more so by NSAIDs such as aspirin and ibuprofen, that leads to prominent inflammatory effects). The other principal way that acetaminophen seems to work is by blocking nerve cell (neuronal) reuptake of a signaling molecule called anandamide, which leads to high levels of anandamide persisting in the spaces ("synapses") between nerve cells, and such levels lead to desensitization of a nerve cell receptor called TRPV1, which is the body's main pain receptor.

Acetazolamide

> "Uh-seet´-uh-zohl´-uh-mīd." Acetazolamide is a medication that inhibits the enzyme carbonic anhydrase, with effects in the kidney leading to excretion in the urine of sodium, chloride, and bicarbonate, which in turn carries more water, too, out into the urine, thus giving the drug its "diuretic" effect that helps reduce blood pressure, intracranial pressure (which can help with some forms of seizure disorder and certain other neurologic illnesses), and intraocular pressure (which can help with glaucoma). Its most common trade name, at least in the U.S., is Diamox.

Activin A

> "Act´-i-vin A." Activin A is a signaling molecule made by certain marrow and blood cells, among other cells, and seems to have a wide range of effects including stimulating red blood cell production.

Acute lymphocytic leukemia

> "Uh-kyoot´ limf´-oh-sit´-ik loo-keem´-ee-uh." Acute lymphocytic leukemia (ALL) is a cancer of marrow stem cells leading to excessive production of the "lymphoid" type of leukocytes, or white blood cells, as opposed to excessive production of the "myeloid" type of leukocytes, which would result in a somewhat similar disease called acute myelogenous leukemia (AML). As the "acute" would imply, both ALL and AML progress rapidly and can easily cause death within weeks to a few months of first emerging.

Acute myelogenous leukemia

> "Uh-kyoot´ my´-el-oj´-en-us loo-keem´-ee-uh." Acute myelogenous leukemia (AML) is a cancer of marrow stem cells leading to excessive production of the "myeloid" type of leukocytes, or white blood cells, as opposed to excessive production of the "lymphoid" type of leukocytes, which would result in a somewhat similar disease called acute lymphocytic leukemia (ALL). As the "acute" would imply, both AML and ALL progress rapidly and can easily cause death within weeks to a few months of first emerging.

Adalimumab

> "Ad´-uh-lim´-oo-mab." As the "mab" at the end of its name indicates, adalimumab is a bioengineered (human) monoclonal

antibody that binds to tumor necrosis factor alpha (TNF-alpha, a major inflammatory mediator that can be produced by mast cells and plenty of other types of cells, too) and thereby prevents TNF-alpha from binding to, and activating, TNF-alpha receptors that sit on the surfaces of a variety of cells, thus blocking all of the downstream effects of such binding which would ultimately result in TNF-alpha's inflammatory effects. The trade name for adalimumab in the U.S. is Humira ("Hyu-meer´-uh").

Adenoidectomy

"Ad´-uh-noid-ect´-uh-mee." Removal (usually by surgery) of the "adenoid" lymph nodes at the back of the throat. Patients who suffer frequent episodes of throat inflammation may find such problems attributed by their doctors (rightly or wrongly) to infection in the "adenoid" lymph nodes and in the "tonsil" lymph nodes (both sets of lymph nodes located at the back of the throat), leading their doctors to remove the tonsils (tonsillectomy) and adenoids (adenoidectomy) (or a "T&A" in slang doctor-speak). This is more commonly done in childhood than adulthood. Of course, if the underlying problem causing such inflammation is mast cell disease, this surgery may not result in significant reduction in the episodic upper respiratory inflammatory issues.

ADHD

"A-D-H-D." ADHD stands for attention deficit hyperactivity disorder, a chronic neuropsychiatric developmental disorder (in which the patient obviously is hyperactive and has difficulty remaining focused on the task at hand) which perhaps is overdiagnosed (especially in kids) but nevertheless is a real disease in at least some patients with some relationship to the chronic anxiety disorders. There are interesting findings emerging in the medical literature showing that the more asthma- and allergic-type disease (likely implying the presence of abnormal mast cell activation) one suffers as a toddler, the higher one's risk for ADHD (and, for that matter, autism). It is tempting, therefore, to speculate that ADHD in some patients (and autism in some patients) is a consequence of MCAS, but far more research must be done to prove such a hypothesis.

Adipose tissue

"Ad´-i-pos tish´-oo." Fat. Seriously, that's what adipose tissue is: fat tissue. Interestingly, we've been learning in the last several years that in addition to mast cells preferentially siting themselves at the body's environmental interfaces and around blood and lymph vessels, there's a significant number of mast cells in the body's adipose tissue, too. And since the prostaglandin D_2 produced by the mast cell, and plenty of other mast cell mediators, have some influence in the development of fat tissue, one wonders whether MCAS might be as much of an underlying issue in the development of obesity (which we now understand to be a chronic inflammatory disease) as much as it might be an underlying issue in the development of other chronic inflammatory diseases such as inflammatory/irritable bowel syndrome, fibromyalgia, and chronic fatigue syndrome. More research to be done, for sure…

Adrenal gland

"Uh-dreen-ul gland." Kind of a thickish disc of an organ, one sitting more or less on top of each kidney, responsible for sensing the state of various systems in the body and pumping out a large assortment of hormones to keep those systems ship-shape. Yes, mast cell disease not only can cause tissue/organ havoc through the mediators it incorrectly directly pumps out, but it also can cause havoc by influencing the adrenal glands to incorrectly pump out various hormones. Again, normal mast cells can affect, and can be affected, by all sorts of bodily processes, and in turn *abnormal* mast cells have the potential to cause abnormalities in every tissue, organ, and system.

Adrenaline

"Uh-dren´-uh-lin." An older name for epinephrine.

Advil

"Ad-vil." One of the most common trade names in the U.S. for ibuprofen.

Albuterol

"Al-byoo´-ter-ol." Albuterol is a medication, usually inhaled, that binds with "beta-2-adrenergic receptors" in the airways to cause the airways to relax, thus relieving the shortness of breath and even wheezing that can come from the tightening and constriction of the airways that can happen in various respiratory diseases such as asthma and chronic obstructive pulmonary disease (COPD). Since inflammation from mast cell disease sometimes drives airway constriction, it shouldn't be surprising that some mast cell disease patients sometimes find albuterol useful when their flares of their disease cause shortness of breath or wheezing. Ventolin (pronounced "Vent′-oh-lin") is the trade name for a commonly used brand of albuterol.

Alemtuzumab

"Al′-em-too′-zoo-mab." As the "mab" at the end of its name indicates, alemtuzumab is a bioengineered monoclonal antibody that binds to "CD52," a molecule found on the surfaces of various types of cells including certain lymphocytes and mast cells. The binding of alemtuzumab to CD52 initiates certain processes that eventually result in the destruction of the CD52-bearing cell. Alemtuzumab can provide temporary benefit in some patients with mastocytosis, but its side effects are significant enough (principally, a very substantial suppression of the immune system) that it doesn't make any sense to use it unless the patient has a relatively aggressive form of mastocytosis. Perhaps there will come a time when alemtuzumab is found useful in particularly severe forms of MCAS (it's unlikely its use could be justified in less symptomatic forms), but it will take much careful research to adequately vet that question. Alemtuzumab's most common trade name, at least in the U.S., is Campath.

Alendronate

"Al-en′-droh-nāt." Also known as alendronic acid, this oral medication is in the class of bisphosphonates (see Bisphosphonates). In the U.S., the most common trade name for alendronate is Fosomax ("Fo′-so-max").

Aleve

"Uh-leev." One of the most common trade names in the U.S. for naproxen.

Allergen

"Al′-er-jen." Any substance (natural or artificial, environmental or food or medication) which provokes an allergic reaction.

Alprazolam

"Al-praz′-oh-lam." A medication in the benzodiazepine class, alprazolam has a short half-life, so although it can help anxiety and other problems soon after taking it, its effects tend to wear off relatively quickly. The most recognized trade name for alprazolam in the U.S. is Xanax (pronounced "zan-ax").

Alzheimer's disease

"Alz´-hy-merz di´-zeez." An eventually fatal condition of chronic degeneration of the brain, clinically causing dementia, but usually with initial emergence of symptoms much earlier than would be expected from "normal" age-related dementia. Alzheimer's is the most common form of dementia. Given that early symptoms are similar to the "brain fog" episodically suffered by mast cell patients, and given that stress (which can cause flares of mast cell activation) makes Alzheimer's symptoms worse, there are unanswered questions about whether activation of (normal or abnormal) mast cells might be playing some role in the development of this disease. Mast-cell-targeted drugs have been, and are being, tried in the treatment of Alzheimer's.

Ambien

See Zolpidem.

Amicar

"Am´-i-car." See Aminocaproic acid.

Aminocaproic acid

"Uh-meen´-oh-cap´-roh-ic ass´-id." Aminocaproic acid is an inhibitor of the coagulation-related process of fibrinolysis, in which strands and networks of a coagulation protein called fibrin – a major part of any clot/scab – are broken down. Fibrinolysis, of course, is a natural process (how else would a scab get broken down?), but when the process is incorrectly "amped up" (as can happen in some patients with diseases like mast cell disease or a variety of rare coagulation system disorders), it results in persistent bleeding because the network of fibrin strands doesn't get enough time to plug the break in the blood vessel before it gets broken down. Mast cell disease seems to cause, at least in some patients, a fibrinolytic state which can be mild (or worse) at baseline – and which can get much worse when there is a flare of the disease, sometimes even leading to spontaneous bleeding/bruising. Aminocaproic acid inhibits fibrinolysis and thus can be helpful in some situations of excessive fibrinolysis and resulting bleeding such as what can be seen with mast cell disease. The danger in using it, of course, is that it will "tip the teeter-totter" of the coagulation system in the other direction and that excessive clotting will then begin to develop. Aminocaproic acid's most recognized trade name in the U.S. is Amicar.

270

Aminocaproic acid is one of the two most commonly used fibrinolytic inhibitors (the other is tranexamic acid).

Amitriptyline

"Am´-i-trip´-tih-leen." An oral anti-depressant medication in the "tricyclic" class, one of the oldest classes of anti-depressants. As with all tricyclic anti-depressants, amitriptyline has some "anti-cholinergic" properties including sedation, a drying effect (in mucosa in the sinuses, mouth, and elsewhere), and a muscle-inhibiting effect such as in the intestinal and urinary tracts where constipation and difficulty urinating might be consequences. The tricyclics also have some histamine H_1 receptor blocking effect, so it can help somewhat with mast cell disease. The most recognized trade name for amitriptyline in the U.S. is Elavil.

Amotivation

"Ā´-mōt-i-vā´-shun." A psychiatric condition in which a patient does not appear motivated to do anything. Amotivation can be a sign of depression.

Anakinra

"An´-uh-kin´-ruh." Anakinra is an expensive drug, administered as a daily subcutaneous injection, which blocks the receptor found on the surfaces of many different types of cells for interleukin-1 (IL-1), an inflammatory mediator which in turn is produced by many different types of cells including the mast cell. Anakinra (also known in the U.S. by its trade name of Kineret, pronounced "Kin´-er-et") is used in patients with rheumatoid arthritis not responding to a number of other drugs, but it appears particularly useful for patients with a certain form of the rare congenital "autoinflammatory" disease called cryopyrin-associated periodic syndrome (CAPS), a disease of chronic IL-1-beta overproduction (principally by mast cells) and resulting chronic inflammation that stems from a mutation in a gene called NLRP3. Because the IL-1 overproduction in CAPS stems principally from the mast cell and causes an inflammatory clinical syndrome virtually indistinguishable from what can be seen in some of the more severely afflicted MCAS patients in whom symptoms begin emerging fairly early in life, one might consider CAPS to be one of the first specific genetic variants of MCAS to be defined. Alternatively, if one wants to restrict the definition of MCAS to include only mutations in mast cell regulatory elements acquired after birth, then CAPS of course would be distinguished from MCAS even though CAPS does create a state of constitutive (i.e., always-on) mast cell activation.

Anaphylaxis

"An´-uh-fil-ax´-is." (Also the adjective form "anaphylactic.") A major, often life-threatening reaction, usually in response to exposure to some trigger in the environment or to a food (or drink) or medication. Symptoms include low (potentially life-threatening low) blood pressure and swelling which, if severe enough and in the right place (for example, the throat) can also be life-threatening. During the first several hundred thousand years of humanity's evolution, anaphylaxis was a useful in teaching us to avoid highly toxic natural substances in the environment, but the problem is that most of the time when it occurs in our modern environment, it is an abnormal reaction in response to exposure to unharmful triggers. Although antihistamines and the glucocorticoid type of steroid medications can help settle an anaphylactic reaction, usually a shot of epinephrine (adrenaline) is needed to truly break such a reaction. Epinephrine's dominant effects, though, take place via the drug's binding to beta adrenergic receptors in blood vessel walls, so when a patient is taking a beta blocker drug (usually for hypertension (high blood pressure)), the beta adrenergic receptors are blocked and epinephrine can't do much, so patients with mast cell disease are often advised to avoid beta blocker drugs when possible, and when such drugs are necessary in such patients, glucagon has to be used instead of epinephrine to settle down anaphylaxis, as glucagon works through a totally different mechanism. Sometimes "anaphylaxis" is used interchangeably with "allergy" or "allergic reaction," but anaphylaxis truly describes just the spectrum of symptoms from the reaction which might be "allergic" if a trigger can be clearly identified. But, if no trigger is clear, we describe the reaction as "idiopathic anaphylaxis."

Anasarca

"An´-uh-sark´-uh." Anasarca is a condition of diffuse, severe swelling ("edema") which usually also includes advanced ascites, or fluid in the abdomen that causes significant distention of the abdomen and possible mechanical compression of abdominal organs. Anasarca can be caused by several different advanced disease processes – yes, including mast cell disease

Anemia

"Uh-neem´-ee-uh." A low concentration in the bloodstream of hemoglobin, the protein in red blood cells that carts oxygen from lungs to tissues and carbon dioxide from tissues to lungs. There usually are no symptoms from mild anemia (that is, mild anemia is usually asymptomatic), but as anemia worsens, common issues that emerge are fatigue and shortness of breath, and the patient becomes progressively more pale. When anemia becomes severe, insufficient oxygen delivery to the body's organs can even lead to a heart attack, stroke, and other major complications. Common causes of anemia (in general, not necessarily just in patients with mast cell disease) include iron deficiency, inflammation, and, of course, major acute bleeding (hemorrhage).

Anemic

"Uh-neem´-ik." A state of having anemia.

Anergia

"An-erj´-ee-uh." Lack of energy, fatigue, tiredness.

Angioedema

"An´-jee-oh-eh-deem´-uh." Like "edema," angioedema refers to swelling in tissues, but angioedema refers more specifically to swelling in tissues coming about from leakage of fluid (not whole blood, but fluid from the blood) from blood vessels. There is a variety of ways this can happen, but they all eventually wind up creating more of a signaling molecule called bradykinin (pronounced "bray´-dih-kyn´-in") which interacts with the wall of the blood vessel to make the wall more permeable to the fluid (but not cellular) component of the blood. And, in case you were wondering, yes, there are ways that mast cell activation can lead to formation of more bradykinin. Angioedema can come on very quickly and, when it happens in the right (or wrong?) places – such as the throat – and is severe enough, it can be lethal.

Angioma

"An´-jee-oh´-muh." Plural "angiomas" or "angiomata." Abnormal but benign blood vessel growth of various forms, sometimes just enlargement (dilation) of a segment of a blood vessel, or sometimes a growth of a collection of blood vessels. Usually small but sometimes can be huge ("cavernous"). When present in the skin, the extra blood accommodated by an angioma of course makes it appear red, and sometimes the term "cherry angioma" is applied to such a lesion. Because mast cell disease can affect normal tissue growth (including normal blood vessel growth), some mast cell disease patients develop angiomata. Cherry angiomata (small red dots in the skin) should be distinguished from "petechiae" (also small red dots in the skin), which are due to tiny amounts of bleeding (escape of blood out of the blood vessels) into the skin. Because the blood that makes cherry angiomata red is contained within blood vessels, when you apply pressure against them, the blood is temporarily squeezed out of the vessel so that when you release the pressure, the angiomata briefly appear to have blanched (turned pale), though they will soon turn red again as blood returns to fill the blood vessels in that area. The blood that has escaped into the skin tissue to form petechiae, on the other hand, is not going to be forced out of the area by applying pressure, so petechiae remain red upon release of pressure on the area.

Anhedonia

"An´-heh-dōn´-ee-uh." Anhedonia is a psychiatric condition, usually a sign of depression, that one can't experience pleasure even when engaged in ordinarily enjoyable/pleasurable activities.

Anorexia

"An´-or-ex´-ee-uh." Anorexia is the $400 medical word for diminished (sometimes even absent) appetite. Many conditions, such as cancers and inflammation and depression (guess what disease can cause any or all of these?), can cause anorexia.

Antibodies

"An´-tee-bod´-eez." See Immunoglobulin.

Anticoagulant

"An´-tee-kō-ag´-yoo-lent." Describing any product or process which impedes coagulation, or blood clotting. Common anticoagulant medications include warfarin and heparin. (Note that heparin also happens to be the very first mast cell mediator ever discovered, back in the 1930s.)

Antihistamines

"An´-tee-hist´-uh-meenz." Describing any product or process which impedes the action of histamine. Antihistamine medications work by blocking one or more of the various types of histamine receptors (there are five of them presently known), so we talk about an "H_1 blocker" or an "H_2 blocker," and so on and so forth. Histamine receptors of one type or another are present on a wide variety of types of cells. In general, there are far more H_1 and H_2 receptors in the human body than receptors of the other types; as a result, the vast majority of antihistamine medications are targeted at blocking the H_1 and H_2 receptors. Very few, if any, drugs are available to block the other types of histamine receptors. The mast cell surface has H_1, H_2, H_3, and H_4 receptors. Docking of histamine (which comes principally from mast cells!) with mast-cell-surface H_1 and H_2 receptors leads to further activation of the mast cell. H_1 blockers are divided into sedating and non-sedating H_1 blockers. One of the most commonly used sedating H_1 blockers in the U.S. is diphenhydramine. The most recognized trade name for diphenhydramine in the U.S. is Benadryl. The most commonly used non-sedating H1 blockers in the U.S. are loratadine, cetirizine, and fexofenadine (the most recognized trade names for these products in the U.S. are Claritin, Zyrtec, and Allegra, respectively). The most commonly used H_2 blockers in the U.S. are famotidine and ranitidine. The most recognized trade names for these H_2 blockers in the U.S. are Pepcid and Zantac, respectively.

Anti-nuclear antibody

"An´-tee-noo´-klee-er an´-tee-bod´-ee." Also frequently abbreviated as "ANA," the term anti-nuclear antibody refers to any of a class of autoantibodies targeted against any component of a cell's nucleus. ANA levels in blood are often found in rheumatologic diseases like lupus, Sjögren's syndrome, scleroderma, etc.

Anti-phospholipid antibody

"An´-tee-fos´-fō-lip´-id an´-tee-bod´-ee." This term generally refers to autoantibodies targeted against various proteins in the coagulation system. Not all anti-phospholipid antibodies cause problems, but when they do cause a problem, that problem tends to be a hypercoagulable state (i.e., an abnormal state of the coagulation system in which clots are prone to abnormally develop in the bloodstream even when there hasn't been a break in any blood vessel leading to bleeding.

Anti-prothrombin antibody

> "An´-tee-proh-thromb´-in an´-tee-bod´-ee." This is a type of anti-phospholipid antibody targeted against the clotting protein prothrombin.

Anti-RANKL

> "An´-tee-rank´-el." Refers to any action or effect that inhibits a signaling molecule called RANKL that gets involved in a lot of different processes including stimulating the normal (i.e., healthy, under the right circumstances) process of dissolving bone. Denosumab is the prototypical anti-RANKL drug, so it helps strengthen bone which is becoming weaker through excessive dissolving due to one disease process or another (including, yes, mast cell disease).

Anti-thyroglobulin antibodies

> "An´-tee-thy´-roh-glob´-yoo-lin an´-tee-bod´-eez." A type of autoantibody directed against the thyroid gland-related protein called thyroglobulin. In some cases, anti-thyroglobulin antibodies can lead to significant destruction of the thyroid gland.

Anti-thyroid antibodies

> "An´-tee-thy´-roid an´-tee-bod´-eez." A class of autoantibodies directed against various components of the thyroid gland. Specific types of anti-thyroid antibodies include anti-thyroglobulin antibodies and anti-thyroid peroxidase antibodies.

Anti-thyroid-peroxidase antibodies

> "An´-tee-thy´-roid per-ox´-i-dās an´-tee-bod´-eez." A type of autoantibody directed against the thyroid gland-related enzyme called thyroid peroxidase. In some cases, anti-thyroid-peroxidase antibodies can lead to significant destruction of the thyroid gland.

Apnea

> "Ap´-nee-uh." (Adjective form "apneic," pronounced "ap´-nee-ik," though the last two syllables are often slurred together to sound more like one syllable "nik".) Cessation of breathing. True, one becomes permanently apneic when one dies, but temporary apnea also can happen (obviously just briefly) during sleep for a variety of reasons, creating a disease called sleep apnea. Sleep apnea is divided into two main subtypes, central

sleep apnea (caused by problems in the brain which stop the diaphragm from driving the breathing process) and obstructive sleep apnea (caused when the nasal passages are obstructed or the throat temporarily collapses, obstructing the flow of air). Obstructive sleep apnea is commonly caused by massive obesity (causing the throat, which is relaxed at night, to literally collapse under the weight of the fat tissue in the neck), but I've also seen it occur in thin, or only mildly overweight, individuals who have MCAS, raising the question of whether certain types of MCAS can release mediators during sleep which cause the throat muscles to become so relaxed that the throat collapses even when there's no significant amount of weight pressing down on it.

Appendectomy

"Ap'-en-dect'-uh-mee." A surgical procedure of removing the appendix, a small part of the intestinal tract where the small intestine joins the large intestine. This is usually done because the appendix has become infected, and an infected appendix (also called appendicitis, pronounced "uh-pen'-dih-sīt'-is") has significant potential to rapidly become lethal.

Arixtra

"Ar-iks'-truh." The trade name in the U.S. for fondaprarinux. See Fondaparinux.

Arthralgias

"Ar-thral'-juhz." Arthralgias is the $400 medical word referring to pains ("algias") in the joints ("arth").

Ascites

"A-sy'-teez." Ascites is a condition in which fluid has accumulated in the abdomen. It usually is present in advanced liver disease or other conditions that cause severe bodily deficiency of protein, but it also can be caused by fluid-secreting tumors in the abdomen – or, yes, by mast cell disease (usually more advanced/aggressive forms).

Aspirin

"As'-pir-in." Aspirin is the prototypical non-steroidal anti-inflammatory drug (NSAID) and thus decreases pain, fever, and inflammation. However, aspirin is different from most other NSAIDs because its inhibition of the cyclo-oxygenase (COX) enzymes which leads to the aforementioned effects is irreversible, whereas the COX-inhibiting effects of almost every other NSAID reverses after several hours. (Even though aspirin's effects are irreversible, the body compensates by simply making fresh COX enzymes, so that's why it's necessary to keep taking aspirin at least once daily to maintain its COX-inhibiting effects.)

Atarax

See Hydroxyzine.

Atorvastatin

"Uh-tor´-vuh-stat´-in." One of the "statin"-class medications which lower cholesterol levels in the blood. Its most commonly recognized trade name in the U.S. is Lipitor.

Atrial fibrillation

"Ay´-tree-ul fib´-ril-ay´-shun." Atrial fibrillation (AF) is an abnormality in the rhythmic beating of the heart's atria (its two upper chambers, the right atrium and the left atrium) in which instead of regular contraction that forces blood into the ventricles (the heart's two lower chambers), there's just a quivering which not only can't force blood into the ventricles but also permits some stasis of blood which can lead to clotting, with disastrous consequences. AF occasionally is an acute problem that comes and goes but much more commonly is ongoing, or "chronic."

Autism

"Aw´-tism." A large spectrum of chronic neuropsychiatric developmental disorders with many potential behavioral consequences and with such symptoms almost always first emerging in childhood. Like ADHD, there appears to be a relationship between how "allergic" a child is (implying the possible presence of abnormal mast cell activation, i.e., some form of mast cell activation disease, much more likely MCAS than mastocytosis) and the child's risk for developing autism or ADHD. Dr. Theoharis Theoharides has been a pioneer in showing that autism occurs nearly ten-fold more often in children with mastocytosis than in children without mastocytosis, so given that MCAS seems to be much more common than mastocytosis, it will be interesting, too, to figure out how much more often autism (and ADHD) occurs in kids with MCAS than kids without MCAS. Another research project to be done by somebody at some point…

Autoantibody

"Aw´-toh-an´-tee-bod´-ee." Any antibody targeted against any natural part of one's body instead of something foreign like a microorganism or transplanted/transfused human tissue.

Autoimmune

"Aw´-toh-im-yoon´." Describing any process in which the immune system (erroneously) targets any natural (human) component of the body. Autoimmune processes work in part by producing autoantibodies.

Autoimmune hemolytic anemia

"Aw´-toh-im-yoon´ heem´-oh-lit´-ik uh-neem´-ee-uh." An autoimmune process in which the immune system erroneously generates an autoantibody targeted against red blood cells, leading to destruction of red blood cells which often outpaces the body's ability to generate new red blood cells to replace the ones that are getting destroyed, with the net effect being an anemia which potentially might be quite severe. I won't belabor the biology here, but autoimmune hemolytic anemia frequently causes not only tiredness due to anemia but also jaundice.

Autoinfarction

"Aw´-toh-in-fark´-shun." Spontaneous shrinkage of an organ, usually because the blood supply to the organ became obstructed for one reason or another. Probably the most common occurrence of autoinfarction is when the spleen becomes autoinfarcted (usually relatively early in life) in patients with sickle cell anemia, a condition in which the sickle cells obstruct the flow of blood in the tiniest blood vessels called capillaries (pronounced "kap´-il-ayr´-eez").

Azathioprine

"Az´-uh-thy´-oh-prin." One of many "immunosuppressant" drugs, or drugs that suppress one or more aspects of the immune system. The most commonly recognized trade name for azathioprine in the U.S. is Imuran ("Im´-yur-an").

Azithromycin

"Ā-zith-roh-my-sin." A type of antibiotic drug. The most commonly recognized trade name for azithromycin in the U.S. is Zithromax ("Zith´-roh-max").

B

Basophil

"Bās´-oh-fil." A type of white blood cell, primarily involved in some types of allergic reactions. Typically about 1-2% of the body's leukocytes are basophils.

Basophilia

"Bās´-oh-fil´-ee-uh." A condition that refers to an increase in basophils in the blood. This might be a relative increase (i.e., an increase in the percentage of basophils relative to the percentages of the other white blood cells in the blood) or an absolute increase (i.e., an increase in the total number of basophils, even if the percentage of basophils relative to other white blood cells remains normal). Intermittent mild basophilia (usually just a modest, relative increase) is not uncommonly seen in MCAD patients.

Behçet's disease

"Beh-shayz´" disease. Behçet's disease is a rare disorder of inflammation of small blood vessels whose clinical manifestations typically are ulcerations in the mucosal membranes (like in the mouth or anus) and in the perineal area, plus an inflammation in the eye called uveitis, but it certainly can affect pretty much every other organ/tissue, too. Its cause is not known – which in my opinion, seeing as how it's a chronic multisystemic polymorbidity of generally inflammatory theme, there ought to be a research project investigating what portion of the Behçet's disease patient population can be found to have a definitive diagnosis of MCAS (and, in particular, what portion can be found to have MCAS in which mutations in various regulatory elements in the mast cells are definitely present).

Benadryl

"Ben´-uh-dril." Benadryl is the most recognized trade name in the U.S. for diphenhydramine. See Diphenhydramine.

Benazepril

"Ben-az′-uh-pril." This is a medication, in the angiotensin-converting enzyme (ACE) inhibitor class, that treats hypertension. Its most commonly recognized trade name in the U.S. is Lotensin ("Loh-ten′-sin").

Benzodiazepine

"Ben′-zoh-dy-ă′-zeh-peen." A class of medications which bind to receptors for such medications which are located on the surfaces of various types of cells in the body, including mast cells. The most common use of benzodiazepines is to decrease anxiety, but – especially in mast cell disease patients – they can have a wide range of other positive effects, too. The most common side effect of benzodiazepines – typically related to the dose of the drug – is sedation. In general, when a benzodiazepine drug engages a mast-cell-surface benzodiazepine receptor, there quickly develops some decrease in the overall level of the cell's activation (i.e., its production and release of various mediators, and its reactivity to various triggers). To be sure, though, some benzodiazepines seem to have little effect on mast cell disease in some MCAD patients, and there's even the occasion in which trying any particular benzodiazepine in a given MCAD patient leads to some worsening of symptoms. (Of course, whenever that happens, one also has to wonder if the patient's abnormal mast cells are reacting to the fillers and dyes in the particular formulation of the medication that was tried, so sometimes simply switching to an alternative formulation, sharing as few of the fillers and dyes with the offending formulation as possible, results in finding benefit from that particular benzodiazepine.) Whether an MCAD patient clinically responds positively, negatively, or not at all to any one particular benzodiazepine doesn't seem to predict (not that we can tell yet, anyway) whether the same patient will clinically respond to any other specific benzodiazepine either positively, negatively, or not at all.

Beta blockers

"Bay′-tuh" blockers. Beta blocker medications are used to treat high blood pressure (hypertension). They block (of course!) the "beta adrenergic" ("bay′-tuh adj′-ren-er′-jik") receptors found on the walls of arteries and on cells in the heart, kidney, airways, smooth muscles, and other tissues.

Beta thalassemia major

"Bay´-tuh thal´-uh-seem´-ee-uh" major. The beta thalassemias are a group of inherited diseases in which one or both of the genes for beta globin ("bay´-tuh gloh´-bin") either are missing or are mutated to the point where they're producing an insufficient amount, or an inoperable form, or beta globin. Since beta globin is a critical component of hemoglobin, and hemoglobin is the principal component of red blood cells, any form of beta thalassemia inevitably leads to significant anemia, which can have a wide variety of consequences depending on the level of anemia. Different forms of beta thalassemia lead to different levels of anemia. In beta thalassemia minor, only one of the two genes for beta globin that are present in every cell in the body is "messed up," usually leading to a mild-moderate level of anemia, whereas in the beta thalassemia major, both of the genes for beta globin are messed up, inevitably leading to severe anemia. Also, since production of hemoglobin is greatly impeded, the size of the red blood cells necessarily decreases – significantly. In beta thalassemia minor, the MCV (normally 80-100 femtoliters, or fL) tends to be in the 60s, and in beta thalassemia major, the MCV tends to be in the 50s. The anemia in beta thalassemia major is so severe and causes such severe other consequences that stem cell transplantation is often recommended to be done as early in life as possible for such patients. Now that you've gotten all that explanation, it shouldn't surprise you that there also is a group of inherited diseases called the alpha thalassemias in which there are problems with one or more of the four genes for alpha globin, which also is a critical component of hemoglobin. When one alpha globin gene is messed up, that's alpha thalassemia minima and the MCV tends to be in the upper 70s. When two alpha globin genes are messed up, that's alpha thalassemia minor and the MCV tends to be in the lower 70s. It's very rare to have all four alpha globin genes messed up, but when that happens in the fetus, it's not survivable and results in miscarriage, or death shortly after birth, with a clinical appearance we call "hydrops fetalis" ("hy´-drops feh-tal´-is"). Having three alpha globin genes messed up is also pretty rare and results in something called hemoglobin H disease.

Biliary dyskinesia

"Bil´-ee-ayr´-ee dis´-kin-eezh´-uh." A condition in which bile does not move normally through bile ducts (inside and outside of the liver) and/or the gallbladder. Biliary dyskinesia can be caused by many diseases – yes, including mast cell disease.

Bipolar affective disorder

"By´-pohl-er ahf-ect´-iv" disorder. Also known as "manic depressive illness," bipolar affective disorder is a psychiatric disorder in which at times the patient seems to have incredible high levels of energy, while at other times the very same patient seems depressed. The cause of bipolar affective disorder is unknown. I wonder what other diseases show such "opposites" of behavior, in the same patient, over the course of time. ☺ Clearly, there is much research yet to be done.

Bisphosphonates

"Bis-fos´-foh-nāts." The bisphosphonates are a class of medications which fight moderate bone weakening called osteopenia and severe bone weakening called osteoporosis, almost regardless of what might be causing such weakening (and there are a lot of reasons why bones might get weak). Some of the bisphosphonates are oral drugs, and some are IV. Bisphosphonates are sometimes used in mast cell disease patients because MCAD (both mastocytosis and MCAS) can cause (focal or diffuse) weakening of the bones which, when advanced, can lead to pain and fractures (which then are difficult to heal). All of the bisphosphonates have the potential to cause a serious degenerative condition of the jawbone (i.e., the mandible) called osteonecrosis of the jaw (ONJ), and ONJ appears more likely in patients who get certain dental procedures done while taking bisphosphonate therapy, so it's important for patients (of any type) to try to get any dental issues "squared away" before starting bisphosphonate therapy.

Blepharospasm

"Bleh´-fer-oh-spasm." A condition in which the eyelids uncontrollably twitch. No doubt it can be caused by many diseases, but I certainly have seen it in association with MCAD, and I've seen it get better with MCAD therapies ranging from trigger identification and avoidance (which sometimes involves relocating to a new residence or locale) to MCAD-specific medication.

Bone densitometry

Bone "den´-sih-tom´-eh-tree." An X-ray study of the bones that puts a number (actually, a couple of numbers, the "T score" and the "Z score") on how dense (or, conversely, how thin) the bones are. Most people go by the Z score, which ranges from the negative end of the scale (abnormally thin bones) to the positive end of the scale (abnormally dense bones), so the more negative your Z score is, the thinner your bones are, and the more positive your Z score is, the denser/thicker your bones are. (Note that either thinning *or* thickening can make your bones weaker in overall strength.) Mild to moderate thinning is called osteopenia (see Osteopenia); moderate to severe thinning is called osteoporosis (see Osteoporosis). Abnormal thickening of the bones is called osteosclerosis (see Osteosclerosis).

Bosutinib

"Boh-soot´-in-ib." A "third-generation" tyrosine kinase inhibitor (see Tyrosine Kinase Inhibitors) that can help some patients with chronic myeloid leukemia (CML), and there is a theoretical basis for thinking it ought to be helpful in at least some patients with MCAD, but so far no such reports (much less formal studies) have appeared in the literature.

Bovine

"Boh´-vyn." An adjective meaning that something (such as some formulations of the anticoagulant heparin) is derived from a cow.

Botulinum toxin

"Boch´-oo-lin´-um tox´-in." Also known by its most recognized trade name in the U.S. of "Botox" (pronounced "Boh´-tox"). This is a paralyzing agent which, when injected under the skin, causes paralysis of the muscles in the area. It is most commonly used for cosmetic purposes (by stiffening muscles through paralysis, it gives somewhat of an appearance that the tissues in the area aren't sagging as much, so it's often used, for example, to treat the wrinkling of the skin that inevitably comes with age), but it also helps in some patients with bothersome focal tics and tremors (e.g., blepharospasm). Sometimes a botulinum toxin treatment yields permanent paralysis of the injected area (resulting eventually in unusual appearance of portions of skin in patients who are old enough that you know there's no way their skin could look that tight on its own), and sometimes the effect just lasts a few months and then has to be administered again.

Brimonidine

"Brih-mon´-ih-deen." In binding with the "alpha 2 adrenergic receptor" (mostly in blood vessel walls), this drug constricts blood vessels, which can help with a form of glaucoma called open-angle glaucoma.

Budd-Chiari syndrome

"Bud Kee-ahr-ee" syndrome. This is a syndrome resulting from obstruction of the veins that drain blood from the liver. It causes abdominal pain, collection of fluid in the abdomen (ascites), and enlargement of the liver. Sometimes the myeloproliferative diseases of polycythemia vera, essential thrombocytosis, or myelofibrosis – and, yes, mast cell disease – can cause the clotting that leads to Budd-Chiari syndrome even before the myeloproliferative disease itself is clinically apparent.

Buerger's disease

"Ber´-gerz" disease. Also called thromboangiitis obliterans ("throm´-boh-an´-jee-īt´-is oh-blit´-er-anz"), Buerger's disease is a rarely seen problem of inflammation and clotting of the arteries and veins of the hands and feet. It's strongly associated with smoking, and its cause is unknown.

Bullous pemphigoid

"Bul´-us pem´-fih-goid." Bullous pemphigoid (BP) is an autoimmune skin disease, usually seen only in the elderly, in which the immune system erroneously generates autoantibodies attacking a very specific and critical molecular component of skin tissue resulting in the breakdown of the normal adhesion between the outer layer of the skin (the epidermis) and the inner layer of the skin (the dermis), all of which results clinically in large, painful blisters. BP, like virtually all autoimmune diseases, is of unknown cause. Sometimes BP is an acute disease that resolves after a few months either on its own or with treatment, and sometimes it becomes a chronic condition.

Bupivacaine

"Byoo-piv´-uh-cayn." Bupivacaine is a numbing agent (i.e., an anesthetic medication) of the "amide" class of anesthetics, similar to lidocaine but a little different from procaine (a.k.a. Novocaine), which is of the "ester" class of anesthetics.

Burning mouth syndrome

Burning mouth syndrome (BMS) is a syndrome in which there comes to be a burning sensation in the mouth (and sometimes also other parts, or all, of the GI tract) most or all of the time. BMS has been in the medical literature since the 1950s, and although there are a few specific diseases that have been found to be at the root of it in a minority of cases, most cases are of unknown cause. I have found (and published) that MCAS appears to be the root issue in at least some cases of BMS.

Butalbital

"Byoo-tal´-bih-tal." Butalbital is a sedating pain reliever in the "barbiturates" class and is sometimes prescribed for pain and headache.

Butorphanol

"Byoo-torf´-uh-nol." Butorphanol is a narcotic pain reliever. It's most commonly used in nasal-spray form for treating migraine headaches.

C

C-reactive protein

Pronounced just as you're reading it, "see"-reactive protein. It's a protein produced by the liver, chiefly in response to mediators released by macrophages and fat cells (adipocytes), and it's regarded as providing a rough indication as to how much inflammation is present in the body – though, to be sure, there still are plenty of patients (including some mast cell disease patients) who are obviously terribly inflamed but who also, for unclear reasons, have a C-reactive protein level in the blood that's well within "normal limits."

Calcitonin

"Kal´-sih-tohn´-in." A hormone, secreted by the thyroid gland, which drives calcium to migrate from the blood into the bones. It opposes the action of parathyroid hormone, so the two hormones in balance exert a major force on bone health.

Campath

"Kam´-path." See Alemtuzumab.

Canakinumab

"Kan'-uh-kyn'-oo-mab." Also known in the U.S. by its trade name Ilaris, canakinumab is a monoclonal antibody medication that binds to and thus inactivates a cytokine, or mediator, called interleukin-1-beta (IL-1-beta) that directly and indirectly stirs up a lot of effects we clinically recognize as "inflammatory." IL-1-beta is one of the inflammatory mediators that can be produced in mast cell activation disease, and it also appears to be the key inflammatory mediator that is abnormally released (principally by mast cells, but also by other types of cells) in the rare inborn autoinflammatory syndrome called cryopyrin-associated periodic syndrome (CAPS). We now understand that, in CAPS, there is a mutation in a gene called NLRP3 which causes the gene to become non-functional, and this effectively removes any "brakes" on the production of IL-1-beta. Canakinumab certainly doesn't fix the underlying genetic mutation, but it at least binds up most of that excessive IL-1-beta, effectively precluding the inflammatory effects it would otherwise cause.

Cannabinoid

"Kan-ab'-in-oid." A class of molecules, including tetrahydrocannabinol (THC), the "active compound" in marijuana, which binds to the body's cannabinoid receptors – including such receptors on the surface of the mast cell. In some patients with mast cell activation disease, engagement of the mast-cell-surface cannabinoid receptors can lead to inhibition of mast cell activation. Cannabinoids are available in natural form, of course, but also in man-made (synthetic) pharmaceutical form.

Carcinoembryonic antigen

"Kar'-sin-oh-em'-bree-on'-ik ant'-ih-jen." Carcinoembryonic antigen (which is a mouthful, so it's usually referred to in writing and speaking as "CEA") is a protein ordinarily found on the surfaces of a lot of different types of cells in the body, more so in abdominal tissues/organs (especially the colon) than elsewhere. There normally is some relatively small amount of CEA that's been shed from these cells and is floating around in the blood, but in some patients who suffer inappropriate excessive growth (principally cancerous growth) of tissues bearing CEA, the amount of CEA in the blood can increase, sometimes hugely so. The CEA level in blood is tested by doctors when they suspect the patient has colon cancer, and in some patients the CEA level (which should return to normal after a colon cancer has been completely removed) can be followed over time as a marker for relapse.

Carcinoid

"Kar´-sin-oid." Carcinoid is the most common of the neuroendocrine tumors (which, as a class, are some of the rarest cancers), arising from the enterochromaffin (EC) or EC-like cells of the body which most commonly are found in the intestinal tract and the lungs. EC cells have receptors on their surfaces for a hormone called somatostatin (which inhibits EC cell activity) and in turn produce a number of hormones and other chemical signals such as chromogranin A and serotonin, whose main breakdown product is 5-HIAA. Therefore, when EC cells become cancerous and excessively reproduce to form a carcinoid tumor, one would expect levels of chromogranin A (in the blood) and 5-HIAA (in the urine) to substantially rise and for the symptoms caused by carcinoid to respond at least somewhat to octreotide, which is chemically similar to somatostatin. Because the common symptoms of carcinoid (unpredictably episodic flushing, diarrhea, and wheezing) partially mimic what's seen in some patients with mast cell disease, patients who are ultimately diagnosed as having mast cell disease sometimes have been previously suspected of having (and have been tested and even treated for) carcinoid.

Cardiac catheterization

"Kar´-dee-ak kath´-eh-ter-ih-zay´-shun." This is a procedure in which a doctor (usually a cardiologist or a cardiac surgeon) inserts a catheter into an artery (usually the femoral artery near the groin) and threads it up the artery (against the normal flow of blood) until it's positioned, near the heart, at the origin of the arteries that feed blood to the heart itself, the so-called coronary arteries, and then the doctor injects into the coronary arteries a dye which can be seen on an X-ray movie that he's taking at the time of the injection. In this fashion, the contours of the interior surfaces of the arteries – most importantly, where the arteries are open and where they're partially or completely blocked – are revealed, thus telling the doctor where he may need to focus his efforts to open up significantly blocked blood flow that's crippling heart muscle.

Cardiology

"Kar'-dee-ol'-oh-jee." Technically, this means study of the heart, but it also refers to the branch of medicine that tends to heart disease.

Cardiomyopathy

"Kar'-dee-oh-my-op'-uh-thee." Refers to any process that results in weakening of heart muscle. Cardiomyopathy is the central issue in the common clinical condition of congestive heart failure.

Carisoprodol

"Kar'-ih-soh'-proh-dol." This is a muscle relaxant medication. Its most widely recognized trade name in the U.S. is Soma (pronounced "Soh-muh").

Cataplexy

"Kat'-uh-plex'-ee." Often triggered by emotionality (laughing, crying, fear, etc.), cataplexy describes an abnormal state of sudden body-wide weakness (sometimes even complete paralysis) without affecting consciousness so much. Cataplexy is typically associated with fairly rapid follow-on onset of narcolepsy (an abnormal, very acute dropping off to sleep – obviously potentially quite dangerous), and while we somewhat understand the cause of narcolepsy (autoimmune destruction of a central nervous system protein called hypocretin), we don't understand what causes cataplexy without narcolepsy – except to say that I've certainly observed some mast cell activation disease patients to exhibit exactly that.

Catecholamines

"Kat'-uh-kohl'-uh-meens." Catecholamines are a small group of natural body chemicals, made by the body from the amino acid tyrosine, critically involved in regulating many key systems in the body. The main catecholamines made in the human body are epinephrine, norepinephrine, and dopamine. Dopamine is the first chemical product of the conversion of tyrosine, and then additional chemical processing steps can be applied by the body to create norepinephrine and then, from norepinephrine, epinephrine. Dopamine (in the right amounts and at the right places and times) is an absolutely crucial molecule for normal nerve cell functioning. Norepinephrine is greatly involved in regulation of blood pressure, among other aspects of bodily functioning. Epinephrine, also still sometimes referred to by its older name of adrenaline, is also involved in regulation of blood pressure (among many other aspects of bodily functioning) and of course is also made as a drug to help treat anaphylaxis.

CD117

Just like it looks: "see-dee" one seventeen. This refers to the part of the KIT protein that sticks up outside of the cell. Medical science has been able to manufacture antibodies against KIT, and since there's a huge number of KIT proteins studding all about the surface of each mast cell (about 50,000 copies of KIT per mast cell in normal circumstances), when we apply those antibodies against some tissue in the pathology laboratory, we're able to identify whether there are any mast cells in that tissue because we have ways to see how many cells have had a lot of that CD117-directed antibody stuck to them. There are other types of cells, to be sure, that also have KIT, but the mast cell bears roughly 10 times as much KIT as any other type of cell, so when the cell "stains brightly" for the CD117-directed antibody (sometimes sloppily referred to as just "CD117," even though that term technically refers not to the antibody but to the extracellular portion of KIT against which the antibody is directed), we know it's almost certain that that cell is a mast cell.

CD2

Just like it looks: "see-dee" two. This refers to a protein that's normally found on the surface of a couple types of immune system cells called T cells and NK (natural killer) cells. CD2 is involved in helping these cells stick, or adhere, to other cells to accomplish various functions. Ordinarily, CD2 should never appear on the surface of the mast cell – but in many patients (though certainly not all) with mastocytosis (and far fewer patients with MCAS), CD2 does indeed – quite abnormally – show up on the surface of the patient's abnormal mast cells, and this can be detected in the pathology laboratory through a technique called flow cytometry, by which we can simultaneously apply antibodies against both CD117 and CD2 to a tissue sample, and if any cells "light up" as showing both CD117 and CD2, we know that has to be an abnormal mast cell.

CD25

Just like it looks: "see-dee" twenty-five. This refers to the "alpha chain" component of the receptor for a "cytokine" signaling protein called interleukin-2 (IL-2) that ordinarily is made by certain immune system cells called T cells in response to virtually any kind of attack against the body. The IL-2 receptor ordinarily is found only on the surface of T cells. Ordinarily, this receptor – and thus CD25 – should never appear on the surface of the mast cell, but in many patients (though certainly not all) with mastocytosis (and far fewer patients with MCAS), CD25 does indeed – quite abnormally – show up on the surface of the patient's abnormal mast cells, and this can be detected in the pathology laboratory through a technique called flow cytometry, by which we can simultaneously apply antibodies against both CD117 and CD25 to a tissue sample, and if any cells "light up" as showing both CD117 and CD25, we know that has to be an abnormal mast cell.

CEA

Just like it looks: "see-ee-ay." See Carcinoembryonic antigen.

Celecoxib

"Sel´-eh-kox´-ib." Celecoxib (still protected in the U.S. by patent and made by only its original maker, marketed in the U.S. under the trade name of Celebrex) is a non-steroidal anti-inflammatory drug (NSAID) with a twist. Virtually all NSAIDs inhibit two critical enzymes in the body's path toward making prostaglandin-type mediators, cyclo-oxygenase 1 (COX1) and cyclo-oxygenase 2 (COX2). It's thought that inhibiting COX1 is what principally leads to the problems that standard NSAIDs cause for the stomach, the kidneys, and platelets. Well, in response the wizards of modern pharmaceutical science came up "COX2-selective" inhibitors, i.e., NSAIDs that only inhibit COX2. As a result of leaving COX1 pretty much alone, the COX2-selective NSAIDs cause less stomach, kidney, and platelet problems than traditional NSAIDs (but don't for a moment think that the COX2-selective NSAIDs can't cause those problems to some (lesser) degree, because they certainly can). There used to be two COX2-selective NSAIDs on the market, rofecoxib and celecoxib, but rofecoxib (Vioxx) was found to have too much of a risk for causing cardiovascular problems like heart attacks, so it was pulled off the market. Celecoxib has that risk, too, but it's less than what was seen with rofecoxib, so celecoxib is still on the market, though most of the doctors who prescribe celecoxib (typically for arthritis, the primary disease for which it's been approved) will caution their patients about this increased risk and the need to take any signs of cardiovascular disease seriously.

With regard to mast cell disease, I've observed (but not yet published in the peer-reviewed literature, so take this with the proverbial grain of salt) that an occasional (certainly not every!) MCAS patient who's intolerant of, or unresponsive to, standard NSAIDs can then be found to be tolerate of, and nicely responsive to, celecoxib.

Celiac disease

"Seel´-ee-ak" disease. Celiac disease is an autoimmune disease leading to a shortening of the microscopic villi, the tiny "absorbent fingers" of intestinal tract tissue, and thus also leading to malabsorption of a range of key nutrients which of course then leads to a whole range of secondary consequences in the GI tract and other systems which mimic many of the symptoms seen in mast cell disease, which is why patients often get suspected of having (and often even incorrectly diagnosed as having) celiac disease long before getting suspected of having, and being proven to have, mast cell activation disease. (Note, of course, that because celiac disease is an autoimmune disease and because mast cell disease can "spin off" virtually any autoimmune disease, it is certainly possible for a patient with MCAD to also have celiac disease, and this may explain, at least in part, why some MCAD patients gain at least some improvement from switching to a gluten-free diet.) Celiac disease occurs in certain genetically predisposed individuals (yes, we know what these genetic markers are and can test for them) and can clinically emerge anywhere from infancy to any later point in life. Because the disease is triggered by exposure to the gliadin component of gluten in wheat, the only standard treatment is to switch to a gluten-free diet.

Cellulitis

"Sell´-yoo-līt´-is." Cellulitis technically refers just to inflammation of the dermis layer of the skin (the layer beneath the very outermost skin layer called the epidermis) and the layer of fat below the dermis, but in practice it's also taken to refer to any infectious process producing such inflammation.

Cerebral vascular accident, or cerebrovascular accident

This quaint term ("accident"? really?), often abbreviated in writing and speaking to simply "CVA," is also known as a "stroke" and basically refers to a process in which one or more areas of the brain die because of a failure of the blood supply to those areas. A CVA or stroke can be a hemorrhagic stroke if the blood supply to those areas "failed" because the blood vessels ruptured and there was bleeding in the area, or it can be a thromboembolic stroke if a blood clot developed (usually in an artery closer to the heart) and eventually got lodged and stuck as it traveled through smaller and smaller arteries, eventually causing the blood supply to that area of the brain to "fail" because it simply gets occluded by the clot.

Cerumen

"Ser-oo´-men." The $400 medical word for ear wax.

Cetirizine

"Seh-teer´-i-zeen." Also known by its popular trade name Zyrtec, this oral-only drug is a non-sedating histamine H_1 receptor blocker (see "histamine" for more information).

Chelator

"Kee´-lay-ter." A medication which has the ability to latch onto iron atoms in the body and carry that iron with it as it eventually gets urinated out of the body. Only two chelators are presently approved for use in the United States, deferoxamine (which has to be injected) and deferasirox (an oral medication).

Chemotherapy

"Kee´-moh-ther´-uh-pee." Medication that kills cancer cells.

Cherry angioma

See Angioma.

Chloride

"Klor´-īd." Essentially, chloride is an atom of chlorine that becomes negatively charged (i.e., becomes a negative ion, or anion) by gaining an electron. Along with sodium, potassium, and bicarbonate ("bicarb"), chloride is one of the "electrolytes" that's intimately involved in maintaining the balance in body fluids between acids and bases, in transmitting nerve impulses, and in regulating the flow of fluid into and out of cells.

Chloroacetate esterase

"Klor´-oh-as´-eh-tāt est´-er-ās." Chloroacetate esterase is a stain, not commonly used any longer, but still occasionally used by pathologists to try to identify whether a given type of cell being seen under a microscope might be a mast cell.

Cholecystectomy

"Kohl´-eh-sist-ect´-oh-mee." Removal (virtually always via surgery via one technique or another) of the gallbladder. Not surprisingly, because mast cell disease can cause abdominal pain and because inflammation of the gallbladder (cholecystitis) can cause abdominal pain, many patients eventually found to have MCAD have previously undergone cholecystectomy based on the presumption, and/or perhaps marginal test results, showing the gallbladder is inflamed. However, since MCAD is capable of causing inflammation in every tissue in the body, it's also possible that there's real, and really symptomatic, gallbladder inflammation that leads to a legitimate cholecystectomy before the underlying MCAD is recognized. (Note this is *not* to say that every case of real gallbladder inflammation is necessarily due, directly or indirectly, to MCAD. This has never been studied, and nobody knows what portion of gallbladder inflammation cases is caused, directly or indirectly, by MCAD. It might be a big portion or it might be a small portion, or somewhere in the middle. Nobody knows – yet.)

Cholecystitis

"Kohl´-eh-sist-īt´-is." Inflammation of the gallbladder. Usually causes abdominal pain in the right upper part (what health care professionals learn to call the "right upper quadrant") of the abdomen. In some cases cholecystitis can get so bad it can literally kill the patient. There are lots of different ways cholecystitis can happen in mast cell disease. For example, misbehaving mast cells in the gallbladder can release inflammatory mediators in the gallbladder, obviously directly causing gallbladder inflammation. As another example, acid-lowering drugs that patients with mast cell disease take to help control stomach discomfort from the disease can reduce the bacteria-killing acid produced by the stomach, leading to an increased risk that potentially harmful bacteria will start growing further downstream in the GI tract from the stomach, including in the gallbladder, and when harmful microorganisms grow, that's an infection, and an infection virtually always induces at least some inflammation. This is not to say that everybody on an acid-lowering drug (such as a histamine H2 receptor blocker like famotidine or ranitidine or a proton pump inhibitor like omeprazole or lansoprazole) should stop taking such drugs. Actually, the risk for infectious cholecystitis developing from use of acid-lowering drugs is pretty low. It's just another example that not every pain or other symptom in a patient with MCAD is necessarily a result of aberrant release of inflammatory mediators from misbehaving mast cells. In a patient with known mast cell disease, every symptom – especially every *new* or *changed* symptom – needs to be regularly evaluated/re-evaluated with careful consideration of everything else besides mast cell disease that might reasonably cause it. Do the testing for everything else first, make sure it's nothing else, and then and only then does it become more reasonable to attribute it to the patient's known mast cell disease.

Cholescintigraphy

"Kōl´-eh-sin-tig´-rah-fee." See Hepatobiliary iminodiacetic acid scan.

Chromogranin A

"Krohm´-oh-gran´-in A." A natural human body chemical made by a relatively small number of types of cells in the human body including not only certain specialized cells which can develop into the rare class of tumors called neuroendocrine cancers, but also mast cells. Chromogranin A levels in the blood almost always rise substantially when a carcinoid tumor is present, and they can also rise when there is heart failure, kidney failure, or use of proton pump inhibitor (PPI) medications. Thus, when there is no heart or kidney failure or PPI use or neuroendocrine cancer present, an elevated chromogranin A level in the blood can be a sign of mast cell activation.

Chromosomes

"Krohm´-oh-sohmz." Long strands of DNA, inside every cell nucleus, divided into shorter strands called genes, each of which contains the instructions for making a particular protein. In the normal human, there are 23 pairs of chromosomes in every cell nucleus, and these pairs are identical in every cell nucleus in the body. 22 of these pairs simply contain a chromosome containing a unique set of genes, plus a duplicate copy of that chromosome, while the remaining pair is either a pair of two (again, duplicates of one another) X chromosomes or an X chromosome paired with a Y chromosome. Having two X chromosome in all of one's cells is what makes a fetus become female, whereas having an X chromosome paired with a Y chromosome in all of one's cells is what makes a fetus become a male. The genes that seem to be key genes in governing normal mast cell behavior, and thus also mast cell disease, are scattered about a wide range of these chromosomes. In particular, the most important mast cell regulatory gene, KIT, is found on chromosome #4.

Chronic atrial fibrillation

See Atrial fibrillation.

Chronic lymphocytic leukemia

"Kron´-ik limf´-oh-sit´-ik loo-keem´-ee-uh." Chronic lymphocytic leukemia (CLL) is a typically slowly progressing leukemia (many patients don't actually run into clinical problems from it (and thus don't need treatment for it) until many years after diagnosis) in which there is excessive production of the "lymphocyte" type of leukocyte, or white blood cell. Similar to the relationship between *chronic* myelogenous leukemia and *acute* myelogenous leukemia, CLL's progression tends to be much slower (over many years) than the rapid (over weeks to months) progression of the far more deadly acute lymphocytic leukemia (ALL).

Chronic myelogenous leukemia

"Kron´-ik my´-el-oj´-en-us loo-keem´-ee-uh." Chronic myelogenous leukemia (CML) (also commonly referred to as chronic myeloid leukemia) is a type of MPN in which there is excessive production of the "granulocyte" type of leukocyte, or white blood cell, but CML tends to progress slowly (over years), in contrast to the rapid (over weeks to months) progression of the far more deadly acute myelogenous leukemia (AML).

Chronic myeloproliferative neoplasms

See Myeloproliferative neoplasms.

Cimetidine

"Sim-et´-ih-deen." The first marketed histamine H_2 receptor blocker, and it's inexpensive and still commonly used (the most recognized trade name in the U.S. is Tagamet), but it has more drug-drug interactions than most other H_2 blockers (which also tend to be quite inexpensive).

Cladribine

"Klă´-drih-been." A chemotherapy (cancer-cell-killing) drug, typically given as a short IV treatment or a shot under the skin every few weeks, that benefits some mastocytosis patients, but it certainly doesn't cure the disease, it only works in a portion of patients, and in those patients in whom it works, it tends to kill only a portion of the malignant mast cells and that improvement tends to last for only several months. Like most chemotherapy drugs, cladribine is too toxic (i.e., causes too many side effects) to be able to take such treatment indefinitely, so most patients take a few to perhaps several rounds, or cycles, of treatment and then have to stop. It's important to note that chemotherapy drugs generally are thought to be helpful in truly cancerous diseases (where one cell type or another is growing out of control), and that describes more aggressive forms of mastocytosis pretty well, but it does not describe mast cell activation syndrome (MCAS), so – at least at present – there doesn't seem to be any sensible role for chemotherapy in the treatment of MCAS.

Claritin

"Klahr´-ih-tin." Claritin is the most commonly recognized trade name for loratadine in the U.S.

Clavicles

"Klav´-ih-kulz." Clavicles is the official anatomical term for what everybody else knows as collarbones.

Clonazepam

"Kloh-naz´-eh-pam." Clonazepam is a type of benzodiazepine drug useful for settling some symptoms in some patients with mast cell disease. It binds with benzodiazepine receptors in the body, including benzodiazepine receptors on the surface of the mast cell, and when that binding takes place, it tends to lead to some quieting of the mast cell's activation. See Benzodiazepines for more information.

Clonidine

"Klon´-ih-deen." Clonidine is an old, inexpensive, oral anti-hypertensive medication (its best recognized trade name in the

U.S. is Catapres) that binds with the alpha-2 adrenergic receptor on blood vessel walls and results in relaxation of the vessel wall and thus a lowering of blood pressure.

Clostridium difficile colitis

"Klos-trid´-ee-um dif´-ih-sil kohl-īt´-is." *Clostridium difficile* colitis is inflammation of the intestinal tract from an infection from *Clostridium difficile* bacteria. ("*Clostridium difficile*," of course, is such a mouthful that it always gets abbreviated, at least in speaking, as "*C. diff.*") (By the way, I'm italicizing it because the names of microorganisms are supposed to be italicized in writing.) C. diff. is a "bug" that one tends to get as a consequence of having other, normal bugs in the intestinal tract wiped out as a side effect of antibiotic therapy given for infection (in the intestinal tract or elsewhere) for some other bug. Its most prominent symptom is diarrhea that can become so severe as to be life-threatening.

Coagulopathy

"Koh-ag´-yoo-lop´-uh-thee." Although this term technically refers to *any* disorder of the clotting system, it's often taken by many doctors to refer just to those clotting system disorders that result in excessive bleeding, leaving the term "hypercoagulability" or "hypercoagulable state" to refer to just those clotting system disorders that result in excessive clotting.

Colitis

"Kohl-īt´-is." This is a general term that simply means inflammation (from any cause) in some or all of the colon (i.e., the large intestine). As mast cell activation disease (both mastocytosis and MCAS) very commonly causes inflammation in multiple parts of the body, it shouldn't be surprising that colitis is a common issue in MCAD.

Colon

"Kohl´-on." Colon is the medical/anatomical term for the large intestine.

Colonoscopy

"Kohl´-on-osk´-oh-pee." A procedure in which a scope is inserted through the anus and rectum and then advanced through the colon to provide the doctor (usually a gastroenterologist, but sometimes a surgeon) a view of the entire interior surface of the colon. Colon cancers and inflammation sometimes can be discovered this way. This is a common test to be performed when the patient has symptoms (for example, blood in the stool, or otherwise mysterious abdominal pain or chronic diarrhea) suggesting the possibility of disease of some sort in the colon.

Computed tomography

Computed "toh-mŏ´-graf-ee," abbreviated CT, also referred to as computed tomographic scanning or CT scanning. A method of X-raying the body (or, in truth, any object) to produce a series of images that represent serial slices through the body, allowing you to see much of what lies inside the body without having to cut open the body, which is sort of what a normal X-ray does, except a standard X-ray picture superimposes all of the "slices" in an imaged field into one relatively blurred picture, whereas CT scanning separates out those slices to provide far clearer pictures which, in a sense, actually provides a three-dimensional picture of the imaged field since the *depth* of where any particular finding resides in the imaged field corresponds to which particular slice(s) show that finding.

Constitutive activation

"Kon-stich´-ih-tiv ac´-tih-vay´-shun." Programmed, constant activation of some protein, molecule, or system. A good thing when the thing that's constantly activated is supposed to be constantly activated, but quite a bad thing when the thing that's constantly activated is *not* supposed to be constantly activated.

Continuous positive airway pressure

Another mouthful of a term, and thus almost always abbreviated CPAP, usually pronounced "see-pap." This refers to both a technique in general, as well as to the machine that applies the technique, to treat obstructive sleep apnea (OSA). CPAP involves placing a mask (usually held in place by straps around the head) over the patient's nose, or nose and mouth, taking care to seal the edges of the mask against the face. The mask is then connected to a hose that in turn is connected to an air pump that pumps air through the hose and mask, and therefore into the patient's airway, at a predetermined pressure. Because the fundamental problem in OSA is collapse of the airway which prevents inhalation of air, pumping air in will prevent that collapse and thus keep air moving smoothly into the lungs. Of course, when the patient exhales, that stream of air has to fight against the air being (constantly) pumped in, but the human diaphragm which powers lung inhalation and exhalation is a powerful muscle and can easily do this. Many modern CPAP machines have the "smarts" built in to sense the various phases of the respiratory cycle to increase pressure during inhalation, decrease pressure during exhalation, and, of course, always maintain some level of pressure to ensure the airway remains open and doesn't collapse. Nevertheless, the pressure of the machine's air supply/flow against the patient's lungs at rest, not to mention the machine's pressure against exhalation, makes CPAP feel weird when first applied, and there are some who simply cannot tolerate it, but it is safe and effective therapy that has helped millions of people with OSA rid themselves of the severe morning fatigue and headaches that come from OSA. This situation is a perfect example of one of the key principles in managing mast cell disease, namely, that it's imperative to ensure, as best as is reasonable to pursue, that no more-obvious issue than mast cell disease is causing any given specific symptom or abnormality, since regardless of whether that more-obvious issue is ultimately rooted in mast cell disease or not, that more-obvious issue needs to be treated with whatever standard therapy exists for that issue. To be sure, *if* the more-obvious issue indeed is ultimately rooted in mast cell disease, then it's likely that the absolute *best* outcome with respect to that issue will come from applying not only standard therapy for that issue but also effective therapy for the underlying mast cell disease. Nevertheless, whatever the established standard therapy is (e.g., CPAP) for that issue (e.g., OSA) absolutely remains the "starting point" for effective treatment of the issue, even in a mast cell disease patient.

Coproporphyrin

"Koh´-proh-por´-fir-in."

Coronary artery disease

"Kor´-oh-nār-ee" artery disease, typically abbreviated CAD.

Corticotropin releasing hormone

"Kor´-tih-koh-trohp´-in" releasing hormone, typically abbreviated CRH.

Coryza

"Kor-ī-zuh." The $400 medical word for discharge of clear fluid from the nose, i.e., when your nose is "running," you've got coryza.

COX1

"Kox" one. One of the types of cyclo-oxygenase enzymes involved in manufacturing certain inflammatory mediators. See Cyclo-oxygenase.

COX2

"Kox" two. One of the types of cyclo-oxygenase enzymes involved in manufacturing certain inflammatory mediators. See Cyclo-oxygenase.

Creatine kinase

"Kree´-uh-teen kī´-nās," often abbreviated CK.

Cromolyn

"Krohm´-oh-lin."

Cronkhite-Canada Syndrome

"Kron´-kīt" (just like the famous old newscaster, which this syndrome has nothing to do with) Canada Syndrome.

Cyropyrin-Associated Periodic Syndrome (CAPS)

"Krī´-oh-pir-in" associated periodic syndrome.

Cutaneous

"Kyoo-tayn´-ee-us." The medical word referring to the skin. A cutaneous lesion is a skin lesion. A subcutaneous injection is an injection under the skin.

Cyanosis (also cyanotic)

"Sī´-uh-nohs´-is." A bluish appearance to the skin, almost always due to insufficient oxygen in the blood for one reason or another.

Cyclobenzaprine

> "Sī′-kloh-benz′-uh-preen." A muscle relaxant medication, often prescribed when patients complain of muscle pain and aching that the doctor thinks might be due to excessive muscle tightness/tension, or spasm. Its most recognized trade name in the U.S. is Flexeril.

Cyclo-oxygenase (COX)

> "Sī′-kloh-ox′-ih-jen-ās" (COX: "kox"). COX (which appears to have been officially renamed by biologists as PTGS (prostaglandin-endoperoxide synthetase, "prost′-uh-gland′-in end′-oh-per-ox′-ih-dās sinth′-eh-tās") since I first learned about it in medical school longer ago than I care to reveal here, except that to this day it still seems to be popularly referred to (amongst members of the medical profession, anyway) as COX) actually refers to a small group of enzymes ("small" as in "2," namely, COX-1 and COX-2) which are found in many (actually, most) types of cells in the body and which are responsible for formation of a large class of important biological molecules called prostanoids ("prost′-uh-noidz") including – yes, you guessed it – the prostaglandin D_2 molecule that's relevant to diagnosis of mast cell disease. In general, prostanoids stir up inflammation, so medications that inhibit their formation have anti-inflammatory effects. Most of the non-steroidal anti-inflammatory drugs (NSAIDs; see the entry for such in this dictionary) temporarily inhibit both COX-1 and COX-2, though the classic NSAID aspirin permanently inhibits both (at least until the aspirin is gone from your system and your cells begin making more COX-1 and COX-2). There also are the relatively new "COX-2 inhibitors" (such as celecoxib; its sister drug rofecoxib, or Vioxx, was pulled off the market when it was found to cause too much heart trouble), which of course inhibit only COX-2, which sometimes provides some advantages over the less expensive combined COX-1/COX-2 inhibitors.

Cyclophosphamide (Cytoxan)

> "Sī′-kloh-fos′-fuh-mīd." A chemotherapy medication commonly used to treat various types of cancer and, somewhat less often, various types of immune system disorders, especially autoimmune conditions. Its most recognized trade name in the U.S. is Cytoxan (pronounced "sī-tox′-an").

Cyclosporine

"Sī′-kloh-spor′-in." This is a medication, available in both oral and IV forms, which suppresses the immune system. It's used very occasionally to treat mast cell disease but far more following transplantation, when you want to keep your immune system from perceiving that wonderful new organ you just got as a foreign invader in your body and attacking and destroying it.

CYP2C9

"Sip"-2-C-9. Before I can explain CYP2C9, I need to back up and explain CYP450 ("sip" four fifty). There is a large family of enzymes in the body, called the CYP450 enzymes, which are responsible for breaking down and otherwise detoxifying lots of substances we take into our bodies, including medications. This family of enzymes is part of the human body's very wide and complex array of mechanisms which enable us to survive for decades in environments that often are pretty harsh, assaultive, and toxic. The CYP450 enzyme family includes many members, generally called isozymes ("ī′-soh-zīmz") with designations such as 2C9 or 2D6 or 3A4 (and thus also called CYP2C9 or CYP2D6 or CYP3A4), each of which is able to detoxify one specific chemical class of toxins or another. You can easily imagine, then, that if one of your CYP450 isozymes is not working properly, there may well be consequences (and by "not working properly," I mean either working poorly or even working too well). Sometimes a CYP450 isozyme won't work properly because of an interaction with a medication, but in the majority of the situations where a CYP450 isozyme is found to not be working properly, the cause is traceable to a mutation in the patient's gene that codes for the protein that is that isozyme. These mutations are called polymorphisms ("pawl′-ee-morf′-izmz"). (Often these polymorphisms are inherited, but sometimes they spring up out of the blue at the time of conception, after which they may be handed down to later offspring.) What are the potential consequences of a CYP450 isozyme not working properly (whether due to an interfering medication or a polymorphism)? Well, if the isozyme is working too well (i.e., a "fast metabolizer"), any medications that normally are broken down by that isozyme will be broken down faster than usual, meaning that to get the usual amount of effect out of the medication, the dosing may need to be higher and/or more frequent. On the other hand, if the isozyme is working poorly (i.e., a "poor metabolizer") (which sometimes means it's not working at all), then any medications that normally are broken down by that isozyme will be broken down more slowly, if at all – which in turn means that the medication will build up in the body, not only causing more of the intended effect but quite possibly also causing a number of unintended effects ordinarily not seen unless unusually high levels of the medicine are seen (like in an overdose). Although many medications interfere with CYP450 isozyme functioning, and although CYP450 polymorphisms are far more prevalent in the human population than most doctors are aware, it is difficult to diagnose CYP450-related problems because it is difficult to *suspect* CYP450-related problems. Why? Principally because the number of medication/CYP450 interactions is vast and can't possibly all be remembered, and because medical training about CYP450-related problems consists of about a minute's worth of in-class lecturing relatively early in the decade or so of training most doctors get (and with no follow-up clinical training), and because the more troublesome CYP450-related problems – the poor-metabolizing ones – tend to result in relatively slow (over weeks to months) build-up of an unmetabolized medication, meaning the toxicities of such build-up show up relatively slowly, and by the time those toxicities become clinically apparent, it's a long way down the road from when the medication was started and thus would require a lot of (typically uncompensated) effort to very carefully dig through the patient's chart, and through the medical literature describing the actions of all of the patient's drugs, to finally pin down that a CYP450-related problem is the *likely* cause of the toxicities, at which point the CYP450-interfering medication needs to be adjusted or stopped and/or special, typically expensive blood testing needs to be done (usually requiring 2-4 weeks to get a result) to prove that a CYP450 polymorphism actually is present. Little wonder, then, that the vast majority of people with CYP450-related problems never get diagnosed as such, eh? And let me make clear that I'm no better than any of my colleagues at recognizing such problems. Yes, I've caught some CYP450-related problems relatively early, but others I've caught only in the nick of time to save the patient's life, and there have been a few times I didn't catch it until I came to be involved in the patient's care too late to save the patient from permanent injury or death – and I'm quite confident there have been lots more times that I never caught it all because I never suspected it, for all the reasons mentioned above. Final lesson of the day on CYP450-related problems: although most such problems that result in toxicities from build-up of unmetabolized medications tend to cause slow such build-ups and thus slow-to-emerge toxicities (over many weeks or months), sometimes the build-ups and toxicities develop more quickly (over mere days to perhaps a few weeks), and because adverse medication reactions within days to a few weeks can be caused by mast cell disease, too, it can be even more difficult than usual to suspect CYP450-related problems in a patient with mast cell disease. In a mast cell disease patient in whom adverse medication reactions emerge within minutes to hours of taking a new medication, it's more likely the patient's dysfunctional mast cells improperly reacting to the new medication that's causing a reaction seen within minutes to hours of trying an "offending" or "triggering" medication, but if the reaction doesn't start to show up until days to a few weeks into the medication trial, it's almost impossible to tell, on clinical grounds alone, whether the problem is a real adverse reaction to the active ingredient or a triggering of the patient's mast cell disease (by either the active ingredient or one of the fillers or dyes in the medication) or a problem related to the metabolism of the drug (whether a CYP450 isozyme issue or an issue with some other drug-metabolizing enzyme involved in the metabolism of that drug). (So at this point you're wondering, "Is there no limit to the complexity that has to be dealt with in mast cell disease patients?" And the answer is "No.")

Cyproheptadine

"Sip′-roh-hep′-tuh-deen." This is a medication in the class of sedating histamine H_1 receptor blockers.

Cystitis

"Sis-tīt′-is." The medical word for inflammation (of any cause) of the bladder. Infection in the bladder certainly can cause cystitis, but when there is sterile inflammation in the bladder (such as often happens with mast cell disease, particularly in women), it is often called "interstitial cystitis" (pronounced "in-ter-stish-uhl" cystitis).

Cytogenetics

"Sīt′-oh-jen-et′-iks." This is a test done on a cell sample in the pathology laboratory to see if there are any major disruptions in the chromosomes in the cells in the sample. Determining a sample's cytogenetics is sometimes also referred to as determining the sample's karyotype ("kār′-ee-oh-tīp"). This is the sort of test that will tell you, for example, whether a baby has Down syndrome (cytogenetics on a sample of white blood cells will show an extra copy of chromosome #21) or an older patient with a hugely elevated white blood cell count and a grossly enlarged spleen has chronic myeloid leukemia (cytogenetics on a sample of white blood cells will show that parts of chromosomes 9 and 22 have abnormally grafted together). Cytogenetics works well at finding gross chromosome disruptions, but the mutations in mast cell disease only rarely cause such gross disruption of one or more chromosomes that they can be seen in cytogenetics testing. Actually, from what I've seen in my own MCAS patients, cytogenetics testing often fails because the lab is unable (for reasons I am very far from figuring out) to get the cells in the sample to grow as much as they need to grow for cytogenetics testing to succeed, but even when cytogenetics testing succeeds in an MCAS patient, the results are virtually always normal. Much more detailed testing for mutations is needed to find the mutations usually present in mast cell disease – and that's a big part of the problem in showing that mast cell disease is usually due to mutations, because such detailed testing is available today only in a very few clinical laboratories around the world. This situation will improve in the years to come, but it still may be more than a decade before this sort of detailed testing is routinely available in most clinical laboratories.

Cytokine

"Sī´-tō-kīn." Cytokines are protein molecules manufactured by cells for the purpose of communicating various messages to other cells, which then adjust their behavior in response to the specific message received. In other words, cytokines are among the array of ways that cells have for signaling other cells. Many of the mediators produced and released by mast cells are cytokines, but there are other types of signaling molecules that mast cells also can produce and release.

Cytoxan

"Sī-tox´-an." See Cyclophosphamide.

D

Daclizumab

"Dah-kliz´-oo-mab." This rarely used medication kills the subtype of lymphocytes known as T cells. It's useful in certain types of T-cell lymphomas.

Darier's sign

"Dār-ee-erz" sign. This is the eponym for dermatographism (see entry for that term in this dictionary) accompanied by hives in the track of the examiner's scratch.

Dasatinib

"Dah-sat´-in-ib." Also known by its trade name Sprycel ("sprī´-sel"), dasatinib is a "second generation tyrosine kinase inhibitor" (essentially, a more powerful version of imatinib) which, just like imatinib, was initially designed for patients with chronic myeloid leukemia but has since been found to help in other diseases, too, including occasional patients with mast cell disease. Like imatinib and all the rest of the tyrosine kinase inhibitors, it's extremely expensive.

Deep venous thrombosis

Deep "veen´-us thromb´-ohs-is," often abbreviated DVT. A DVT is a blood clot in a deep-seated vein. Aside from the discomfort in the local area of the clot, a DVT is A Bad Thing To Have because it often poses a risk for a portion of the clot breaking off and traveling along with blood flow until it gets stuck in the lungs, at which point it's called a pulmonary embolus (a "PE") with lethal potential.

Deferoxamine

"Def´-er-ox´-uh-meen." Probably more widely known by its most common trade name of Desferal ("dez´-fer-al"), deferoxamine is a medication, typically administered as an infusion either into a vein or under the skin, that leeches (a.k.a. "chelates" (pronounced "kee-lāts")) excess iron out of the body via the urine. This is something that becomes important to do when the body comes to have too much iron in it, since otherwise the excess iron will – over many years – essentially rot out most of the body's major organs. Although there's a relatively uncommon genetic disease called hemochromatosis that results in a build-up of iron in the body, the more common way to get to a state of excessive iron in the body (a state called "hemosiderosis," pronounced "hee´-moh-sid´-er-ōs´-is") is by getting a large number of red blood cell transfusions. It takes only a single unit of red blood cells being transfused to give you all the iron you need for a year, so a patient who becomes seriously anemic may get lots of red blood cell transfusions and thus may become seriously iron-overloaded, especially when the anemia is a chronic condition (for example, sickle cell anemia) rather than an acute condition (say, an accident causing major bleeding).

Denosumab

"Den-ohs´-oo-mab." Also called by its two brand names Xgeva and Prolia, denosumab is the first of a new class of medications for treating elevated levels of calcium in the blood and impeding the bone weakening seen in many cancerous and non-cancerous diseases. (There were plenty of medications for such problems in the past, but they were in other chemical classes and they worked differently from how denosumab works to achieve the same end effect.)

Deoxyribonucleic acid

"Dee-ox´-ee-rīb´-oh-noo-clā´-ik" acid, usually abbreviated as just DNA. DNA, of course, is a chain of organic molecules called nucleic acids. There are five basic types of nucleic acids. Four of them get used in making up chains of DNA, and it is the specific order they're placed in in a chain of DNA that defines our genes which instruct our cells how to make the proteins that, well, are a large part of what makes us living beings. We all share more than 99% of our DNA in common; it is tiny differences (scattered all about the 23 pairs of chromosomes in each of our trillions of cells) in the order of the nucleic acids in the remaining 1% of our DNA that make each individual look and act differently than all the rest of the people who have ever lived and will ever live.

Dercum's disease

"Der-kumz" disease. A rare disease in which abnormal nodular deposits of fat accumulate under the skin.

Dermatographism

"Derm-at´-oh-graf´-ism," sometimes also called dermatographia (pronounced "derm-at´-oh-graf´-ee-uh"). An abnormality in the skin in which redness emerges in the track of a light scratch. There is little other than mast cell activation that can cause this. Everybody normally gets a little bit of redness, briefly, in the track of a vigorous scratch, but dermatographism refers to the abnormal state of a scratch producing more than just a little bit of redness, and for a much longer period of time, than normally seen. Most patients with mast cell disease of one type or another show at least some dermatographism.

Dermatology

"Derm´-uh-tol´-oh-jee." Study of the skin, or the specialty to which doctors who specialize in skin diseases and research belong.

Dermatomyositis

"Derm-at´-oh-mī´-oh-sīt´-is." A chronic inflammatory disease of unknown cause, classically producing inflammation chiefly of the skin and muscles. I have occasionally seen dermatomyositis in the long list of problems a mast cell disease patient has accumulated long before his/her mast cell disease is diagnosed.

Dermatopathic

"Derm-at-oh-path-ik." Describing a state in which there exists some abnormality in the skin.

Desferal

"Des´-fer-al." The most commonly recognized trade name in the U.S. for deferoxamine. See Deferoxamine.

Desferasirox

"Des´-fer-as´-ir-ox." Known more widely by its common U.S. trade name of Exjade ("Eks´-jād"), desferasirox is, like deferoxamine, an iron-chelating agent, except deferoxamine is only available as an infusion and desferasirox is only available as a pill.

Diagnostic Phlebotomy

See Phlebotomy.

Diamox

"Dy´-uh-mox." See Acetazolamide.

Diaphoresis

"Dī´-ah-for-ees´-is," also the adjective form diaphoretic (pronounced "dī´-ah-for-et´-ik"). A word that simply describes a state of profuse sweating.

Diastolic

"Dī'-ah-stol'-ik." The phase of the blood-pumping cycle in which the heart has relaxed, thereby resulting in lower pressure of the blood in the bloodstream. Therefore, in a blood pressure reading, the bottom, lower number is the diastolic blood pressure.

Diazepam

"Dī-ah'-zeh-pam." Diazepam, known more widely by its most popular U.S. trade name of Valium ("val'-ee-um"), is a benzodiazepine which, by engaging benzodiazepine receptors on different types of cells throughout the body (including neurons, intestinal tract cells, and mast cells) can settle down anxiety and inflammation quite well in some patients. Diazepam has a much longer half-life in the human body than some other benzodiazepines such as lorazepam (Ativan) and clonazepam (Klonopin).

Diflucan

"Dī'-floo-can." Diflucan is the trade name for fluconazole, a widely used anti-fungal type of antibiotic.

Diphenhydramine

"Dī'-fen-hī'-drah-meen." Far better known by its dominant U.S. trade name Benadryl, diphenhydramine is the prototypical histamine H_1 receptor blocker (in the sedating class). It's potent and it goes to work quite fast, but it doesn't last long, only a few hours, so it's not an ideal drug for keeping the H_1 receptors in the body (including on the mast cell) continuously blocked.

Diverticulitis

"Dī'-ver-tik'-yoo-līt'-is." Simply put, diverticulitis is inflamed diverticulosis, and like diverticulosis, I not uncommonly find diverticulitis on the prior problem list of a patient who comes to be diagnosed with MCAS.

Diverticulosis

"Dī'-ver-tik'-yoo-lōs'-is." A condition in which there are outpockets, or outpouchings, of the intestinal wall at one or more points along the intestinal tract. It obviously is an abnormality of intestinal tissue growth, and although the presence of diverticulosis certainly doesn't prove the presence of mast cell disease, I have nevertheless seen diverticulosis as a previously established diagnosis in a lot of mast cell disease patients.

DNA

See Deoxyribonucleic acid.

Dopamine

"Dōp´-uh-meen." Dopamine is not only a major hormone with many different functions in different organs in the human body, but it also serves as a major neurotransmitter in the human nervous system. Dopamine-related problems are at the root of many human diseases, probably the most famous being Parkinson's disease, in which loss (still of unknown cause) of dopamine-secreting neurons in a particular region of the brain leads to characteristic neurologic abnormalities.

Doxepin

"Dox´-eh-pin." Doxepin (sometimes also referred to by its trade name of Sinequan) is an anti-depressant that also has sedating histamine H_1 blocking abilities.

Doxycycline

"Dox´-ih-sīk´-lin." Although most doctors learn about doxycycline's antibiotic properties, few are also taught that it has anti-inflammatory properties.

Duloxetine

"Doo-lox´-eh-teen." Known more commonly by its popular U.S. trade name Cymbalta, duloxetine is an "SSRI" (selective serotonin reuptake inhibitor) type of antidepressant.

Duodenum

Pronounced either as "Doo´-oh-dee´-num" or "Doo-ŏd´-en-um." Coming after the stomach, the duodenum is the first part of the small intestine, followed by the jejunum and then the ileum – and then the large intestine.

Dysacusis

"Dis´-uh-cyoo´-sis." Alteration in hearing.

Dysarthria

> "Dis-arth′-ree-uh." A state of difficulty in speaking clearly, dysarthria can result from both neurological issues affecting the movement of the body parts that help us talk to physical issues (e.g., deformities) affecting those body parts (such as the vocal cords, tongue, or lips).

Dysautonomia

> "Dis′-aw-toh-nohm′-ee-uh." Also known as autonomic dysfunction or autonomic neuropathy, dysautonomia is just a general term for describing a state in which the autonomic nervous system – that is, the parts of the nervous system that are supposed to always be on autopilot – is not working properly. Dysautonomia can result in one or more of a wide assortment of symptoms including lightheadedness, blood pressure fluctuations, abdominal bloating, problems going to the bathroom (#1 and #2), abnormalities in sweating, heat intolerance, sexual problems, etc. There are lots of known causes of dysautonomia, but in a substantial minority of such patients, a specific cause is never found. So guess what type of cell, when dysfunctional, can also cause dysautonomia, but which few doctors are ever trained to know much about? That's right: the mast cell. I long ago lost count of the number of patients whose long lists of diagnoses included "dysautonomia" and who eventually proved to have MCAS as the cause of all of their problems. Again, please note that the diagnosis of dysautonomia in these patients is not wrong. Rather, it's a matter of whether "dysautonomia" is a good explanation for *all* or just *part* of the patient's symptoms. If dysautonomia explains only part of their symptoms but mast cell disease (or some other disease) explains all of their symptoms, then it's most likely that the "dysautonomia" is just another aspect of a more all-encompassing disease.

Dysfunctional

> "Dis-funk′-shun-al." Simply put, not working properly.

Dysmotility

> "Dis′-moh-til′-ih-tee." This word is used to describe muscles that aren't moving correctly. For example, when the muscles in the intestinal tract aren't working properly (typically resulting in constipation), we call that intestinal dysmotility.

Dyspnea

"Disp'-nee-uh." Simply put, shortness of breath.

Dystonia

"Dis-tōn'-ee-uh." A neurologic condition, of potentially many causes (including (of course!) mast cell disease), in which central and/or peripheral nerves abnormally send signals to one or more muscles (usually within one specific muscle group or another) to contract, resulting in odd movements the patient cannot control – at least, not without the help of some sort of treatment to suppress the abnormal signaling. In patients in whom mast cell disease causes dystonia, mast-cell-directed treatment sometimes can effectively suppress this signaling and thus suppress the (often quite uncomfortable) movements. For example, dystonia affecting muscles in the arm might cause strange arm movements, while dystonia affecting the muscles controlling the shape of the vocal cords can cause difficulty speaking, dystonia affecting the muscles in the intestinal tract can cause uncomfortable bowel contractions, and dystonia affecting the diaphragm can cause hiccups or difficulty breathing.

Dysuria

"Dis-yur'-ee-uh." A condition in which the passing of urine causes pain. The way most doctors are trained, they come to reflexively think that just about the only cause of dysuria is infection, but in truth it is inflammation in the bladder and urethra (the tube passing urine from the bladder to outside of the body) that causes dysuria, and inflammation can result from both infectious and non-infectious causes – and guess what one non-infectious cause of inflammation in the bladder and urethra can be? That's right, you guessed it: mast cell disease. So when mast cell disease is the cause of dysuria (a sterile inflammation called interstitial cystitis), you should expect a urine culture (looking for infection in the urine) to be negative, and you should expect antibiotics to work poorly, if at all.

E

ECG

See Electrocardiogram.

Echocardiogram

"Ek′-oh-card′-ee-oh-gram." Also, echocardiography (pronounced "Ek-oh-card-ee-ŏ-graf-ee"). An echocardiogram (or just "echo" for short) is an ultrasound picture of the heart providing the doctor with all sorts of useful information about heart structure and function.

Eculizumab

"Ek′-yoo-liz′-oo-mab." Also known by its U.S. trade name Soliris, eculizumab is an extraordinarily expensive drug (roughly four times as expensive as the extremely expensive tyrosine kinase inhibitors; so expensive that some countries with nationalized health care systems have made a decision they're not going to buy the drug, leaving patients in those countries who need the drug to find on their own some way to access the drug), usually given IV every couple of weeks, that works fairly well to control a couple of rare blood diseases called paroxysmal nocturnal hemoglobinuria ("PNH") and atypical hemolytic uremic syndrome ("aHUS"). PNH is caused by any of a number of possible mutations in a stem cell in the marrow which lead to defects in an important protein called – well, it's enough biological gobbledygook that we'll just call it by its abbreviation, GPI. Copies of the GPI protein ordinarily are studded all about the surface of blood cells – especially red blood cells – and they serve a critical role as anchors for other proteins which protect blood cells – especially red blood cells – from being destroyed by the immune system. So when blood cells aren't making enough normal GPI protein, the protecting proteins can't remain attached to the blood cells, and the immune system attacks and destroys them– especially red blood cells – with its own special conglomeration of proteins called the membrane attack complex, a key component of which is a protein called C5. Well, eculizumab latches on to C5, preventing formation of the membrane attack complex, so even though PNH patients have blood cells that are "wide open" to attack by the immune system, eculizumab prevents that attack from happening. As a result, PNH patients need fewer transfusions and suffer fewer blood clots, two of the key consequences of PNH. As I said before, PNH is incredibly rare, but I've found it interesting that the three patients I've seen so far with it all met criteria for MCAS, too. One wonders if the same epigenetic-mutation-driven genetic fragility that might predispose to development of MCAS also might predispose to development of PNH. Eculizumab also treats another rare disease of acquired mutational origin, aHUS, where

314

inhibition of C5 again provides a critical advantage for controlling the breakdown of red blood cells seen in the disease. aHUS is so rare, though, that I've only seen one case of it, and that was so long ago (well before I started recognizing MCAS) that I can't say whether MCAS might also be present in cases of aHUS.

EEG

"Ee-ee-jee." See Electroencephalogram.

Effexor

"Ef-fex´-or." The most common trade name for venlafaxine. See Venlafaxine.

Ehlers-Danlos syndrome

"Eh´-lerz dan´-lōs" syndrome (EDS). EDS refers to a group of disorders, almost all traceable to congenital mutations in various genes that govern how cells build connective tissue proteins, thus resulting in assorted connective tissue abnormalities that can cause all sorts of different clinical problems depending on what the specific connective tissue abnormality is in a given patient. Now, where this gets really interesting is that although researchers have identified the specific mutation causing almost all the different types of EDS, there's one particular type of EDS – type III, also known as the hypermobility type because it predominantly features weak joints that let affected patients flex and extend their joints way beyond what normal people can do – for which decades of research have completely failed to clearly find a causative mutation in any of the connective tissue proteins. And what makes the situation even odder is that Type III is the most common type of EDS by far. So how could it be that researchers have managed to find the mutations underlying every form of EDS except the most common type? And when you further add in the observation that there seem to be an awful lot of EDS Type III patients who have symptoms of mast cell activation, you begin to wonder if maybe what's going on in EDS Type III is that there indeed *isn't* any mutation in any connective tissue protein. Instead, maybe what's going on is that all of the connective tissue proteins in EDS Type III patients are normal, but since mast cells, through their mediators, are integrally involved in guiding the normal growth and development of all tissues, maybe there are variants of MCAS that put out a particular aberrant pattern of mediators that leads to the misassembly of normal connective tissue proteins into abnormal connective tissue of a sort that clinically behaves such as we see in EDS Type III – sort of how (maybe!) some other particular variants of MCAS put out particular aberrant patterns of mediators that lead to misguided growth of brain cells so as to result in autism, or attention deficit/hyperactivity disorder, or how (maybe!) some other particular variants of MCAS put out particular aberrant patterns of mediators that lead to misguided growth of uterine lining cells throughout the abdomen (i.e., "endometriosis"). All of this, of course, is total conjecture at this point, but I haven't observed anything yet in the EDS Type III (or autism) cases that I've seen that would be inconsistent with the possibility that MCAS might underlie at least some portion of the populations with these disorders. Time (and much research) will tell, eh?

EKG

See Electrocardiogram.

Elavil

"El-uh-vil." The most common trade name in the U.S. for amitriptyline. See Amitriptyline.

Electrocardiogram

"Ee-lec'-troh-card'-ee-oh-gram" (ECG). A common test providing the doctor a tracing, or diagram, of the heart's electrical activity. To the layman it looks like a bunch of squiggly lines, but each squiggle reveals something important about the structure and/or function of the heart. ECGs (to this day often still called EKGs because the Greek word for "heart" begins with a "k": "kardia") can diagnose heart attacks (a.k.a. myocardial infarctions), heart rhythm problems, and other heart problems.

Electroencephalogram

"Ee-lec'-troh-en-cef'-uh-loh-gram" (EEG). A common test providing the doctor a tracing, or diagram, of the brain's electrical activity. To the layman itlooks like a bunch of squiggly lines, but each squiggle reveals something important about the structure and/or function of the brain. EEGs are most commonly used to diagnose seizure disorders, but they can help diagnose other brain disorders, too.

Emphysema

"Emf´-ih-see´-muh." Emphysema is a lung disease in which there is breakdown of lung tissue due to inflammation in a way that still allows air to get in to the lungs relatively easily but makes it more difficult for air to get out. As a result, excess volumes of air get trapped in the lungs and the lungs get to be chronically expanded, sometimes even physically making the chest get (chronically) bigger. Although emphysema technically refers to the inflammatory breakdown of lung tissue and chronic obstructive pulmonary disease (COPD) technically refers to the state – produced by emphysema – of excess air getting chronically trapped in the lungs, in practice the two terms, emphysema and COPD, are used pretty much interchangeably. In the vast majority of cases, emphysema/COPD is caused by chronic exposure to tobacco smoke, though other causes of emphysema do exist (such as rare congenital mutations leading to deficiency of alpha-1-antitrypsin, a protein critical to the health of many organs including the lungs) – and, you guessed it, I have seen COPD in a small portion of MCAS cases in whom no other known cause of COPD could be found, making me wonder whether there is a particular variant of MCAS that can result in the production of just the right (or wrong?) pattern of inflammatory mediators needed to make the lungs deteriorate in ways similar to what we see in emphysema.

Endocrinology

"End´-oh-crin-ol´-oh-jee." The study of, or the medical specialty focusing in, the body's hormones.

Endodontics

"End´-oh-dont´-iks." Endodontics is the dental specialty focusing on diseases of dental pulp, the soft tissue (blood vessels, nerves, etc.) at the center of every tooth. Because many MCAS patients suffer (presently inexplicable) deterioration of teeth no matter how much attention they pay to dental hygiene, such patients often come to need the attention of an endodontist.

Endometriosis

"End´-oh-mee´-tree-ohs´-is." Endometriosis is a chronic idiopathic condition in which there is abnormal growth – there's that theme again! – of the cells that line the uterus (endometrial cells) at places outside of the uterus. Oh, and I should mention that endometriosis most definitely is an inflammatory condition, too. Of course, nobody knows what causes endometriosis, and there may well be multiple conditions that can lead to abnormal growth and inflammation, but I'll bet by this point in your reading of this book you can identify at least one such condition, eh?

Endoscopic retrograde cholangiopancreatography

"End-oh-scop-ik" retrograde "kōl-anj-ee-oh-pank-ree-uh-toh-graf-ee," which certainly is a heck of a mouthful, so it's usually abbreviated as ERCP. ERCP is a procedure somewhat similar to an EGD in that a scope is inserted through the mouth of a sedated patient, down through the esophagus, stomach, and duodenum just as is done with an EGD, but the main purpose of an ERCP is to find the point in the duodenum where the main bile duct coming from the liver and gall bladder, and the main pancreatic duct coming from the pancreas, come together and dump into the duodenum, and once that point has been found, some dye that can be seen on X-rays is injected (through the scope, up into the main bile and pancreatic ducts) and then X-ray pictures are taken which show the outlines of these ducts, potentially revealing abnormalities in the courses and shapes of these ducts which might be the cause of various biliary and pancreatic disorders.

Endoscopy

"En-dosk´-oh-pee." Technically, this is a general term for taking a look at some internal part of the body by inserting a scope (which typically allow visualization of the area at the end of the scope by means of fiber optic technology), but in practice the word usually is taken to mean specifically the EGD type of endoscopy.

Enoxaparin

"Ee-nox´-uh-par-´in." Known more commonly by its U.S. trade name Lovenox ("Loh-ven-ŏks"), enoxaparin is the prototypical drug in the drug class known as the low molecular weight (LMW) heparins, which basically are chemically modified forms of the basic anticoagulant drug heparin. Typically injected under the skin (subcutaneously), the LMW heparins have an anticoagulant effect that typically lasts for 12-24 hours, far longer than what's seen with heparin, which has to be given intravenously to get a strong enough effect to treat a clot. There are lots of LMW heparin drugs now on the market; their names all end in "parin" (for example, dalteparin).

Enzyme

"En´-zīm." Think back to your middle-school biology days and you'll probably remember that an enzyme is a protein that catalyzes (speeds up) a specific chemical reaction. There are thousands of enzymes that human cells are capable (by the genetic programming in their chromosomal DNA) of making, and each one catalyzes a specific reaction that's important to normal body functioning. Mess up an enzyme in any way that interferes with its ability to catalyze its target chemical reaction and there *will* be consequences.

Eosinophil

"Ee´-oh-sin´-oh-fil." A type of white blood cell, primarily responsible for fighting less common types of infection such as parasitic infections. Eosinophils also are involved in some allergic reactions. Typically about 1-5% of the body's leukocytes are eosinophils.

Eosinophilia

"Ee´-oh-sin´-oh-fill´-ee-uh." This word refers to either the state of having more eosinophils than normal or the state of a tissue, being examined by pathologists, absorbing more of the standard "eosin" stain than usual and thus appearing redder than usual.

Epigastrium

"Ep´-ih-gast´-ree-um." This is the anatomical term for the central upper part of the abdomen, basically where the stomach is.

Epigenetics

"Ep´-ee-jen-et-iks." To put it in a grossly oversimplified manner, epigenetics is the study of the processes that govern the transcription of genes into proteins. Think about it. The DNA that's in each of your genes (long strings of which make up the chromosomes that are present in most of your cells) is a code for directing the protein-assembling machinery in your cells as to the *structure* of the proteins that the cells need to make in order to survive and function properly and contribute to the body's health. So, fine, the "protein assembly line" is in place, but what *regulates* it? If you have a car assembly line, and all the parts and tools needed to make a car, but there's no *regulation* of the assembly line, then you can imagine the chaos that would quickly result and the dysfunctional junk that would eventually be produced. Unsurprisingly (given how many proteins have to be produced in just the right amounts, at just the right times, and in just the right cells), there are lots of regulatory mechanisms, and the study of this whole mélange of genetic transcription regulatory mechanisms is collective called epigenetics – though in practice many take this word to specifically refer to just one such (major!) mechanism, namely, the pattern with which methyl groups (think back to your high school chemistry days: methyl is a carbon atom with three attached hydrogen atoms) are attached all about the genes. It turns out that the pattern of how methyl groups are laid out around the genes has a huge influence on how actively those genes are transcribed and translated into proteins, and the same way you can have a DNA mutation in a gene that results in a gene producing a dysfunctional protein or producing no protein at all, you also can have an epigenetic mutation in which a methyl group is present where it shouldn't be, or absent from where it should be, and this error can wind up having an effect on how actively the cell goes about producing protein from that gene. So even if the gene itself is completely normal, if the epigenetic *regulation* of that gene is messed up, you can get too much protein, or too little protein, or no protein at all from that gene, and any of those situations has potential for causing clinical problems of one sort or another. We've been studying epigenetics for a lot shorter period of time than we've been studying genetics, so we understand a lot less about epigenetics than we do about genetics, but there certainly are a lot of researchers in this area who are trying to make up for lost time, as they say.

Epigenome

"Ep´-ee-jeen´-ohm." Just as the word "genome" refers to the total set of genes that define an individual (or a species), the word "epigenome" refers to the total set of regulators (methyl groups attached to chromosomes, and other regulators) which, working in concert with a given genome, defines an individual (or a species).

Epinephrine

"Ep´-ih-nef´-rin." Both a natural molecule made by the human body and available in much greater amounts as a drug, epinephrine interacts with the beta adrenergic receptors in blood vessel walls to cause contraction of those vessels, thereby raising blood pressure and countering the potentially life-threateningly severe drop in blood pressure resulting from blood vessel dilation that occurs in anaphylaxis.

Epistaxis

"Ep´-ee-stax´-is." This is the $400 medical word for a nosebleed. Some people suffer recurrent epistaxis for no apparent reason, and given that MCAS can cause bleeding (due in part to release of heparin from dysfunctional mast cells, which as you know tend to site themselves at the environmental interfaces, which certainly includes the nasal passages), I have to wonder if MCAS is what's underlying "idiopathic epistaxis" in at least some portion of the population that suffers that problem. It would be interesting testing the blood from such nosebleeds for levels of mast cell mediators, wouldn't it?

ERCP

See Endoscopic retrograde cholangiopancreatography.

Erythema

"Ehr´-ih-theem´-uh." This is the $400 medical word for a visualized redness to any part of the body. For example, when you lightly scratch an MCAS patient and you see redness popping up in the track of the scratch (see the entry in this dictionary for "dermatographism"), you can call that redness "erythema."

Erythrocyte sedimentation rate

"Ehr-ith-roh-sīt"sedimentation rate, which is yet another medical mouthful, so it almost always gets abbreviated as ESR. The ESR is an old, simple, cheap blood test that has long been thought to be a general indicator of how inflamed a person is. If you draw a blood sample from a person and set it upright in a tube and then measure how high (in millimeters) a column of red blood cells accumulates in the bottom portion of the tube in one hour, that's the ESR. The funny thing is, even though it's been used for many decades and has been extensively researched, we still don't really understand why it's abnormally high in some inflammatory states in some patients and totally normal in the same inflammatory states in other patients. So it turns out that when it's abnormally high, it's a pretty reliable indicator that inflammation is present (though it doesn't even begin to identify what the cause of that inflammation might be), but if it's normal, it does a poor job of discriminating between those who truly aren't inflamed vs. those who are inflamed but, for whatever reason, just aren't showing a high ESR.

Erythrocytosis

"Ehr-ith´-roh-sī-tohs´-is." This is the medical word that describes the state of their being more red blood cells in the body than there should be – a state which I often see in MCAS, and when I see erythrocytosis in MCAS, I've observed that there's a good chance that imatinib will be able to help improve at least some of the patient's symptoms somewhat (and a few patients even achieve spectacular improvement).

Erythromycin

"Ehr-ith´-roh-mīs´-in." This is an old, cheap antibiotic that's still good for treating lots of different types of infections, but it also has a reputation for causing stomach upset in a lot of the people who try it.

Erythropoiesis/erythropoietic

"Ehr-ith´-roh-poh-ees´-is,"also known by the adjective form erythropoietic (pronounced "ehr-ith´-roh-poh-et´-ik"). Erythropoiesis is the process of red blood cell production, a process which in most people takes place exclusively in the bone marrow but which in certain diseases (such as myelofibrosis) can relocate to other organs like the spleen or liver.

Erythropoietin

"Er-ith´-roh-poh´-ih-tin." A hormone made principally by the kidneys which, upon traveling through the bloodstream to the bone marrow, stimulates marrow cells to produce more red blood cells. Because it's a mouthful and a tongue-twister, "erythropoietin" is often shortened (in writing and speech) to just "epo" (pronounced "ee´-poh"). Because the kidneys have the ability to sense how much oxygen is in the blood, they crank out more epo when the patient is anemic (with less blood in the blood vessels, there's less oxygen there, too). This is the principal mechanism by which those who live at higher altitudes come to have higher hemoglobin levels and more red blood cells than those who live at lower altitudes.

Esomeprazole

"Ees´-oh-mep´-ruh-zōl." Known much more widely by its common U.S. trade name Nexium, esomeprazole (like all of the drugs whose names end in "prazole") is one of the proton pump inhibitors (PPIs), a class of drugs which does a spectacularly good job of inhibiting acid production in the stomach.

Esophagitis

"Ee-sof´-uh-jīt´-is." The way to make the medical word describing the presence of an inflammatory state in any part of the body is to state the medical word for that part of the body and then follow it with "-itis." Therefore, esophagitis simply means inflammation of the esophagus.

Esophagogastritis

"Ee-sof´-uh-goh-gas-trīt´-is." As per my explanation for "esophagitis," esophagogastritis simply means inflammation of both the esophagus and stomach.

Esophagogastroduodenoscopy

"Ee-sof´-uh-go-gas´-troh-doo´-oh-den-osk´-oh-pee," usually abbreviated as EGD. This is a procedure in which a scope (through which the field of view at the "business end" of the scope can be seen by the operator at the other end of the scope via fiber optic technology) is inserted through the mouth and then into the esophagus, stomach, and duodenum. If the operator is using the simplest form of an endoscope for performing this procedure, then he can only see what's going on in the scope's field of view, but most endoscopes these days have lots of other technological trickery built into them so that the operator not only can see the field of view but also can perform tests on tissues in the field of view, obtain samples of the tissues in the field of view, and even apply treatments to tissues in the field of view.

Essential thrombocytosis

"Ee-sen´-shul throm´-bo-sy-toh´-sis." A type of MPN (see "myeloproliferative neoplasms") in which the causative mutations drive excessive production of blood cells, especially (and, often, only) platelets. The natural history of essential thrombocytosis (ET) tends to parallel that of polycythemia vera (PV), i.e., it's a blood cell cancer that usually progresses very slowly, over many years. When (if ever) it causes clinical problems, issues with abnormal clotting (and sometimes even bleeding, in spite of the high platelet count) tend to dominate. In general, it's not curable, but there are several treatments available to help control it (hydroxyurea is what's most commonly used). The JAK2-V617F mutation (see JAK2-V617F mutation) is found in about 60% of patients with ET, and recently it was found that any of a range of mutations in a gene called CALR is present in most of the rest of the patients with ET.

Etanercept

"Eh-tan´-er-cept." Known much more widely by its common U.S. trade name Enbrel, etanercept is an inhibitor of a mediator (produced by many types of cells including the mast cell) called tumor necrosis factor alpha, or TNF-alpha. Because the production and release of TNF-alpha leads to inflammation, etanercept has anti-inflammatory effects and is used in inflammatory diseases (such as rheumatoid arthritis and ankylosing spondylitis) in which TNF-alpha appears to have a major role in causing the effects of the disease. Etanercept has been shown safe and helpful in treating ankylosing spondylitis in patients with systemic mastocytosis, but it has not been specifically studied as a treatment for mastocytosis, much less MCAS – though since MCAD certainly can produce excessive amounts of TNF-alpha, there's certainly a good theoretical reason for thinking etanercept ought to be able to help tone down at least some symptoms somewhat in at least some MCAD patients. Just add it to the pile of MCAD-related research projects that need to be done.

Exjade

"Eks-jād." The trade name in the U.S. for desferasirox. See Desferasirox.

Ezetimibe

"Eh-zeht´-ih-mib." Known much more widely by its common U.S. trade name Zetia, ezetimibe is a cholesterol-lowering drug that works by binding to a protein ("NPC1L1," most commonly found on cells lining the intestinal tract and cells in the liver) that has a major effect on absorption of cholesterol.

F

Factor V Leiden

Factor 5 "Lī´-den." This is a mutated form of an important blood clotting protein called Factor V ("Factor 5"). As with every protein in the body, each cell in the body has two genes coding for that protein, so if one of the genes is mutated significantly enough (a so-called "heterozygous" mutation), then half of the Factor V that gets made will be mutated, and if both of the genes are mutated significantly enough, then all of the Factor V that gets made will be mutated. (If both of the genes are mutated in the same way, that's called a "homozygous" mutation, but if the two genes are mutated in different ways, they're called "compound heterozygous" mutations.) The particular mutation called Factor V Leiden results in a mutated form of Factor V that tilts the see-saw of the coagulation system toward the clotting end of the spectrum. Most people who have heterozygous Factor V Leiden will never suffer a blood clot unless they also develop some other risk factor (such as smoking, use of hormonal birth control interventions, immobilization for any significant period of time (like sitting for a long time on a road trip or a flight), trauma/surgery, etc.), but people with homozygous Factor V Leiden have a high risk of spontaneously clotting even without any other risk factors. Because some patients with mast cell disease also have a propensity to spontaneously clot, and because most doctors don't know that, many a patient ultimately shown to have MCAS who develops a spontaneous clot (called a deep venous thrombosis or a pulmonary embolus) will be tested for Factor V Leiden (which just about every doctor knows about) long before he/she will be tested for MCAS.

Factor VIII

"Factor 8." This is another protein with an important role in the coagulation system. You almost certainly have heard of a disease related to Factor VIII: hemophilia, which is what you get when you have mutations in one or both of the genes for Factor VIII, resulting either in production of insufficient amounts of Factor VIII or in production of a mutated form of Factor VIII that doesn't work as well as normal Factor VIII to drive blood clotting. Either way, such Factor VIII problems result in an insufficient amount of *normally functioning* Factor VIII, and this tilts the see-saw of the coagulation system toward the bleeding end. However, there also are conditions where *excessive* amounts of (normal) Factor VIII are produced on a chronic basis, and in the last decade or so we have begun to get a sense that such patients might have a tendency to excessive clotting, though it's not so clear a situation that it's been settled yet. Although most of the Factor VIII in the body and in the circulation gets made in cells in the liver and cells that line blood vessels, mast cells (some of which are located directly adjacent to blood vessels) can manufacture Factor VIII, too, and I have definitely seen significant elevations in Factor VIII levels in the blood in MCAS patients (some of whom have had problems with excessive clotting, and some not). At present, though, it's impossible to know whether the excess Factor VIII in such patients is coming directly from the patient's dysfunctional mast cells or coming from liver and blood vessel cells that have been stimulated to release excess Factor VIII as a direct or indirect consequence of certain mediators being inappropriately released by the patient's dysfunctional mast cells.

Famotidine

"Fuh-mōt´-i-deen." Also known by its most popular trade name Pepcid, the drug famotidine is a histamine H_2 receptor blocker (see the entry for "histamine" for more information). Famotidine has the fewest drug-drug interactions of all the presently available H_2 blockers.

Fasciculations

"Fah-sik´-yoo-lā´-shunz." This is the medical word for fine tremors.

Ferritin

"Fer´-ih-tin." Ferritin is an important protein in our bodies (heck, *every* protein in our bodies does *something* important in our bodies, or else the gene for that protein wouldn't still be in our genetic make-up; evolution is fairly (though not perfectly) efficient like that) and is primarily responsible for storing iron until it's needed (mostly for making the hemoglobin that goes into red blood cells). As more iron gets absorbed by the body than is needed right away, the body will make more ferritin, so the level of ferritin in the body is a good measure – in some people – of how much iron is stored up. Unfortunately, where it gets complicated is that the body also starts making more ferritin whenever there is inflammation around, so although a ferritin level below normal is a pretty reliable indicator of iron deficiency (due to any one or more of a wide range of potential causes), it's difficult to tell, in an inflamed patient, how much of a normal or elevated ferritin level is due to inflammation and how much is due to iron storage.

Fexofenadine

"Fex´-oh-fen´-uh-deen." Also known by its popular trade name Allegra, this oral-only drug is a non-sedating histamine H_1 receptor blocker (see "histamine" for more information).

Fibrinolysis

"Fī´-brin-ol´-ih-sis." (Sometimes alternatively pronounced as "fĭ´-brin-ol´-i-sis," i.e., with a short "i" sound rather than a long "i" sound in the first syllable. Adjective form "fibrinolytic," pronounced "fy-brin´-oh-lit´-ik or "fĭ-brin´-oh-lit´-ik.") Fibrinolysis is the natural coagulation system process in which strands of fibrin, or networks of such strands (which comprise the majority of any clot/scab), are broken down. In some patients, mast cell disease can amplify fibrinolysis, leading to abnormal bleeding/bruising. Medications called fibrinolytic inhibitors (see the entries in this dictionary for Aminocaproic acid and Tranexamic acid) are given when fibrinolysis and associated bleeding becomes clinically significant.

Fibroid

"Fīb´-roid." A fibroid is a common tumor of smooth muscle cells most commonly found about the uterus, and though we describe it as "benign" because it doesn't have any potential to metastasize, it still has potential to cause significant trouble both from mechanical effects (i.e, pressing on other structures as it grows) and bleeding. Given that it's an abnormality of tissue growth and development, it's not surprising that many women with MCAS have fibroids. What's unknown, though, is what percentage of women who have fibroids also have MCAS and whether, in those patients, it's the MCAS that's the primary driver of fibroid development. More research projects for the "to be done" pile…

Fibromyalgia

"Fīb´-roh-mī-al´-jee-uh." This is both a medical word that can mean either just general pain in connective tissues and muscles or a chronic condition/disease of such pain. For a long time, my profession didn't even acknowledge that such a condition existed. Now, at least, most doctors acknowledge it exists, and there are drugs touted to help it somewhat, even though we still haven't a clue what causes it. Many patients with mast cell disease have been previously diagnosed with fibromyalgia, raising the possibility that mast cell disease might underlie the condition in at least a portion of the patients who have it. And it is interesting that it's been shown that there are roughly ten times as many mast cells found in random skin biopsies in patients with fibromyalgia compared to patients without fibromyalgia. But there hasn't yet been any study that's taken a group of fibromyalgia patients and has specifically run the diagnostic work-up for mast cell activation disease in them to see what portion of them harbor previously unsuspected MCAD (whether SM or, far more likely, MCAS). Yet another research project for the "to be done" pile…

Fibrous myositis

"Fīb´-rus mī´-oh-sīt´-is." Inflammation of one or muscles (myositis) that's accompanied (somewhat unusually) by development of scar tissue ("fibrous") in those muscles. Given that mast cell disease can cause both inflammation and fibrosis, one has to wonder whether development of fibrous myositis in a patient might be due to (recognized or, more likely, unrecognized) mast cell disease.

FLAER

Pronounced just like the word "flair," this stands for FLuoroscein-labeled proAERolysin ("floor´-oh-seen"-labeled "pro-air´-oh-lys´-in"), a particular application of a common lab technology called flow cytometry that's useful for helping to diagnose a rare disease called paroxysmal nocturnal hemoglobinuria (PNH, which can cause life-threatening (and -shortening) problems with breakdown of red blood cells and excessive blood clotting) because proaerolysin binds to the "GPI anchor" protein which is a critical part of the surface of blood cells (especially red blood cells), and in PNH the GPI anchor is absent from a substantial proportion of blood cells, so if you mix a fluorescent form of proaerolysin (i.e., FLAER) with the patient's blood and then find, by running the sample through a flow cytometry test that a significant portion of the blood cells *don't* have the FLAER attached to them, congratulations, you've just diagnosed PNH.

Flecainide

> "Flek′-uhn-īd." This is a medication that can help stabilize a heart that has a tendency to switch into certain types of abnormal rhythms.

Flexeril

> "Fleks′-er-il." See Cyclobenzaprine.

Florinef

> "Flor-ih-nef." The most commonly recognized trade name in the U.S. for fludrocortisone.

Flow cytometry

> Flow "sī-tom′-uh-tree." This is a pretty slick lab test in which a cell sample is prepared into a fluid state (a lot easier to do when it's already a fluid, like blood) and mixed with various molecules (or "tags," usually antibodies of one sort or another, each specially prepared to glow with one color or another) which specifically bind with particular cellular parts (some of which are common to many cells, and some of which are found only in very specific types of cells), and then the sample is pushed with high pressure through a channel so narrow that only one cell at a time can fit through it. There's a set of glass windows at roughly the mid-point of the channel, and a laser is fired into the channel through one of the windows with the intention of crossing the channel. A portion of the laser light (called the "forward scatter") penetrates through the window directly opposite from the window where the laser light is fired into the channel, while another portion of the laser light (called the "side scatter") comes out through a window in the channel that's off to the side of the straight line in which the laser is fired. So, other than the fact that anything done with lasers is inherently cool and fun to play with, what's the point of all of this? Well, it turns out that as cells pass through the part of the channel where the windows are, they affect how much of the laser light comes out as forward scatter and how much of the laser light comes out as side scatter – and based on the tags that have been used and careful measurement of the forward and side scatter seen as any given cell passes through the channel, you can tell an awful lot about what *type* of cell has just passed through the channel. For example, because big cells in general impede forward scatter more than small cells (think about it), you can tell the difference, when running a blood sample through flow cytometry, between the large white blood

cells in the sample, the medium-size red blood cells in the sample, and the small platelets in the sample. Furthermore, the more *internal complexity* there is in the cell, the more of the laser light (which ordinarily shoots in a very straight line) gets deflected off to the side and shows up as side scatter. So, using the same blood sample as an example, the very complex white blood cell (which always contains a cell nucleus and often contains granules full of important proteins for white blood cell functioning) produces a lot of side scatter, while the very simple red blood cell (normally just a bag of hemoglobin, nothing more) produces little side scatter. Furthermore, the tags that are mixed with the sample before it's shoved through the machine have the interesting property that they glow a very specific color (i.e., they emit light of a certain frequency) when struck by laser light of a specific frequency. In fact, if there are a bunch of copies on a cell's surface of the molecule that a given tag binds with, then more of that tag will bind to that cell, so when that cell passes through the channel and is struck by the laser light that's tuned to the right frequency, that cell will glow more brightly (producing more intense light as forward and side scatter) compared to a cell that has less of that tag (or none of that tag) attached to it, so you can even tell with flow cytometry how many copies of a given molecule is on the surface of each cell that passes through the machine. And the final piece of this machine that you need to understand is that there are light detectors that sit beyond the windows in the channel that can measure not only the brightness of the light that's hitting them but also the frequency, or color, of that light. (Actually, each detector picks up a single frequency, so if you're looking for multiple colors, you need to have multiple detectors, and you wind up having to use prisms and mirrors to split and reflect the light beams so that multiple detectors can be used to look simultaneously for different colors.) So, if you put all of this science together, you get a machine (a flow cytometer) and a process (flow cytometry) that can give you pretty accurate counts of the different types of cells in any cell sample. Flow cytometry has a huge number of applications. Just to start with, it's the basic technology in automated blood cell counting, so when a sample of your blood gets drawn and processed for a "complete blood count" (CBC), it is virtually certain that it's an automated count that's being done and that it's a flow cytometer that's doing that automated counting, in merely a few seconds, of the many thousands of blood cells found in the tiny portion of your blood sample that the machine sucks in. Now that you understand the basics of flow cytometry, you can see how one of its valuable applications is to identify whether certain rare types of cells are present in a cell sample. This becomes helpful in trying to diagnose mast cell disease because it turns out that the surface of a normal mast cell is supposed to feature lots of CD117 (the extracellular portion of the KIT protein) – more copies of CD117, actually, by a ten-fold difference compared to any other type of cell in the human body. It also turns out that normal mast cells do not feature the molecules CD2 and CD25 on their surface, while some forms of mast cell disease do. So when you perform "multi-color" flow cytometry, mixing the tags for CD117, CD2, and CD25 with the sample and running it through the machine, you find out really quickly not only how many mast cells are in the sample (by counting the cells that showed super-bright glowing of the color used in the tag that binds to CD117) but also how many of them have abnormal, mast-cell-disease-defining "co-expression" of CD117 together with either CD2 and/or CD25 (by counting the cells that glow simultaneously with the color that marks for CD117 and either or both of the colors that mark for CD2 and CD25.

Fluconazole

"Floo-con´-uh-zōl." Also known widely by its most common U.S. trade name Diflucan ("dī´-flū-can"), this is an antibiotic that's specifically able to fight certain fungal microorganisms (like some types of *Candida*).

Fludrocortisone

"Floo´-droh-cort´-ih-sōn." Also known widely by its most common U.S. trade name Florinef ("flor´-ih-nef"), fludrocortisone is used to treat postural orthostatic tachycardia syndrome (POTS), a chronic disease of unknown cause in which you get lightheaded when you transition from a mostly horizontal position to a more vertical position. Just like "fibromyalgia" and "chronic fatigue syndrome" and "irritable bowel syndrome" and "dysautonomia" and lots of other diagnoses of chronic idiopathic diseases of a vaguely inflammatory nature, POTS, too, is commonly diagnosed in MCAS patients before they get diagnosed with MCAS (though it's never explained in such POTS patients how POTS accounts for their also getting lightheaded even when they haven't changed position), and since fludrocortisone is used to treat POTS, you wind up with a situation in which some MCAS patients have been treated with, or are being treated with, fludrocortisone by the time they have MCAS diagnosed. Of course, since fludrocortisone is a steroid and steroids help some patients with mast cell disease, it's not surprising that fludrocortisone given for POTS winds up providing some help to some mast cell disease patients whose "POTS" is actually just one more manifestation of their mast cell disease.

Flunitrazepam

"Floo´-nih-traz´-eh-pam." Known more widely by its most common U.S. trade name Rohypnol ("Roh-hip´-nol") or its "street name" of "roofie," flunitrazepam is yet another benzodiazepine medication which can be helpful in calming down mast cell disease. (When your doctor decides that a trial of flunitrazepam is appropriate for your (proven!) mast cell disease, do not use illegally obtained roofies. Medication purity and specific dosing are important to gain a medication's benefit while avoiding troublesome side effects. With any illegally obtained substance, of course, you have no idea of the purity of what you're getting, much less the dose you're self-administering. So do yourself a favor and always obtain your medications through legal, authorized medication dispensaries such as licensed pharmacies.

Fluticasone

"Floo-tik´-uh-sōn." Known more widely by its most common U.S. trade name Flonase ("Floh´-nās"), this is a steroid, usually taken as a nasal spray or in inhaled form, that – as you'd expect from the anti-inflammatory properties of most steroids – decreases inflammation and therefore is used most commonly as a treatment for inflammation of the nose, or rhinitis ("rīn-īt´-is"). Of course, since mast cells tend to sit at the environmental interfaces (such as in the nose) and since dysfunctional mast cells are always pumping out mediators (many of which cause inflammation), rhinitis is a common problem in mast cell disease patients and many such patients have taken fluticasone or similar drugs at some point during the many years they have suffered symptoms before they finally get to the point of figuring out the mast cell disease that truly underlies their problems. Note I'm not saying that all rhinitis is necessarily due to mast cell disease. I'm just saying that rhinitis that's due to mast cell disease often has been treated with fluticasone before (and even after) the mast cell disease has been diagnosed.

Folate

"Fohl-āt," also known as folic acid. This is an essential vitamin for life because you can't have life without replication of DNA and you can't have replication of DNA without folate. When it gets to be severe enough, folate deficiency leads to decreased production of all blood cells (and the red blood cells that do get produced are much bigger than normal).

Folliculitis

"Fol-ik´-yoo-līt-´is." This is an acne-like rash.

Fondaparinux

"Fon´-duh-par´-ih-nuks." This is a blood-thinning (or "anti-coagulant") drug somewhat similar to enoxaparin and the other low-molecular-weight heparins except that it's got a pretty different molecular structure from the low-molecular-weight heparins, so it really can't be classified as a low-molecular-weight heparin even though it works the same way that heparin and the low-molecular-weight heparins work.

Fosomax

"Fos´-oh-max." See Alendronate.

Fuchs corneal dystrophy

"Fooks corn´-ee-ul dis´-troh-fee." This is an eye disease in which there's slow thickening of a part of the corneas that eventually leads to distortion and deterioration of vision. Its cause is unknown. I've seen it in a few of my MCAS patients, but I have no idea whether it's a potential consequence of MCAS or not.

Furosemide

"Fyur-ohs´-em-īd." Far more widely known by its most common U.S. trade name Lasix ("Lā-siks"), furosemide is a diuretic medication, meaning it makes the patient's kidneys produce more urine than usual and that makes the patient urinate more than usual, which can be useful when there are disease states that lead to more water in the body than there should be

G

Gabapentin

"Gab´-uh-pent´-in." Known more widely by its most common U.S. trade name Neurontin, gabapentin is a drug that was originally developed to treat seizures but now is more commonly used to treat "neuropathic pain," i.e., pain of unknown origin – plus it's also used to treat a whole rafter of other odd neurological syndromes of unknown cause such as restless leg syndrome, anxiety, insomnia, and bipolar affective disorder (all of which, interestingly, are seen in various patients with mast cell disease). Interestingly, it is chemically similar to the natural brain chemical GABA that binds to benzodiazepine receptors, except that gabapentin is different enough from GABA that it doesn't actually bind to benzodiazepine receptors at the doses used, so if it doesn't work that way, then it must work some other way(s), except nobody has yet figured out what any of those other ways are.

Galactorrhea

"Gal-act´-oh-ree´-uh." This is a condition in which the breasts (virtually always female) secrete milk when they shouldn't. It's driven by various hormone imbalances, most commonly an excess level of prolactin which most commonly comes about due to an abnormal growth of the particular area of the pituitary gland (up in the head near the brain) that's the major source for prolactin in the body. Interestingly, I've seen elevated prolactin levels in some MCAS patients, but I have no idea whether in those patients it's coming from the mast cells directly or coming from the pituitary gland or someplace else in the body due (directly or indirectly) to influences from dysfunctional mast cells – or whether it has absolutely nothing at all to do with the MCAS in those patients.

Gastrin

"Gas´-trin." This is a hormone, released by certain parts of the stomach, duodenum, and pancreas, that stimulates secretion of gastric acid by the stomach. I've seen elevated gastrin levels in some MCAS patients, but I have no idea what combination(s) of mediators put out by the dysfunctional mast cells in such patients might be leading, directly or indirectly, to the increased gastrin levels in those patients.

Gastrinoma

"Gas´-trin-oh´-muh." This is a rare type of cancer that grossly overproduces gastrin without any regulation at all. Not only does it grow and spread as usual for cancer, the extra gastrin that it produces of courses causes excess secretion of gastric acid and, consequentially, ulcers in the stomach and duodenum.

Gastritis

"Gas-trīt´-is." Inflammation of the stomach. This is commonly seen in MCAS patients – though when it's found there's (understandably) almost never any suspicion that mast cell disease might be driving it. Sometimes, if there actually is suspicion that mast cell disease might be driving gastritis, biopsied stomach tissue can be specially processed in the pathology laboratory to reveal more mast cells in the tissue than seemed to be there based on standard processing.

Gastroenterology

"Gas´-troh-ent´-er-ol´-oh-jee." The study of, or the medical specialty focusing in, the stomach, intestinal tract, and related organs such as the esophagus, liver, and pancreas.

Gastroesophageal reflux

"Gas´-troh-ee-sof´-uh-jee´-ul ree´-flux," often abbreviated as GERD when referring to the common disease of excessive gastroesophageal reflux called gastroesophageal reflux disease. GERD is a very common phenomenon and is a diagnosis commonly acquired by MCAS patients long before they get diagnosed with MCAS. (Note this doesn't mean that MCAS is what's underlying GERD in every case of GERD. Nobody really knows what percentage of cases of GERD have an underlying MCAS. Yet another research project…)

Gastrointestinal

"Gas´-troh-in-test´-in-al." An adjective referring to the stomach and intestinal tract.

Genes

"Jeenz." Genes are long strands of DNA which code for proteins that your cells need to make to keep you alive and healthy. Genes themselves are linked end to end to make even longer strands of DNA called chromosomes. There are two copies in each human cell of each human chromosome. Every time a cell divides, each "daughter cell" gets one of the two chromosomes in each pair, and then a copy gets made to get the daughter cell back up to having two of each chromosome (and thus two of each gene).

Genome

"Jeen´-ohm." This word means the full set of genes in a person (or a species).

Genitourinary

"Jen´-it-oh-yur´-in-ār´-ee." An adjective referring to any parts of the urinary tract or the genitals or genital tract.

GI

See Gastrointestinal.

Giemsa

"Gim´-suh." This is one of the many stains used by pathologists to tell what kinds of cells are present in a tissue sample. Giemsa "lights up" many different types of cells – yes, including mast cells.

Gleevec

"Glee´-vek." See imatinib.

Globus

"Glohb´-us." This is an uncomfortable condition of a sense of a lump at the back of the throat, made all the more disturbing to the patient by the fact that doctors who investigate it almost never can find any lump back there. I suspect it's a sensation one gets from subtle edema in the throat tissue caused by dysfunctional mast cells, but that's just a hypothesis. Add it to the list of research projects to be done.

Glucocorticoids

"Gloo´-coh-cort´-ih-coidz." A large class of drugs that mimic the action of cortisol, a powerful hormone produced by the adrenal gland that causes a huge range of effects in the human body.

Glucocorticoids are members of an even larger class of drugs called steroids, and often the word "steroids" is substituted for the bigger mouthful "glucocorticoids" even though they're not precisely the same. Glucocorticoids are helpful in settling down inflammation in many situations, but when given chronically they cause a wide range of adverse effects.

Glucose

"Glu´-cōs." This is the main type of sugar in the human body.

Granuloma inguinare

"Gran´-yoo-loh´-muh in-guin-ar´-ee." This is a dermatologic condition, a particular skin lesion that I have seen in some MCAS patients, though I'll be careful to note that there's no evidence yet that it's produced by dysfunctional mast cells. Funny, though, how I've seen it reliably rapidly disappear once MCAS is diagnosed and effective treatment for settling down the MCAS is found.

Graves disease

Pronounced just like it looks. This is a type of overactivity of the thyroid gland, or hyperthyroidism, caused by erroneous production by the immune system of an antibody that stimulates the thyroid gland, leading to excess thyroid hormone in the body, which basically results in a state in which the whole body is chronically "revved up," resulting in a very wide range of problems.

Grover's disease

Pronounced just like it looks. This is a dermatologic condition, a particular skin rash that I have seen in some MCAS patients, though I'll be careful to note that there's no evidence yet that it's produced by dysfunctional mast cells. Funny, though, how I've seen it reliably rapidly disappear once MCAS is diagnosed and effective treatment for settling down the MCAS is found.

GU

See Genitourinary.

H

Halitosis

"Hal´-ih-tōs´-is." The medical word for bad breath. Typically caused by chronic oral infection, I've seen this as a symptom in some MCAS patients that "magically goes away" once the underlying problem (i.e., the MCAS) gets diagnosed and once effective (though, as usual, individualized) mast-cell-directed treatment is found. Get the underlying problem under control and then the immune system will start working better and get rid of chronic bacteria and fungi that shouldn't be in our microbiome.

Hashimoto's thyroiditis

"Hash´-ih-moh´-tohz thy-roid-īt-is." Hashimoto's is an autoimmune disease in which the immune system attacks and largely destroys the thyroid gland (usually first by erroneously manufacturing an antibody against one part of the thyroid gland or another, and then the rest of the immune system follows the antibody's lead and further attacks the gland), causing hypothyroidism. There are lots of symptoms from hypothyroidism which overlap with symptoms from mast cell disease, and many patients ultimately diagnosed with MCAS are often first diagnosed with hypothyroidism of one cause (e.g., Hashimoto's) or another, often in spite of there being only a trivial elevation in thyroid stimulating hormone (TSH) level, which should be markedly elevated in true, clinically significant hypothyroidism. Many such patients drive their endocrinologists crazy because it seems that no matter what adjustments are made to their thyroid medications, there just doesn't develop any stable settling of the elevated TSH and the presumed "thyroid disease." (Maybe that's because there wasn't any thyroid disease to begin with and the TSH is being driven slightly up for some other (reactive) reason. For example, since thyrotropin releasing hormone (TRH), the hormone that's the dominant stimulus for TSH production, is produced not only in the brain but also in the gastrointestinal tract and pancreas, maybe dysfunctional mast cells in the brain *and/or* the intestinal tract *and/or* the pancreas, by release of inflammatory mediators, are provoking nearby cells to produce and release more TRH than normal, and from there it's virtually inevitable that TSH levels are going to go up, regardless of whether there's any autoimmune attack going on against the thyroid gland or not. And since there are mast-cell-surface receptors for thyroid hormone, if it were the case that engagement of these receptors by thyroid hormone would further activate the mast cell, then it would kind of make sense that giving such a "hypothyroid" patient supplementary thyroid hormone (instead of finding and cooling down the mast cell disease that's at the root of it all) would only make things worse. Note this is all just conjecture, trying to envision a scenario to explain what I've observed in my patients.) What makes this whole situation even more complicated is that I've seen a number of MCAS patients who have sky-high levels of anti-thyroid antibodies – and no clinical or other laboratory signs of hypothyroidism whatsoever. Bottom line: if a patient is manifesting symptoms and signs of hypothyroidism but the TSH level is not substantially (many-fold) elevated, then clinically significant hypothyroidism is unlikely and another cause for those symptoms and signs (such as MCAD) should be sought. Also, just because a patient has a high level of any particular autoantibody doesn't necessarily mean the patient has the disease that's classically associated with that autoantibody.

Helices

"Heel´-ih-seez." This word generically means a spiral, but it is more specifically used to refer either to the spiral shapes taken by strands of DNA or to the external portions of the ear that feature spiral-like ridges of tissue.

Helicobacter pylori

"Heel´-ih-coh-bac´-ter pī-lor´-ee," frequently abbreviated to just "*H. pylori*." This is a particular, common species of bacteria which can cause various diseases in humans including stomach and duodenal ulcer disease and immune thrombocytopenic purpura (ITP). When somebody has chronic epigastric pain and an EGD is done to examine the stomach from inside, many times a biopsy will be done which will show inflammation, and because *H. pylori* so commonly is the cause of such inflammation, special pathology testing will be done to try to see if *H. pylori* is present in the tissue. Unsurprisingly, then, many patients who ultimately come to be diagnosed with MCAS have had *H. pylori* testing in the past which, more often than not, is negative. In fact, in some of these cases, doing the special pathology testing required to see mast cells will reveal that some of the cells that were originally thought (on routine testing) to be "standard" inflammatory cells actually are mast cells instead. Of course, since infiltration into an infected area by mast cells is normal, it's hard to say, when *H. pylori* is present, whether any increased numbers of mast cells also found in the stomach or duodendum are normal mast cells normally reacting to the *H. pylori* or are primarily abnormal mast cells that might well have been there long before the *H. pylori* showed up.

Hemangioma

"Heem-anj´-ee-ohm´-uh." A benign tumor of excess blood vessel growth (which, as is the case with any "benign" tumor, can eventually come to cause problems even though it doesn't metastasize, or spread to other areas). Hemangiomas can cause problems principally by growing big enough to press on other structures and/or by bleeding.

Hemiparesis

"Hem´-ee-par´-eh-sis." A devastating consequence of a major stroke in which half of the body is paralyzed, or at least greatly weakened.

Hemochromatosis

"Hē´-mō-krō´-muh-tō´-sis." A relatively rare, usually inherited disease in which the intestinal tract absorbs into the body too much iron from ingested food. The body uses iron to make hemoglobin, the principal component of red blood cells, and the body needs to always be making a lot of red blood cells, so it's important for the body to keep a good supply of iron in storage. However, when the body's usual iron storage sites get filled up and the intestinal tract erroneously keeps absorbing iron anyway, iron then starts getting stored in odd locations including many organs such as the heart, lungs, pancreas, and kidneys – locations where too much iron will eventually (after many years) cause the organ to fail. The human body has lots of ways of getting rid of lots of things that are harmful to it – but it has absolutely no (normal) way of getting rid of extra iron. (Presumably the human body evolved this way because, up until meat became a readily available part of the average human diet just within the last few hundred years, iron-containing foods used to be very hard to come by, so it actually would have been an evolutionary disadvantage if the human body had ways to normally get rid of iron.) Fortunately for hemochromatosis patients, we have two main ways of getting rid of excess iron: therapeutic phlebotomy and a few medications, called chelators, which literally latch on to iron before they get urinated out of the body, carrying the iron with them.

Hemoglobin

"Hē'-mō-glō-bin." About 280 million copies of this protein are contained in each of the 200 billion new red blood cells made by the bone marrow every day to replace the 200 billion old red blood cells that are cleared out of the blood every day. (It's an incredibly – but necessarily – exquisitely well-balanced equation of creation and destruction. Think what would happen, over an individual's lifetime, if there were even the slightest imbalance in red cell creation vs. destruction.) Hemoglobin latches onto oxygen (and unloads waste carbon dioxide) as the red blood cell circulates through the lung, and then that oxygen gets unloaded (and waste carbon dioxide gets picked up) as the red blood cell arrives at other tissues throughout the body. This cycle is really quite a remarkable feat of chemistry that goes on and on and on, in incredibly reliable non-stop around-the-clock fashion, a few thousand times each day for each copy of hemoglobin in each red blood cell which, in its 120-day lifespan, travels 300 miles through the body's blood vessels, tumbling roughshod through larger blood vessels, jostling up against vessel walls and other red blood cells, and squeezing through the smallest blood vessels (capillaries) whose width is actually smaller than the width of an (unsqueezed) red blood cell.

Hemophagocytic lymphohistiocytosis

"Hee'-moh-fāg'-oh-sit'-ik limf'-oh-hist'-ee-oh-sīt-is," a real mouthful that usually gets abbreviated simply as HLH. This is a terrible, pretty acute, life-threatening, *severe* inflammatory disease of unknown cause (though a few viruses have been associated with it) in which a key feature is that a relatively uncommon type of white blood cell known as a histiocyte starts engulfing ("phagocytic") red blood cells ("hemo"), destroying so many of them that the bone marrow just can't keep up (especially what with all of the inflammation suppressing the marrow), so the patient often dies from severe anemia and one consequence or another of all that inflammation. I have seen hemophagocytosis in bone marrow biopsies in occasional MCAS patients, and anytime you see that you have to wonder about HLH, but even though those patients have tended to be among the sicker MCAS patients I've seen, their overall presentation and chronic course is far more consistent with MCAS than HLH.

Hemophagocytosis

"Heem´-oh-fāg´-oh-sī-tōs´-is." This is the medical term for engulfing of a red blood cell by a histiocyte (or a macrophage, which is simply a histiocyte that's out in the peripheral tissues rather than in the blood or marrow).

Hemorrhage

"Hem´-or-uj." Major bleeding, acute in onset.

Hemosiderosis

Heem´-oh-sid´-er-ōs´-is." Accumulation of too much iron that's not due to hemochromatosis. Hemosiderosis is usually due to lots of red blood cell transfusions.

Heparin

"Hep´-er-in." The very first mast cell mediator to be discovered (in the 1930s!), heparin's principal function is to inhibit blood clotting. As a result, in some mast cell disease patients, a flare of their mast cell disease can result in a micro-flood of heparin being released by their abnormal mast cells into the surrounding tissues, causing bleeding which often seems quite mysterious to the doctor (and patient!) because all of the usual tests for bleeding disorders don't show anything wrong with the coagulation system. This is because these tests look for systemic bleeding disorders, whereas mast-cell-heparin-related bleeding usually is just a local bleeding disorder confined to the particular tissue in which the abnormally activated mast cells are abnormally making and releasing heparin – so there truly isn't anything wrong with the coagulation *system*. There are tests for detecting the level of heparin in the bloodstream, but only a tiny fraction of the heparin that gets released by mast cells into the surrounding tissues eventually gets into the bloodstream and therefore the detected bloodstream heparin level in a patient with mast cell disease often is much less than the actual level of heparin in the tissues where the patient's abnormal mast cells are situated. Further complicating the detection of elevated levels of heparin is the fact that heparin also degrades very quickly (within minutes) when exposed to heat (even room temperature, let alone body temperature), so unless care is taken to keep the blood sample continuously chilled and to expedite analysis for the sample's heparin level, it can be very difficult to *detect* an elevated heparin level in the blood even when the level is elevated at the time the blood sample is drawn.

Hepatic steatosis

"Hep-at´-ik stee´-uh-tohs´-is." Infiltration throughout the liver of fat globules. This is seen in a lot of MCAS patients, and it's also seen in a lot of other liver conditions of unknown cause (such as "metabolic syndrome"), thereby raising the question of whether any of those other conditions might actually be unrecognized MCAS.

Hepatobiliary iminodiacetic acid scan

"Hep´-at-oh-bil´-ee-ār´-e im´-in-oh-dī´-uh-seet´-ik" acid scan, usually abbreviated as HIDA scan, also known as cholescintigraphy (pronounced "kōl´-eh-sin-tig´-rah-fee"). This is a special test that radiologists can do to help define whether there might be gallbladder disease present, and since mast cell disease patients, by virtue of their abdominal pain, are often suspected of having gallbladder disease, such patients commonly come to have HIDA scans done. In a HIDA scan, a special chemical with a very faint amount of radioactivity attached is injected IV. This chemical gets filtered out of the blood by the liver and dumped into the bile, so if everything is working properly, the radioactivity ought to show up in the area of the gallbladder within an hour after the injection. If less radioactivity than normal shows up in the area of the gallbladder, then that's a sign of gallbladder disease, possibly inflammation of the gallbladder, possibly blockage of the bile duct by a gallstone.

Hepatomegaly

"Hep-at´-oh-meg´-uh-lee." Enlargement of the liver. There can be a zillion reasons for this, but mast cell disease is one of them.

Heterozygous

"Het´-er-oh-zī´-gus." Describes a condition in which a given mutation in a gene (any gene) is found in only one of the two copies of the gene that are found in every cell that has a nucleus. Heterozygous stands in contrast to homozygous (see this dictionary's entry for that term, too), in which the mutation is found on both copies of the gene.

HIDA scan

"Hī´-duh" scan. See Hepatobiliary iminodiacetic acid scan.

Hidradenitis suppurativa

"Hī-drad´-en-īt´-is sup´-er-uh-teev´-uh." Hidradenitis suppurativa is a rare chronic inflammatory disease of unknown cause in which cysts and abscesses (often painful) develop in areas where most of our sweating takes place, such as under the arms (i.e., in the axillae), under the breasts, and in the buttocks, groin, and inner thighs. There is no known consistently effective therapy. Merely the fact that it is a chronic inflammatory disease of unknown cause raises the question of whether it might be a particular variant of MCAS.

Histamine

"Hist´-uhm-een." A mediator produced and released by mast cells and a few other cells, histamine then binds to histamine receptors on the surfaces of various cells (including mast cells!) to cause, directly or indirectly, a variety of effects include itching and swelling. There are at least five types of histamine receptors, H_1 through H_5, but H_1 and H_2 seem to be the most common types, and that's a large part of why we only have drugs to block the H_1 and H_2 receptors, though drugs to block some of the other receptors are in development. The H_1 and H_2 receptors on the mast cell surface are activating receptors; in other words, when histamine (which, yes, gets released by the mast cell) binds with an H_1 or H_2 receptor on the surface of the mast cell, the mast cell gets activated, though in ways somewhat different from what happens when KIT or other activating elements of the mast cell get activated. H_1 blocking drugs are divided into sedating and non-sedating H_1 blockers. Sedating H_1 blockers include diphenhydramine and hydroxyzine (among others) and are available in many forms including oral and IV; non-sedating H_1 blockers include loratadine, cetirizine, and fexofenadine and are available only in oral form for reasons related to their chemistry. H_2 blockers include famotidine and ranitidine and are available in many forms. Most patients with mast cell disease gain at least some improvement by taking H_1 and/or H_2 blockers.

Histiocyte

"Hist´-ee-oh-sīt." A relatively uncommon type of white blood cell that plays a particular role in the immune system of sensing the presence of foreign invaders and then marshaling the rest of the immune system to the attack.

Hodgkin's disease

"Hoj´-kinz" disease. Also known as Hodgkin's lymphoma or just Hodgkin lymphoma. This is a particular class of lymphomas that usually feature a relatively unique kind of (abnormal) cell called the Reed-Sternberg cell which, under the microscope, has a nucleus that kind of looks like a pair of owl's eyes staring out at you. Since mast cell disease causes increased risk for malignancy, especially hematologic malignancy, and since lymphoma is a type of hematologic malignancy, Hodgkin's lymphoma is sometimes seen in the setting of mast cell disease .

Holter monitor

Pronounced just like it looks: Holter monitor. This is a heart test in which the patient is hooked up to EKG leads in a fashion very similar to what's done when an EKG is taken, except the wires from the leads are plugged into a small portable computer which records much of the heart's electrical activity, usually for at least a day, sometimes longer. Later, the recording can be analyzed to see if there are any concerning irregularities in the heartbeat at times other than when the patient just happens to be hooked up to an EKG machine in the doctor's office.

Homocidality

"Hoh´-moh-sī-dal´-ih-tee." A psychiatric condition for sure, homocidality describes a tendency/desire to kill people.

Homocysteine

"Hoh´-moh-sist´-een." Homocysteine is a precursor of the critical amino acids cysteine and methionine. Increased levels of homocysteine can result from deficiency of vitamin B12 or another vitamin, folic acid, or from mutations in a critical enzyme called methyltetrahydrofolate reductase (a real mouthful, so everybody calls it by its abbreviation MTHFR). Modest increases in homocysteine probably have no significant clinical impact, but stark increases have been associated with excess inflammation and blood clotting and blood vessel injury that may lead to a variety of consequences such as development of cholesterol-laden atherosclerotic plaque in arteries, which in turn can lead to arterial obstruction (such as what happens in a heart attack, or myocardial infarction, when the affected arteries are the coronary arteries that supply blood to the heart muscle). All of this becomes potentially relevant to mast cell disease because people with mast cell disease sometimes have abnormal excessive blood clotting, and elevations in homocysteine are associated with excessive blood clotting, and mast cell disease patients sometimes have MTHFR mutations, so it becomes a really complex mess trying to figure out what's really causing the excessive blood clotting in a mast cell disease patient with a mild MTHFR mutation.

Homovanillic acid

"Hoh´-moh-van-il´-ik" acid. More commonly abbreviated as HVA, homovanillic acid – similar to vanillylmandelic acid (VMA) – is a metabolite (i.e., a breakdown product) of catecholamines such as epinephrine, norepinephrine, and dopamine. Since excess catecholamine production is a major feature of a rare neuroendocrine malignancy called pheochromocytoma that causes episodic hypertension and flushing, and since episodic hypertension and flushing are also seen in mast cell disease, many patients ultimately shown to have mast cell disease have previously been tested for VMA and HVA to check for pheochromocytoma. Where it gets complicated is that I have observed that many patients with mast cell disease also have mildly (generally no more than twice the upper limit of normal) elevated levels of norepinephrine (less so dopamine, whereas epinephrine levels tend to be low or somewhere around the lower limit of normal), and such elevated levels may lead to modest elevations in HVA and VMA, certainly nowhere close to the marked elevations typical for pheochromocytoma, but when a patient is presenting with strange symptoms, any testing abnormalities at all can be confusing to interpret, so it's not surprising that some patients ultimately shown to have mast cell disease have previously been strongly suspected of having a pheochromocytoma, leaving their doctors very confused as to why the special radiology tests done to find the location of a pheochromocytoma keep turning out negative.

Homozygous

"Hoh´-moh-zī´-gus." This adjective describes the state in which a given genetic finding (usually a particular mutation) is present on *both* of the pair of genes harboring that sequence of DNA. Homozygous stands in contrast to heterozygous (see this dictionary's entry for that term), in which the genetic finding is present on only one gene or the other of the pair of genes harboring that sequence of DNA.

Humira

> "Hyoo-meer´-uh." Trade name in the U.S. for adalimumab. See Adalimumab.

HVA

> See Homovanillic acid.

Hydralazine

> "Hī-dral´-uh-zeen." An old drug, hydralazine treats high blood pressure, or hypertension, by relaxing the smooth muscle in the walls of blood vessels, especially arteries. It is usually reserved to treat severe hypertension resistant to treatment by more commonly used drugs, and thus you can begin to understand why some patients with mast cell disease come to be treated with hydralazine before their mast cell disease is discovered.

Hydrochlorothiazide

> "Hī´-droh-klor´-oh-thī´-uh-zīd." Hydrochlorothiazide, much more commonly referred to as "HCTZ" (pronounced simply as the four letters in sequence), is an old medication that functions as a diuretic (i.e., increases urine production by the kidneys), and since the place from which kidneys get the water they put into the urine is the blood, HCTZ decreases (modestly) the amount of water in the blood, and since water is the major component of blood, decreasing the amount of water in blood decreases blood volume, and therefore HCTZ can function in some patients to bring down blood pressure by a mild-moderate degree.

Hydrocodone

> "Hī´-droh-coh´-dōn." Hydrocodone is a narcotic medication that's commonly used to treat pain, and since many mast cell disease patients have problems with chronic pain, hydrocodone is a drug that's often been prescribed at one point or another for such patients – virtually always without the doctor recognizing the mast cell disease, much less the fact that narcotics actually trigger flares of mast cell disease in many patients (which may at least partly explain why some of the most common side effects of narcotics are nausea and vomiting).

Hydroxyurea

"Hī-drox´-ee-yer-ee´-uh." A chemotherapy drug, considered to be only mildly powerful but nevertheless useful (in some patients, anyway) in treating certain types of blood cancers, sickle cell anemia, and mast cell disease. Its principal action seems to be inhibiting a key element of the cell's protein-assembling machinery called RNA synthetase, and when a cell can't make proteins, it can't perform its normal functions, and it may even die as a result. Although hydroxyurea (like most chemotherapy drugs) exerts its actions on all types of cells, including normal cells, the effect is far greater in cells – typically cancer cells – that are making protein at a much greater rate than normal, and that's why cancer cells are more susceptible to being inhibited and killed by hydroxyurea compared to normal cells.

Hydroxyzine

"Hī-drox´-ih-zeen." A histamine H_1 receptor blocking of the sedating type. Its most commonly recognized trade names in the U.S. are Atarax ("At´-er-ax") and Vistaril ("Vist´-er-il"). Doctors commonly prescribe this for complaints of itching, usually doing so without giving much thought to *why* the patient is itching (again bespeaking the limitations on the modern practitioner subject to the modern health care financing system).

Hypercholesterolemia

"Hī´-per-kohl-est´-er-ol-eem´-ee-uh." "Hyper" means too much (as opposed to "hypo," meaning too little), and "-emia" means blood, so hypercholesterolemia means too much cholesterol in the blood, or an elevated blood cholesterol level. I have seen hypercholesterolemia (including a subtype known as hypertriglyceridemia in which just the type of cholesterol known as triglyceride is elevated in the blood) in many mast cell disease patients that has improved (sometimes even fully normalized) simply upon treating the mast cell disease.

Hypercoagulable state

"Hī´-per-coh-ag´-yool-uh-bul" state, also known as hypercoagulability (pronounced "Hī´-per-coh-ag´-yool-uh-bil´-ih-tee"). This is a state in which there is an abnormal, increased tendency to develop clots in the bloodstream, which obviously can have devastating consequences. There are lots of potential causes of a hypercoagulable state, ranging from inherited (genetic) causes to acquired causes.

Hypereosinophilia

"Hī′-per-ee′-oh-sin′-oh-fil′-ee-uh." Hypereosinophilia
(sometimes just referred to as eosinophilia, or "eosinophil-
loving") is a state in which there are too many eosinophils in the
blood or tissue of interest. There are lots of potential causes of
hypereosinophilia, ranging from certain malignancies to allergic
phenomena (essentially, mast cell disease) to certain adrenal
diseases to certain autoimmune diseases (some of which may be
mast cell disease in disguise) to certain infections.

Hypereosinophilic syndrome

"Hī′-per-ee′-oh-sin′-oh-fil′-ik" syndrome, often abbreviated as
HES. HES refers to specific hypereosinophilic disease that
doesn't seem to be reactive to any other identifiable cause and is
either found to be due to, or is presumed to be due to, some
marrow stem cell mutation that results in overproduction of
eosinophils. HES most commonly causes problems – potentially
fatal – in the heart and nervous system.

Hyperglycemia

"Hī′-per-glī-seem′-ee-uh." Hyperglycemia is the medical word
for an elevated glucose level in the blood (i.e., an elevated "blood
sugar" level).

HyperIgE (Job) syndrome

"Hī′-per" I-G-E ("Jōb") syndrome. HyperIgE syndrome, also
known as Job syndrome, is a rare disease, typically due to
inherited mutations, in which a number of developmental and
inflammatory abnormalities develop, including very high levels
of immunoglobulin type E (IgE) in the blood. Probably the most
consistent feature of HyperIgE syndrome is recurrent skin
abscesses, particularly with Staphylococcus bacteria.

Hyperlipidemia

"Hī′-per-lip′-id-eem′-ee-uh." Hyperlipidemia refers to elevation
in blood level of any type of fat such as cholesterol or
triglyceride. The word is sometimes used interchangeably with
hypercholesterolemia, though in fact hypercholesterolemia refers
just to an increase in blood level of cholesterol, whereas
hyperlipidemia includes both hypercholesterolemia and
hypertriglyceridemia.

Hyperpigmented

"Hī′-per-pig-ment′-ed." Simply, too much pigment (coloring). A lesion (in skin or any other tissue) is hyperpigmented if it has more color to it than surrounding normal skin.

Hypertension

"Hī′-per-ten′-shun." Elevation in blood pressure. Many conditions – including, yes, mast cell disease – can cause hypertension.

Hyperthermia

"Hī′-per-therm′-ee-uh." Elevation in temperature. Although infection, of course, is the most common cause of an elevated body temperature, there are many other potential causes, too – including, yes, mast cell disease.

Hyperthyroidism

"Hī′-per-thy′-roid-ism." Excessive production of thyroid hormone. Hyperthyroidism can come about from many potential causes. Probably the most common cause is an erroneously generated antibody (i.e., an autoantibody) that binds with cells in the thyroid gland in such a way as to stimulate production of thyroid hormone. Because thyroid hormone has a wide range of effects in the body, hyperthyroidism can have a wide range of effects including – are you ready? – nervousness, irritability, increased perspiration, heart racing, tremors, anxiety, insomnia, thinning of the skin, fine brittle hair and hair loss, muscular weakness (even paralysis), diarrhea, weight loss, vomiting, lighter menstruation, tachycardia, palpitations, low cholesterol, increased appetite, anxiety, intolerance to heat, muscle aches, weakness, fatigue, hyperactivity, irritability, hyperglycemia, excessive urination, thirst, delirium, edema, panic attacks, inability to concentrate, memory problems, psychosis, paranoia, depression, atrial fibrillation, shortness of breath, loss of libido, breast enlargement (in women and men), osteoporosis, bulging eyes, and double vision. So now you probably understand why so many doctors focus so much attention on looking for thyroid problems when presented a not-yet-accurately-diagnosed mast cell disease patient, especially since doctors are trained that thyroid disease is common and mast cell disease is rare.

Hypertriglyceridemia

"Hī´-per-trī-glis´-er-ih-deem´-ee-uh." Elevation in blood level of the "triglyceride" type of lipid, or fat. There are may potential causes of hypertriglyceridemia, including inherited mutations, but clearly there is some mechanism by which some type(s) of mast cell disease can cause hypertriglyceridemia because I have seen mast-cell-targeted therapy immediately normalize otherwise utterly treatment-refractory severe hypertriglyceridemia.

Hyphema

"Hī-feem´-uh." This is the medical word for a bleed in the sclera (i.e., "the white") of the eye. There obviously are lots of potential reasons why hyphemas can develop, but since mast cell disease can lead to an increased likelihood for bleeding in some patients, it shouldn't be surprising that hyphemas will be an occasional problem in some patients with mast cell disease.

Hypoalbuminemia

"Hī´-poh-al-byoom´-in-eem´-ee-uh." Too little albumin (the major type of protein in human blood) in the blood. There are lots of reasons why hypoalbuminemia can develop, but malnutrition and chronic liver disease probably are the most common.

Hypoglycemia

"Hī´-poh-glī-seem´-ee-uh." A low level of blood glucose ("blood sugar").

Hypomania

"Hī´-poh-mān´-ee-uh." Hypomania is a state of excessive energy, i.e., abnormally low fatigue, that can be a component of many disease states (such as hyperthyroidism). The hypomanic patient is usually able to productively channel such energy and is distinguished from the frankly manic patient, whose seemingly boundless energy is handicapped by impaired thought processes leading to poor decision-making. Since I've seen mast cell disease drive any given parameter of any given system in totally opposite directions in different patients, and since fatigue (and even depression) is certainly a potential consequence of mast cell disease, I wouldn't be surprised if there are other mast cell disease states that can drive hypomania (or even mania).

Hypoparathyroidism

> "Hī′-poh-par′-uh-thy′-roid-ism." A state of too little generation of parathyroid hormone by the four parathyroid glands abutting the thyroid gland in the front part of the neck, hypoparathyroidism has many causes, but the end effects are largely the same with low levels of calcium in the blood and excessive generation of bone since hypoparathyroidism leaves parathyroid hormone's principal balancing "opponent," calcitonin, unchecked, and since calcitonin drives calcium into the blood, excessive calcitonin activity is going to result in lowered calcium in the blood and increased bone formation which, because of the architecture of bone, can lead to weakness in the bone, and often a good amount of bone pain, too.

Hypopigmentation

> "Hī′-poh-pig′-men-tā′-shun," also the adjective form hypopigmented. The opposite of hyperpigmentation, hypopigmentation means too little coloring. For example, when an area of skin bears less color than in surrounding normal skin (such as in the autoimmune disease of vitiligo, which pop singer Michael Jackson was widely believed to have suffered), we describe that lighter area of skin as hypopigmented.

Hypoproteinemia

> "Hī′-poh-proh′-tin-eem′-ee-uh." A state in which there is too little protein in the blood.

Hypothermia

> "Hī′-poh-therm′-ee-uh." A state of inappropriate low temperature.

Hypothyroidism

> "Hī′-poh-thy′-roid-ism." A state of inappropriately low production of thyroid hormone which can lead to fatigue, malaise, depression, and many, many other symptoms also commonly seen in mast cell disease, so – just as with hyperthyroidism – it's not surprising that many doctors (trained to know that thyroid disease is very common and mast cell disease is very rare) spend a lot of time and money evaluating and testing for hypothyroidism when a not-yet-diagnosed mast cell disease patient presents.

Hysterectomy

"Hist′-er-ect′-ohm-ee." An operation in which the womb (uterus) is removed. One of the most common operations performed on women, typically for purposes of birth control, though it may well also be done to address bleeding fibroids caused by (usually unsuspected) mast cell disease.

I

Ibuprofen

"Ī′-byoo-proh′-fen." Ibuprofen, as you probably know, is one of the most commonly used non-steroidal anti-inflammatory drugs (NSAIDs) in the world, and because NSAIDs can help some patients with mast cell disease (especially as regards pain), some such patients wind up using a lot of ibuprofen – which then can lead to stomach and duodenal ulcers and kidney failure.

IC

See Interstitial cystitis.

Idiopathic

"Ih′-dee-oh-path′-ik." A classic medical adjective that allows a doctor to sound ultra-intelligent, and to charge a lot of money, for saying, essentially, "we have no idea what the cause is." The common joke, of course, is that only "idiots" – insufficiently schooled and trained and unable to think more intelligently – diagnose something as "idiopathic." I suspect we'll eventually discover that most cases of idiopathic anaphylaxis actually are just assorted variants of MCAS, although occasionally a case of idiopathic anaphylaxis turns out to be mastocytosis or some rare eosinophil or basophil disease.

IgA

"Ī-jee-ay." A fairly common type of antibody produced by the immune system (making up about 15% of all human immunoglobulin), usually found along the body's mucosal surfaces (like the respiratory and gastrointestinal tracts), that helps prevent invasion of microorganisms at those sites.

IgD

"Ī-jee-dee." One of the most uncommon types of antibody
produced by the immune system (just 1% of all immunoglobulin),
IgD is a bit of a mystery, as its true primary function in the body
remains unclear even today, half a century since its discovery in
1964. We know it assists with activation of B lymphocytes,
basophils, and yes, mast cells, but much of its biology remains to
be discovered.

IgE

"Ī-jee-ee." The rarest type of antibody produced by the immune
system in response to exposure to allergens (normally just 0.05%
of all immunoglobulin), IgE interacts principally with eosinophils
and mast cells, causing activation of those (normally quiescent)
cells.

IgG

"Ī-jee-jee." The most common type of antibody produced by the
immune system (about 75% of all immunoglobulin), usually
found throughout the body's tissues, that helps kill infection that
has managed to penetrate into the tissues. IgM is similar in
location and function, except IgM antibodies are produced by the
immune system earlier in the response to infection and IgG
antibodies are produced by the immune system later in the
response to infection. IgG antibodies interact not only with
infecting microorganisms but also with many different types of
human cells including mast cells.

IgM

"Ī-jee-em." Normally the third most common type of antibody
produced by the immune system (just under 10% of all human
immunoglobulin), IgM is usually found throughout the body's
tissues and helps kill infection that has managed to penetrate into
the tissues. IgG is similar in location and function, except IgG
antibodies are produced by the immune system later in the
response to infection and IgM antibodies are produced by the
immune system earlier in the response to infection.

Ileum

"Il´-ee-um." This is the third and final part of the small intestine
that ends where the large intestine begins. Many important
absorptive processes take place in the ileum, including the

absorption of vitamin B12, so you can see how inflammation in the ileum, or surgery that removes part or all of the ileum, can lead to malnourishment in a variety of ways.

Imatinib

"Ih-mat′-ih-nib." Also known by the trade name Gleevec, the oral drug imatinib was the first tyrosine kinase inhibitor to be brought to market. Originally developed around the turn of the century as an extraordinarily effective treatment for chronic myeloid leukemia (CML), it was soon found to be very helpful (and at low doses, at that) in many of the few patients with mastocytosis who don't have the KIT-D816V mutation. It since has been found helpful in many cases of MCAS, too (of note, most cases of MCAS don't have the KIT-D816V mutation). Imatinib is thought to work in mast cell disease principally by inhibiting the activation of the regulatory protein KIT (see the entry for "KIT"). Some of imatinib's sister drugs developed over the last decade (again, primarily to treat CML) have now been shown to be helpful in some mastocytosis and MCAS patients, too.

Imidazopyridines

"Im′-ih-daz′-oh-pir′-ih-deenz." This is a class of drugs which, while chemically dissimilar from the benzodiazepines, nevertheless have the ability to bind to benzodiazepine receptors. The imidazopyridines tend to function as sleeping agents. The most widely used imidazopyridine by far is zolpidem (Ambien).

Immune thrombocytopenic purpura

Immune "thromb′-oh-sīt′-oh-peen′-ik per′-per-uh", often abbreviated as ITP or AITP (with the "A" standing for "auto," as in "autoimmune thrombocytopenic purpura).

Immunoglobulin

"Im′-yoo-noh-glob′-yoo-lin." A large class of proteins, also known as antibodies, produced by the immune system to aid in defense against attacks on the body. The immunoglobulin, or antibodies, normally produced by the body can "recognize" things that shouldn't be there – such as infecting microorganisms – and help marshal the rest of the immune system to mount a multi-pronged attack to wipe out the thing that shouldn't be there. However, when the immune system is diseased (as can happen in mast cell disease), it also can (erroneously) produce antibodies that target normal/healthy human tissue. Sometimes these incorrectly produced antibodies are unable to marshal the rest of the immune system to attack the antibody's target and thus prove relatively harmless, while at other times they indeed are able to marshal a full-scale immune system attack against one healthy component of the body or another and wind up causing true "autoimmune" disease. Autoantibodies (antibodies directed against one's own normal tissues instead of against "foreign" things) are common in mast cell disease and can be directed against *any* normal tissue, but they often present a confounding situation in which their levels *typically* are mild and insignificant but *sometimes* can be substantial and yet, even so, don't often seem to cause the expected associated autoimmune disease. Furthermore, autoantibody levels in mast cell disease also can confusingly fluctuate quite significantly within relatively short periods of time and sometimes even completely go away for periods of time. Again, though, sometimes true autoimmune disease can develop as a consequence of the effect of mast cell disease on the immune system, much the same as how mast cell disease's impact on the immune system can also cause increased susceptibility to infection, increased difficulty recovering/healing, and increased risk for cancer.

Imuran

"Im´-yur-an." See Azathioprine.

Infiltrate

"In´-fil-trāt." An infiltrate is a material or tissue that intrudes into another material or tissue.

Infliximab

"In-flix´-ih-mab." Known more commonly by its U.S. trade name Remicade, infliximab is an expensive, "monoclonal antibody" drug typically administered IV every 6-8 weeks that binds to, and thus inhibits the action of, the inflammatory mediator tumor necrosis factor alpha (TNF-alpha) that can be produced by many types of cells – including, yes, the mast cell. Infliximab is approved by the U.S. Food and Drug Administration (FDA) for use in the inflammatory skin condition psoriasis (of unknown cause), the inflammatory joint condition ankylosing spondylitis (of unknown cause), and a range of inflammatory GI tract conditions (all of unknown cause), and since TNF-alpha is also produced by the mast cell, there is increasing suspicion that it may be able to help at least some mast cell disease patients, too, but its potential side effects – especially infection – need to be considered cautiously and require careful monitoring.

Insulin

"Ins´-oo-lin." This is a critical hormone, made by the pancreas, which "pushes" glucose from the blood into cells and prevents blood glucose ("blood sugar") levels from getting too high. Loss of insulin-secreting "beta cells" – located only in the pancreas – is what leads to diabetes mellitus.

Integument

"In-teg´-yoo-ment." This is the fancy word referring to our body's covering tissues, protecting us from the environment, such as skin, hair, nails, and teeth.

Interferon-alpha

"In´-ter-feer´-on alf´-uh." Interferon alpha is a signaling molecule that has a very wide variety of effects on the immune system and other parts of the body. Levels of interferon alpha escalate in particular when the body is trying to fight off a viral infection. Interferon alpha is also available as a drug for treating a wide variety of conditions such as the chronic viral infection hepatitis C and chronic myeloproliferative neoplasms such as chronic myeloid leukemia, polycythemia vera, and mastocytosis. Interferon alpha (which has to be injected and is typically done so either daily or multiple times a week) can have a lot of side effects (similar to how the flu virus makes you feel), but there is a long-lasting, "pegylated" form (requiring injection just once a week) that seems to have fewer side effects.

Interleukin-1-beta

"In´-ter-loo´-kin" 1 "bay´-tuh." This is a type of interleukin (see this dictionary's entry for Interleukins), produced by many types of cells including the mast cell, which participates in many processes including inflammation and cell proliferation, maturation, and death.

Interleukins

"In´-ter-loo´-kinz." This word refers to an entire class of molecules used by cells (typically white blood cells) to send various signals to other cells (typically white blood cells).

Internal jugular vein

Internal "jug´-yoo-lar" vein. The "IJ" is a major vein, coursing through the neck, returning blood from the head to the heart.

Interstitial cystitis

"In´-ter-stish´-uhl sis-tīt´-is." See Cystitis.

Intra-abdominal

"In´-tra-ab-dom´-in-al." Simply, inside the abdomen.

Iron sulfate

Iron "sul´-fāt." This is the most common form of oral iron supplementation used to treat a patient who is iron-deficient (from whatever cause, and there certainly are a lot of them).

Ivabradine

"Ī-vab´-ruh-deen." This drug, available in Europe for several years now and possibly to become available in the U.S. within the next few years, helps control excessive heart rate, a problem that sometimes rises to clinically significant degrees in mast cell disease patients. In fact, I have seen some mast cell disease patients who take this drug and find that it controls their mast-cell-disease-driven tachycardia quite well.

J

JAK inhibitors

"Jak" inhibitors. The JAK inhibitors – of which only one a few are presently available on the market – are a new class of medications which inhibit one or more of the JAK regulatory proteins found in many cells (see this dictionary's entry for JAK2 for more discussion). In general, JAK inhibitors seem to have potential for helping to control some chronic myeloproliferative neoplasms (such as how the JAK inhibitor ruxolitinib is now the standard of care for advanced myelofibrosis) and some inflammatory diseases (such as how the JAK inhibitor tofacitinib is now used to treat resistant rheumatoid arthritis). Because abnormally activated KIT is found in almost every patient with mast cell disease, and because activated KIT leads to activation of JAK and activated JAK leads to production of inflammatory mediators, there is reason to suspect that JAK inhibitors may be able to help some patients with mast cell disease, but at present none of the pharmaceutical companies marketing or developing JAK inhibitors have recognized this possibility, much less that the size of the population suffering mast cell disease is far, far larger than the sizes of the populations bearing the diseases for which JAK inhibitor development has targeted to date. (Yes, I've been trying to educate them, but keep in mind the doctors and scientists at the drug companies are trained the same way all other doctors and scientists are trained, so they continue to think that mast cell disease is very rare and is solely the disease of mastocytosis, so why bother spending the hundreds of millions, or even billions, of dollars to develop a drug for a rare disease?)

JAK2

"Jak" 2. JAK2 is one of a large number of regulatory proteins in the mast cell (and other blood and non-blood cells, to be sure) that gets activated when KIT is (normally or abnormally) activated. The JAK proteins in general help drive production of a number of inflammatory mediators, and JAK2 also helps drive survival and reproduction of the cell. Obviously, then, excessive JAK2 activity will contribute to the production of excessive inflammatory mediators and excessive survival and reproduction.

JAK2-V617F mutation

"Jak-2-vee-6-17-eff" mutation. This is the most common mutation (found so far, anyway) in JAK2. It is found in almost every case of polycythemia vera (one of a class of blood cell cancers, or hematologic malignancies, called the chronic myeloproliferative neoplasms) and in about half the cases of essential thrombocytosis and myelofibrosis (which also are chronic myeloproliferative neoplasms). Because some mast cell disease patients present with the excess red blood cells seen in polycythemia vera or the excess platelets seen in essential thrombocytosis or the excessive fibrosis seen in myelofibrosis, it is unsurprising that many not-yet-accurately-diagnosed mast cell disease patients have previously been checked for the JAK2-V617F mutation.

Janeway lesions

"Jān´-wā" lesions. Janeway lesions are tiny thin dark short lines aligned longitudinally along the nails. They're what you see when a tiny blood clot has been generated somewhere in the arterial bloodstream and floats downstream, ultimately getting stuck in a finally-too-small nailbed arteriole.

Jejunum

"Jeh-joo´-num." This is the second part of the three parts of the small intestine and is responsible for a number of important nutrient absorption processes. As such, inflammation of the jejunum, or surgical removal of the jejunum can lead to significant nutritional deficiencies.

K

Karyotype

"Kār´-ee-oh-tīp." The karyotype, or "cytogenetics," of a cell is the layout of the cell's chromosomes. Usually this is performed on a sample of cells from a cancer, a bone marrow, or a fetus, i.e., cells that are actively dividing, as the process for determining a karyotype requires catching cells in the process of dividing. Usually the karyotype of a human cell simply shows the normal 22 different chromosome pairs plus either a pair of "X" chromosomes that programs the person to be female or an X chromosome and a Y chromosome that programs the person to be male. Sometimes, though, specific abnormalities will be seen that either are known to drive, or at least are associated with, specific diseases. For example, the abnormal joining of the tail end of chromosome 22 to chromosome 9 creates an abnormal chromosome, sometimes called the Philadelphia chromosome, that drives chronic myeloid leukemia. It is important to understand that karyotyping can pick up *major* chromosomal abnormalities, but tiny, point changes in the sequence of DNA that make up a gene cannot be identified by karyotyping (no matter how big an effect on the cell such changes may ultimately come to have) and instead require more sensitive testing such as polymerase chain reaction (PCR). Since most mast cell disease is born of such tiny changes, karyotyping in most mast cell disease patients is normal, a result which can seem at odds with the statement that most mast cell disease is mutationally rooted until one understands what the limits of karyotyping are vs. what the types of mutations are that drive mast cell disease. Interestingly, for reasons that have not yet been investigated (to my knowledge), I have observed that in the great majority of instances of attempting to karyotype marrow in MCAS patients, the procedure fails because the marrow cells will not divide adequately for the procedure. (They obviously divide adequately in the patient, but they just won't divide adequately outside of the body.)

Keppra

"Kep´-ruh." The most commonly recognized trade name in the U.S. for levetiracetam. See levetiracetam.

Ketotifen

"Keh-tot´-ih-fen." Ketotifen is a medication – very inexpensive in most places in the world except for the U.S. – for helping control mast cell disease. The precise mechanism(s) by which it achieves such control are unclear. It appears to have some anti-inflammatory and some anti-histamine properties. Although it is readily, inexpensively available in eyedrop and oral forms outside of the U.S., it is routinely commercially available only in eyedrop form in the U.S., and thus patients in the U.S. who want to try it in oral (systemically absorbed) form need to obtain it from a compounding pharmacy, at which the labor required to custom-package the pure drug powder obtained from the manufacturer necessarily adds substantially to the basic, low drug cost. As of late 2014, there are developing expectations that oral ketotifen will become readily commercially available in the U.S. within the next few years.

Kineret

"Kin´-er-et." See Anakinra.

KIT

"Kit." There are roughly 50,000 copies of the key regulatory protein KIT dotting the surface of the normal mast cell. KIT is a "transmembrane" protein, meaning it penetrates the cell membrane, with part of KIT sticking out of the cell, part of KIT embedded in the cell membrane, and the majority of KIT inside the cell. (The part of KIT that sticks out of the cell is called CD117, and we have ways of detecting CD117. This becomes useful because even though other types of human cells also have transmembrane KIT, there's far more of it in the mast cell than any other type of human cell, so when a test for CD117 finds a cell has a lot of it, we know that cell is a mast cell. Finding a lot of CD117 in a cell is just one of many ways to identify a cell as a mast cell, but it certainly is one of the more convenient ways.) Under normal circumstances, the binding of a signaling molecule called stem cell factor (SCF) to the extracellular portion of KIT (again, CD117) causes the intracellular portion of KIT to change shape – this change is the so-called "activation" of KIT – in a way that triggers the activation, in falling-dominoes chain-reaction fashion, of multiple other important pathways in the cell that result in the mast cell producing and release its own mediators which then influence the behaviors of other cells. In mast cell disease, though, KIT usually is mutated in any of a large number of ways that result in the protein *always* being activated, regardless of whether SCF has bound to it or not, and thus such a diseased mast cell starts constantly producing and releasing mediators which cause the same behavior adjustments in other cells that they would have caused under normal circumstances. Of course, when cells make behavior adjustments at times and in places where they have no need to be making such adjustments, that brings illness, not wellness, and the particular symptoms seen in any mast cell disease patient are dependent on the particular mediators abnormally produced by the patient's abnormal mast cells – and the particular abnormal mediator production pattern in any mast cell is dependent on the particular pattern of mutations (in KIT and other mast cell regulatory proteins) in that mast cell.

KIT-D816V mutation

"Kit-dee-8-16-vee" mutation. This is the one mutation that has been most commonly found in any form of mast cell disease thus far. Deciphered, this coded representation means a mutation in the KIT protein (implying a mutation in the KIT gene) in which the type of amino acid found at the 816th position in the chain of amino acids that define the KIT protein has been changed from aspartic acid (amino acid code letter D) to valine (amino acid code letter V). The KIT-D816V mutation is found in about 90% of patients with systemic mastocytosis and is known to be resistant to treatment with imatinib (though since some mastocytosis patients *also* bear other, imatinib-sensitive mutations, the presence of KIT-D816V does not guarantee clinical insensitivity to imatinib). A polymerase chain reaction (PCR) "probe" for the KIT-D816V mutation is widely available, and when mastocytosis is suspected, it is common to perform PCR for the KIT-D816V mutation on bone marrow samples taken from such a patient. If the mutation is found, it is a strong hint that mastocytosis is present – but one needs to be careful in adhering strictly to the full set of criteria for diagnosing mastocytosis because it also is known that there are some individuals who carry this mutation who appear to be completely normal. In other words, although the KIT-D816V mutation appears to contribute to the development of mastocytosis, it does not appear to be able to cause any disease all by itself, and it has not yet been discovered precisely which other mutations (in KIT or other genes of importance to the mast cell), working in combination with KIT-D816V, are truly necessary for the disease state that we recognize as mastocytosis to emerge.

Kounis syndrome

"Koo-nis" syndrome. Kounis syndrome, named after the doctor who first identified it, is a phenomenon in which there is a sudden arterial spasming which partially or wholly occludes the artery, thus significantly impairing blood flow to the tissue served by that artery. There is increasing evidence that Kounis syndrome is caused by abnormal acute release of blood-vessel-constricting (i.e., "vasoconstrictive") mediators from mast cells in the immediate vicinity of the affected artery. Kounis syndrome was first recognized in coronary arteries, causing mysterious heart attacks in which by the time the patient underwent cardiac catheterization (usually just a few hours after the chest pain began), no obstruction in the coronary arteries could be found (in distinct contrast to the situation found in the vast majority of heart attacks). It is thought that cardiac-focused Kounis syndrome (sometimes called "allergic angina") accounts for about 1% of all heart attacks, but Kounis syndrome is now coming to be recognized in other organs, too, such as in cerebral arteries in the brain (causing stroke) and in mesenteric arteries in the intestinal tract (causing a variety of intestinal and abdominal problems including pain). There probably is no artery in the body that is immune to Kounis syndrome. It only takes a few minutes of significantly impaired blood flow to a given organ, or part of an organ, to cause the cells in that region of the blood supply to die, and by the time an arterial occlusion is suspected and investigated, the causative spasm is virtually always long gone. Thus, a high index of suspicion is required to diagnose Kounis syndrome, and when the clinical circumstances lead to such suspicion, then testing for mast cell disease is appropriate.

L

Lamotrigine

"Lah-moh´-trih-jeen." Often known by its most popular U.S. trade name Lamictal, lamotrigine was originally developed as an anti-seizure drug but has also come to be used for depression and bipolar disorder. Given that the range of clinical problems seen in some mast cell disease patients includes seizures (or pseudo-seizures), some such patients come to be on lamotrigine chronically.

Langerhan's histiocytosis

"Lan´-ger-hanz hist´-ee-oh-sī-tōs´-is." A rare disease that's more commonly seen in children and adolescents than adults, and more commonly in boys than girls, Langerhan's histiocytosis (a.k.a. Langerhans cell histiocytosis, or LCH) is a type of cancer of histiocytes, yet another population of white blood cells involved in the immune system. The growths of histiocytes in LCH sometimes are found (and easily treated) in isolated bone lesions but sometimes are widespread and can become fatal. Given that mast cells have the ability, on routine pathologic examination, to mimic the appearance of histiocytes, it happens sometimes that Langerhan's histiocytosis is initially suspected in some patients with lesions in bones or other organs, but usually on further, specialized pathologic evaluation, the difference between true histiocytes and mast cells becomes apparent.

Lansoprazole

"Lan-soh´-prah-zōl." Lansoprazole is one of many proton pump inhibitors currently available on the market for inhibiting acid formation in the stomach. It is manufactured by many drug makers and is marketed worldwide under a huge array of brand names.

Lap-band

Pronounced just like it looks. A lap-band is a device, usually placed via minimally invasive laparoscopic surgery, that is placed around the upper part of the stomach and physically constricts that part of the stomach, making it more difficult for food to pass into the stomach and thereby slowing the consumption of food and hopefully stabilizing or even reversing obesity. Since mast cell disease can drive accumulation of fat and therefore obesity in some patients, some mast cell disease patients have undergone a lap-band procedure (or other stomach-limiting surgical procedure) to treat their obesity before their mast cell disease is diagnosed. Of course, even once mast cell disease is diagnosed, it can still be difficult to stabilize and reverse associated obesity simply via mast-cell-directed therapy, so gastric surgical therapies may still be warranted, though probably the outcome will be better if an associated mast cell disease is successfully concurrently treated.

Larynx

"Lar´-inks," also the adjective form laryngeal (pronounced "lar´-in-jee´-ul"). The larynx is the relatively short segment of the respiratory tract, located in the lower neck that connects the pharynx (throat) to the trachea (windpipe). The larynx also contains the vocal apparatus including vocal cords and associated soft tissue. Inflammation of the larynx (which has many causes, including mast cell disease) can lead to soreness and hoarseness.

Left upper quadrant

Standard English words there, nothing tricky about the pronunciation. Commonly abbreviated as "LUQ," the left upper quadrant simply refers to the left upper quarter of the abdomen. The principal organ in this location is the spleen, though parts of the intestinal tract, stomach, and pancreas are also in the LUQ. Although the abdominal pain experienced (intermittently and/or fluctuating) by some mast cell disease patients often migrates around the abdomen, some such patients experience pain (or sometimes just "discomfort") more consistently in the LUQ, and though there are no studies proving why this is so, my suspicion is that release of inflammatory mediators by dysfunctional mast cells in the spleen is the dominant source of the recurrent LUQ discomfort seen in some mast cell disease patients.

Leukocyte

"Lūk´-oh-sīt." A white blood cell, made in the bone marrow along with all the rest of the body's blood cells. There are many types of leukocytes including neutrophils, lymphocytes, eosinophils, basophils, and mast cells, among others. Each type of leukocyte is responsible for attending to a different set of functions in defending and repairing the body.

Leukopenia

"Lūk´-oh-peen´-ee-uh." Leukopenia is the medical word for a low white blood cell count.

Leukoplakia

"Lūk´-oh-plāk´-ee-uh." Leukoplakia is a whitish coating. This word is usually applied to such coatings on the tongue and may be due to sterile inflammation or infection.

Leukotrienes

"Lūk´-oh-trī´-eenz." Leukotrienes are a particular class of inflammatory mediators all sharing a particular base chemical structure. One of the effects caused by leukotrienes is triggering of contraction of small airways called bronchioles, a state that can cause wheezing, and thus you can see how overproduction of leukotrienes can contribute to asthma. Leukotriene receptor blockers such as montelukast, and leukotriene synthesis inhibitors such as zileuton, can help combat the effects of overproduction of leukotrienes. Mast cell disease can (directly and/or indirectly) cause overproduction of leukotrienes, so you can see why drugs such as montelukast and zileuton can help control some of the inflammatory effects of mast cell disease.

Leukotriene inhibitor

"Lūk´-oh-trī´-een" inhibitor. A leukotriene inhibitor is any drug (such as montelukast or zileuton) that prevents leukotriene-mediated effects (which are usually inflammatory in nature).

Levaquin

"Lev´-uh-kwin." The most commonly recognized trade name in the U.S. for levofloxacin. See Levofloxacin.

Levetiracetam

"Leh-veet´-er-as´-eh-tam." Known much more widely by its most popular trade name in the U.S., Keppra, levetiracetam is an anti-seizure drug. Given that the range of clinical problems seen in some mast cell disease patients includes seizures (or pseudo-seizures), some such patients come to be on levetiracetam chronically.

Levofloxacin

"Lee´-voh-flox´-uh-sin." Levofloxacin is a relatively old, fairly inexpensive antibiotic which, like ciprofloxacin, is of the fluoroquinolone class. The fluoroquinolones are commonly used since they kill many of the most common infection-causing bacteria, but the downside of such profligate use is that bacterial resistance to the fluoroquinolones has really been on the upswing for the last decade, and now there are many common bacteria which can no longer be killed by fluoroquinolones.

Levothyroxine

"Lee´-voh-thy-rox´-in." Known much more widely by its most popular U.S. trade name Synthroid, levothyroxine is an old, inexpensive, man-made form of the natural thyroid gland hormone thyroxine that is used principally to treat hypothyroidism, i.e., a disease or state in which too little thyroxine is produced and released by the thyroid gland.

Lichen planus

"Līk´-en plan´-us." Lichen planus is a disease of the skin and/or the mucosa of the gastrointestinal tract in which lichen-like patches develop, possibly as an autoimmune reaction, though the trigger is not known. The most common clinical issue with such lesions is cosmetic difficulty, though the inflammation can progress to the point of causing discomfort, pain, and/or scarring/fibrosis. Some patients who eventually come to be diagnosed with mast cell disease have been previously diagnosed with lichen planus (usually amongst many other problems, too), raising the question of whether lichen planus, in at least some patients, might be a consequence of a particular variant of mast cell disease.

Lidocaine

"Līd´-oh-cān." Lidocaine is a local anesthetic (pain-reliever) drug whose effect comes on very quickly in the treated area (generally within a minute) and lasts about 10-20 minutes. It also is used – usually in emergency situations – to treat some heart rhythm abnormalities, or dysrhythmias. Many patients with mast cell disease develop acute or delayed adverse reactions to various -caine anesthetic drugs, including lidocaine. However, development of reactivity to one -caine drug does not necessarily guarantee reactivity to all other -caine drugs, and some mast cell disease patients who develop reactivity to one -caine drug then undergo specific testing (usually by an allergist) with other -caine drugs to identify at least one other such drug that can safely be used in such a patient when a local anesthetic is needed.

Lipitor

"Lip´-ih-tor." The most common trade name in the U.S. for atorvastatin. See Atorvastatin.

Lipoma

"Lī´-poh-muh." A lipoma is a benign growth of fat cells (adipocytes). Sometimes it can be tiny, and sometimes it can grow to a very large size, but most commonly they're no bigger than roughly golfball-size. Although very occasionally a lipoma can grow so big as to exert significantly problematic mechanical effects upon one organ or another, usually the only issues resulting from lipomas are cosmetic effects. When necessary, treatment virtually always consists of surgery to simply remove the lipoma. In the vast majority of cases, the cause of a lipoma remains unknown – but since mast cells are intimately involved in the regulation of normal growth and development of all tissues, and since fat tissue is a known reservoir of mast cells, one can be forgiven for wondering whether at least some lipomas develop as a consequence of mast cell disease.

Lisinopril

"Lī-sin´-oh-pril." Lisinopril is an old, inexpensive, oral anti-hypertensive drug (i.e., a drug for treating elevated blood pressure). Since mast cell disease often causes hypertension, some mast cell disease patients come to be on lisinopril long before their underlying mast cell disease is discovered.

Livedo

"Lih-vee´-doh." Livedo is a particular pattern of discoloration. Livedo reticularis is the most common form.

Livedo reticularis

"Lih-vee´-doh reh-tic´-yoo-lar´-is." Livedo reticularis is a form of livedo in which the skin develops a mottled, lacy/reticulated (sort of like a vascular pattern) purplish discoloration resulting from swelling of small veins usually due to microscopic clots in the capillaries feeding into those veins. There's a very wide array of conditions that can cause it, including simple exposure to the cold. It's a pattern that's definitely seen in some patients with mast cell disease, but what portion of livedo patients in whom the condition is due to mast cell disease is yet another project for the to-be-researched pile.

L-methylfolate

"L-meth´-il-fōl´-āt." L-methylfolate is the form of folate used by cells in the critical processes to make certain amino acids and to make DNA. The synthetic folate that we take in in much of our diet needs to be chemically transformed, via the methyltetrahydrofolate reductase (MTHFR) enzyme, to the active L-methylfolate form, but mutations in MTHFR that impede this transformation to varying degrees are fairly common. Thus, some patients who need folate supplementation would do better specifically taking L-methylfolate, which is available under various brand names including Deplin.

Loratadine

"Lor-at´-uh-deen." A non-sedating histamine H_1 receptor blocker, this oral-only drug (also known by its most popular trade name Claritin) has the fewest drug-drug interactions amongst all of the non-sedating histamine H_1 receptor blockers.

Lorazepam

"Lor-az´-eh-pam." Probably known more widely by its most popular U.S. trade name Ativan, lorazepam is a member of the benzodiazepine class of anxiety-relieving drugs. Like all the rest of the benzodiazepines, lorazepam also can help control seizures and muscle spasms in some patients. It is available, inexpensively, in oral and IV forms. In contrast to diazepam (Valium and other brand names), lorazepam has a much shorter duration of action, typically only about 3-6 hours (depending on dose, of course). Benzodiazepines were first discovered in the 1950s and were initially thought to just affect the brain, but over time benzodiazepine receptors were found on many other types of cells, too – including, eventually, the mast cell. Because nerve cell activity can drive mast cell activity and vice versa, and because both nerve cells and mast cells bear benzodiazepine receptors, it is difficult to say how much of the benefit any one person, in any one incident, is receiving from a benzodiazepine dose (whether of lorazepam or any other benzodiazepine) is due to effects on nerve cells, mast cells, or other types of cells.

Lupus anticoagulant

"Loo´-pus an´-tee-coh-ag´-yoo-lint." Lupus anticoagulant is a type of anti-phospholipid antibody, an abnormal autoantibody that targets the coagulation system in a way that causes a propensity for inappropriate clot formation in either veins or arteries. Because lupus anticoagulant usually increases clot formation, the "anti" in the name "lupus anticoagulant" could be seen as a bit of a misnomer, but in fact it comes from the reliable finding that in the artificial conditions in the laboratory in which testing of the coagulation system is done, the primary screening test for lupus anticoagulant (the prothrombin time, or PTT) actually does usually show an elevated result, the same kind of result as is seen with some true anticoagulants like heparin. Because mast cell disease can lead to formation of autoantibodies of potentially any type, it's possible for a lupus anticoagulant, and the clotting consequences thereof, to develop in the setting of mast cell disease.

Lymph node

"Limf" node. Lymph nodes are normal parts of human anatomy. Stationed at various points along the "lymphatic channels" (or lymph vessels) that provide another way to drain waste products from tissues, lymph nodes are organized collection of lymphocytes and related cells which help process the waste and thereby protect the body. The cells from many metastasizing cancers (including lymphomas) tend to "get stuck" (at least temporarily) in lymph nodes, and when such malignant cells then grow, the entrapping node becomes enlarged (to the point where one can easily feel, or even see, the more superficially located ones), and sometimes quite hard and sometimes quite tender. Lymph node biopsy (of either an entire node or a part of a node (usually via a needle)) can be very helpful in diagnosing why a lymph node is enlarged.

Lymphadenopathy

"Limf´-ad-en-op´-uh-thee." Sticking "-opathy" ("something wrong") on the end of an anatomical word is simply the way in medical terminology to say there's something wrong with that part of the anatomy, so lymphadenopathy simply means an abnormality in one or more lymph nodes, and while it's possible that such an abnormality might not cause enlargement of the node, in practice the word "lymphadenopathy" is usually equated to "enlargement" of a lymph node.

370

Lymphocyte

"Limf´-oh-sīt." A type of white blood cell, primarily responsible for fighting less common types of infection such as fungal infections. Lymphocytes are the second most common type of leukocyte in the human body. Typically about 20-40% of the body's leukocytes in the blood are lymphocytes. Lymphocytes generally are divided into T-type lymphocytes (or T-lymphocytes, or sometimes simply T-cells, about 70% of all lymphocytes), B-cells (about 25% of all lymphocytes), and NK-cells (about 5% of all lymphocytes), and there are subtypes of each of those, each with a specific set of roles in making for a properly functioning immune system. Without going into too much detail, NK-cells, like mast cells, are part of the "innate immune system" and are pre-programmed from conception to recognize, and have the ability to kill, certain types of abnormal cells (e.g., cancerous cells or infected cells) all by themselves. T- and B-cells, on the other hand, are parts of the "adaptive immune system" and aren't initially programmed to recognize anything in particular but in fact learn, fairly early in life, to distinguish "self" from "non-self," thereby giving them an ability to recognize foreign cells and material, though usually they are not capable, in and of themselves, of killing such recognized foreign cells/material. Instead, they call in a variety of reinforcements, so to speak, that help actually kill foreign cells and dispose of foreign material. Activated T-cells usually assist with killing by calling in other types of cells to attack, whereas activation of B-cells leads to the development (from those B-cells) of plasma cells which produce specialized proteins called antibodies that are tailored very specifically to recognize and latch on to the foreign cell/substance, and once an antibody has latched onto something foreign, there are other mechanisms in the body (related to T-cells, macrophages, and other cells) that can help actually kill and dispose of the "something foreign." Lymphocytes, like any other type of cell, can develop mutations that lead to inappropriate functioning and malignant growth, and we call a malignant growth of lymphocytes a lymphoma (see this dictionary's entry for Lymphoma).

Lymphoma

"Lim-fohm´-uh." It's easy to say that lymphoma simply is cancer of lymphocytes, but such a statement obscures the truth that, like most types of cancer, lymphoma is a very heterogeneous (highly variable) disease almost certainly because of the great menagerie of mutations underlying it. Lymphoma generally consists of abnormal accumulations – i.e., development of masses – of lymphocytes, usually at sites where lymph nodes are normally found (e.g., around the neck, under the arms, on either side of the groin, and deep in the chest and belly) but potentially at any other site about the body, too. Although surgery is often used to obtain a lymph node biopsy to diagnose lymphoma, treatments for lymphoma generally consist of chemotherapy (drugs that directly kill lymphoma cells), immunotherapy (antibodies that bind specifically to lymphoma cells and activate the immune system to then destroy those cells), and radiation therapy (essentially, killing the lymphoma cells by aiming a radiation beam at them that has enough power to kill most lymphoma cells but not enough power to kill most normal cells). There are two main subdivisions of lymphoma, Hodgkin's lymphoma and non-Hodgkin's lymphoma, and there are many, many subtypes of each of those general types, each with its own prognosis and its own therapeutic approach. It has long been recognized that mast cell disease confers an increased risk for developing cancer, particularly hematologic malignancy, and lymphoma is one of those hematologic malignancies. It also has long been recognized that concurrent treatment of a malignancy with any co-morbid mast cell disease that may be discovered yields better outcomes with the malignancy, so it's important to recognize (even though at present it almost never happens) when symptoms are present in the setting of overt malignancy that are difficult to attribute to the overt malignancy but might be easier to attribute to covert co-morbid mast cell disease.

Lymphopenia

"Limf´-oh-peen´-ee-uh." Lymphopenia simply is low lymphocyte count, or a state of having too few lymphocytes.

Lymphoplasmacytic lymphoma

"Limf´-oh-plas´-ma-sit´-ik lim-fohm´-uh." Sometimes abbreviated as LPL, this is a type of lymphoma that is also called Waldenstrom's macroglobulinemia. In lymphoplasmacytic lymphoma there is aberrant proliferation of both malignant lymphocytes and malignant plasma cells (which are derived from B-type lymphocytes), and these plasma cells usually produce excessive amounts of IgM-type immunoglobulin. At an advanced stage, there can be so much IgM in the blood that the blood literally starts sludging and becomes difficult to flow, leading to a host of (potentially fatal) complications from the inability to deliver as much oxygen and nutrients as the tissues need and usually expect to receive via the blood. Like all other forms of lymphoma, too, LPL is a hematologic malignancy for which one's risk increases when one also has mast cell disease.

Lymphoreticular infiltrate

"Limf´-oh-reh-tic´-yoo-lar in´-fil-trāt." This is a somewhat outdated term that describes a situation in tissue in which "lymphoreticular" cells – meaning histiocytes, macrophages, dendritic cells, lymphocytes, plasma cells, neutrophils, and mast cells – have invaded (or infiltrated) into the tissue for some (benign or malignant) reason.

Lysis (of adhesions)

"Lī-sis" of adhesions. Scarring inside the body can develop for all sorts of reasons, sometimes as a consequence of trauma or the controlled trauma that is surgery, and sometimes as a consequence of inflammation even without any inciting trauma. And sometimes such scars (or fibrosis) comes to cause mechanical problems by fixing in place, and thus preventing normal movement of, various tissues such as the intestinal tract. When such restrictive adhesions develop, surgery to break/cut/remove them becomes necessary, and that sort of surgery is what lysis of adhesions is.

M

MAC

"Mak." See *Mycobacterium avium intracellulare*.

Macrophage

"Mak´-roh-fāj." A macrophage is the term we apply to a histiocyte that has left the bloodstream and gone into the peripheral tissues. A mast cell sometimes can take on the appearance of a macrophage, and it may not be clear that a cell under consideration is not a macrophage but actually a mast cell until special procedures are undertaken in the laboratory to make that distinction.

Macular

>"Mac´-yoo-lar." Basically, this is the $400 medical word for "flat." A skin lesion, for example, is described as macular if it is flat (i.e., not raised).

Magnetic resonance cholangiopancreatography

>"Mag-net´-ik rez´-oh-nens kōl-anj´-ee-oh-pank´-ree-uh-tŏ´-graf-ee." Typically abbreviated as MRCP, this is a radiologic technique using magnetic resonance imaging (MRI) that accomplishes a large part of what endoscopic retrograde cholangiopancreatography (ERCP) can accomplish in taking a look at the biliary and pancreatic ducts for disease. MRCP is sometimes used instead of ERCP when the patient's condition brings into question the tolerability of an ERCP procedure.

Magnetic resonance imaging

>"Mag-net´-ik rez´-oh-nens" imaging. Virtually always referred to by its "MRI" abbreviation, magnetic resonance imaging is a radiologic technique in which the patient is bombarded with pulsations of magnetism which stimulate the hydrogen atoms in the body in a way that causes them to give off radio frequency waves that can be detected by the MRI machine. Because hydrogen is a critical component of water, and because every tissue in the body contains water (with different tissues containing different amounts of water, and a diseased portion of any tissue containing a different amount of water than a healthy portion of that tissue), it becomes possible by measuring the emitted radio frequency waves to construct a pretty accurate picture of both the healthy parts of the body's tissues and the diseased parts of the body's tissues.

Malaise

>"Muh-lāz." Not necessarily just a matter of fatigue, malaise is a general sense of discomfort or uneasiness, often expressed by patients as "I just don't feel well" or "I just don't feel right, but I can't tell you specifically what's wrong."

Malar rash

>"Mā-lar" rash. A malar rash – classically seen in lupus – is an erythematous (red) rash that spreads across the bridge of the nose to involve at least one and usually both facial cheeks.

Masitinib

"Mah-sit´-in-ib." Masitinib is yet another tyrosine kinase inhibitor (TKI). As of the time of this writing, it's still not yet available on the market, though late-stage (Phase III) studies in aggressive mastocytosis have been completed and approval for that condition is expected soon, all while the drug's French maker, AB Sciences of Paris, continues explorations of the drug's utility in other forms of mast cell disease as well as certain other inflammatory diseases.

Mast cell activation disease

Standard English words there, no trickiness to the pronunciation. Sometimes alternatively called mast cell activation disorder, often abbreviated MCAD. Generic term now used to refer to all mast cell diseases since we now understand that all mast cell diseases first and foremost feature inappropriate mast cell activation.

Mast cell activation syndrome

Standard English words there, no trickiness to the pronounciation, often abbreviated MCAS. This is a form of mast cell activation disease (MCAD), likely far more prevalent than the other principal MCAD form called mastocytosis, in which there is inappropriate mast cell activation (with accompanying mast cell mediator production and release) but relatively little to no inappropriate mast cell proliferation (a feature prominently seen in most cases of mastocytosis).

Mastitis

"Mast-īt´-is." Don't be fooled: the only connection between this term – which means inflammation of the breast – and mast cell disease is that since mast cell disease potentially causes inflammation *anywhere* in the body, and since mastitis is inflammation of the breast, then it's always possible that any given case of mastitis *might* be due to mast cell disease.

Mastocyte

"Mast´-oh-sīt." Mastocyte is an alternative, more "medical-sounding" word for mast cell, but mastocyte has three syllables and mast cell has two syllables, so even most mast cell specialists simply say "mast cell" instead of "mastocyte."

Mastocytosis

> "Mast´-oh-sī-tōs´-is." A rare form of mast cell activation disease (MCAD), recognized since the late 1800s, that features not only inappropriate mast cell activation but also inappropriate reproduction/growth/proliferation of mast cells. It's this latter feature that the "osis" part of "mastocytosis" means.

MDS

> See Myelodysplastic syndrome.

Mean corpuscular volume

> Mean "cor-pus´-cyoo-lar" volume. Often referred to by its abbreviation MCV, the mean corpuscular volume, simply put, is the average ("mean") size ("volume") of the red blood cells ("corpuscular") in the bloodstream.

Medrol

> "Meh´-drol." One of the most commonly recognized trade names in the U.S. for methylprednisolone. See Methylprednisolone.

Medullary thyroid carcinoma

> "Med´-yoo-lar´-ee thy´-roid car´-cin-ohm´-uh." Sometimes abbreviated as MTC, medullary thyroid carcinoma is an uncommon type of thyroid cancer in which the thyroid gland's parafollicular, or "C," cells have turned malignant. As the C cells are responsible for the thyroid gland's manufacturing of calcitonin, and since calcitonin drives calcium from the blood into the bones, MTC symptoms often include the symptoms of low blood levels of calcium such as muscular weakness and even the very painful tetany (sustained muscular spasm). Manufacturing of excessive amounts of calcitonin, and the associated calcitonin-gene-related peptide (CGRP), is also thought to lead to flushing, diarrhea, and itching, which of course are symptoms commonly seen in mast cell disease, too. One of the earliest patients in whom I eventually recognized what today we would call a co-morbid MCAS was an unfortunate middle-aged man with an unusually aggressive, metastatic MTC that was not going well with treatment, and I was even more disturbed by his frequent presentations with a variety of symptoms (such as sudden hypotension) that even the often-bizarrely-behaving MTC couldn't possibly explain. Eventually I found signs in him of mast cell activation (well before I made my first "official"

diagnosis of MCAS) and found that simple antihistamines not only acutely resolved most of his strange symptoms but also significantly slowed the progression of his cancer (though he did eventually die from it). Today, given that CGRP is now clearly understood to be a cause of mast cell degranulation, I have to wonder whether many of the symptoms long attributed to MTC might simply be consequences of mast cell activation from MTC-released CGRP – and that perhaps other mast cell mediators released by such activation might (directly or indirectly) boomerang/ricochet back to further stimulate growth of the cancer. It will take a careful examination in the research laboratory of mast cells from MTC patients with possibly mast-cell-related symptoms to figure out which of them harbor normal mast cells normally reacting to CGRP vs. which of them harbor abnormal, mutated mast cells which might even be the instigator and primary driver of the MTC.

Megacolon

"Meh´-guh-kōl´-on." A condition in which the large intestine (i.e., the colon) has become dilated, sometimes massively so. This can be a life-threatening condition that can result from a wide variety of causes including infections, toxins, medications, and a range of inborn and acquired neurologic and metabolic diseases.

Megaloblastic anemia

"Meh´-guh-loh-blast´-ik uh-neem´-ee-uh." An illness in which, usually due to severe deficiency of vitamin B_{12} or folic acid which in turn greatly impedes the basic DNA replication process necessary for cell reproduction, the bone marrow becomes incapable of producing normal numbers of mature blood cells, in the end leading to low blood counts (anemia, leukopenia, and thrombocytopenia) and all the expected consequences thereof. Tellingly, in megaloblastic anemia the red blood cells become very large and thus the average size of the red blood cells (i.e., the mean corpuscular volume, or MCV) rises greatly compared to normal, and many of the neutrophils take on an odd appearance with five or more lobes to their nuclei instead of the usual three or four. The blood cell precursors in the megaloblastic bone marrow can look so weird that doctors sometimes can be fooled into thinking that a leukemia is present.

Megestrol acetate

"Meh´-ges-trol as´-eh-tāt." Probably more widely known by its most popular U.S. trade name Megace ("Meg´-ās"), megestrol acetate is a drug that has some chemical similarity, and thus some similarity in biological action, to the natural hormone progesterone. Megestrol acetate is commonly used to help stimulate appetite in patients who suffer from poor appetite for various reasons, but it's not entirely clear that this effect on appetite is reliable, and megestrol acetate has other disadvantages including increasing the risk for abnormal clotting.

Melanoma

"Mel´-uh-nohm´-uh." Melanoma is a cancer of the pigment-bearing cells in the skin called melanocytes ("mel-an´-oh-sīts"). It has always been a very difficult cancer to fight, especially once it grows large or spreads (metastasizes), but in just the last few years new drugs have been developed and brought to market which are starting to have much more of an impact on this cancer than we've ever seen in the past.

Menarche

"Men´-ar-kee." The point in a woman's life when menstruation begins.

Meningitis

"Men´-in-jīt´-is." Inflammation of the meninges ("men-in´-jēz"), the thin tissue linings surrounding the brain and spinal cord. Meningitis is often assumed to be infectious in origin, but various inflammatory diseases (such as you-know-what) can cause sterile meningitis.

Menorrhagia

"Men´-er-aj´-ee-uh." An abnormal state of menstruation in which there is inappropriate, excessive loss of blood.

Meperidine

"Meh-per´-ih-deen." Better known by its most popular U.S. trade name Demerol, meperidine is a narcotic drug that can help control pain, but there are certain aspects to its metabolism that make it a poor choice of narcotic to use in situations of chronic pain.

Mesial temporal sclerosis

"Meez'-ee-ul temp'-or-al scler-ōs'-is." Mesial temporal sclerosis is a sclerotic (or fibrotic, or scarring) process affecting the temporal lobe of the brain that frequently results in dementia (which can lead to misdiagnosis of Alzheimer's disease) and/or odd types of seizures as the neurons in that section of the brain are progressively lost through the sclerosing process. Classically seen as a result of trauma to that part of the brain, mesial temporal sclerosis also appears to develop in some patients subsequent to other brain insults such as infections and febrile seizures, though in a significant fraction of patients, a cause is not apparent, begging the question of whether other diseases which have a potential for causing fibrosis (such as you-know-what) might be the root of the problem in at least those cases.

Messenger ribonucleic acid

Messenger "rī'-boh-noo-clā'-ik" acid (abbreviated "mRNA"). mRNA is the form of RNA which carries a gene's "message" (its coding sequence) from the nucleus where the cell's chromosomes reside to the cell's protein-making machines, the ribosomes, located out in the cell's cytoplasm. A ribosome "reads" the strand of mRNA formed from the template of DNA in a gene and strings together a corresponding chain of amino acids (at a rate of about 200 amino acids per minute) to form a completed protein.

Messenger RNA

See Messenger ribonucleic acid.

Metanephrine

"Meh'-tuh-nef'-rin." Metanephrine is a metabolite of epinephrine, and this is why metanephrine levels are assessed when investigating whether a patient might have a pheochromocytoma, a rare tumor in which a principal consequence is overproduction of epinephrine.

Methadone

"Meth'-uh-dōn." Methadone is a synthetic narcotic that is used not only for pain control but also to help wean narcotic-addicted patients off the narcotics to which they are addicted.

Methicillin-resistant *Staphylococcus aureus*

"Meth´-ih-sil´-in" resistant "Staf´-il-oh-kok´-us awr´-ee-us," often abbreviated MRSA. *Staph. aureus* is a type of bacteria that is ubiquitous in our environment and often causes infection when our immune system is not working well for one reason or another. MRSA is a type of *Staph. aureus* that, simply, is resistant to the antibiotic methicillin, which usually means it's resistant to many other antibiotics, too, making it a difficult infection to treat and thus a potentially fatal infection. In the last decade or two, MRSA has become a much more common infection.

Methotrexate

"Meth´-oh-trex´-āt." Methotrexate is a drug that can help fight certain types of cancer (particularly certain types of leukemia and lymphoma) and immune system diseases. It that can be given orally or injected into the veins or even into spinal fluid. As is the case with most chemotherapy drugs, patients need to be monitored fairly closely when receiving methotrexate.

Metaiodobenzguanidine scan

"Met´-uh-ī-oh´-doh-benz-gwan´-ih-deen" scan, also abbreviated as a MIBG scan (sometimes pronounced as a "mib-jee" scan and sometimes pronounced just by enunciating each of the four letters in the abbreviation). A MIBG scan is a radiology test performed in a radiology department's nuclear medicine section to help find the location of a pheochromocytoma or a neuroblastoma that might be situated somewhere in the patient. Because mast cell disease patients often are suspected of possibly having a pheochromocytoma before their mast cell disease is diagnosed, it's not uncommon to find that such patients have already undergone a MIBG scan.

Methylprednisolone

"Meth´-il-pred-nis´-oh-lōn". Better known by its common U.S. trade name "Solu-Medrol" ("Sol´-yoo-med´-rol"), methylprednisolone is a type of steroid (more specifically, glucocorticoid) medication that can help settle down inflammation, including in flares of mast cell disease.

Methylsulfonylmethane

"Meth´-il-sul-fon´-il-meth´-ān" (sometimes abbreviated as MSM). Though not approved for any medical uses, MSM is marketed widely as a dietary supplement that can help control stress and inflammation. Interestingly, the parent compound DMSO (metabolized in the body to MSM) was approved long ago by the U.S. Food and Drug Administration for instillation into the bladder to treat interstitial cystitis, an inflammatory ailment of the bladder that is increasingly coming to be seen as due in many cases to mast cell activation syndrome.

Methyltetrahydrofolate reductase.

"Meth´-il-teh´-truh-hī´-droh-fōl´-āt ree-duct´-ās," often abbreviated as MTHFR. MTHFR is a critical enzyme in the chain of biochemical processes needed to make DNA. Certain mutations in the gene for MTHFR are common, but most of the time such mutations have no clinical consequence. Certain uncommon mutations have been associated with increased atherosclerosis and the consequences thereof (e.g., heart attacks).

Metoclopramide

"Meh´-toh-cloh´-prah-mīd." Better known by its most common U.S. trade name Reglan, metoclopramide is in the class of "phenothiazine" drugs and is principally used as an anti-nausea drug, though it also can be considered a sedating histamine H_1 receptor blocker.

MGUS

While this can legitimately be pronounced as simply its four initials M-G-U-S, it much more commonly is pronounced "em´-gus." See Monoclonal gammopathy of undetermined significance.

MIBG scan

Sometimes pronounced as an "M-I-B-G" scan and sometimes as a "mib-jee" scan. See Metaiodobenzguanidine scan.

Microangiopathic

"Mī´-croh-anj´-ee-oh-path´-ik." This is an adjective referring to a state of abnormality ("-pathic") in small and microscopic ("micro-") blood vessels ("angio").

Microcytosis

"Mī´-croh-sī-tōs´-is." A condition in which the average size of the red blood cells in a person is less than the lower limit of normal for this parameter (generally around 80 femtoliters, or 80 quadrillionths of a liter). Microcytosis is most commonly found to be a result of an acquired state of iron deficiency or a congenital state called thalassemia in which one or more mutations in the alpha globin or beta globin genes (which help make the hemoglobin protein that's the principal component of a red blood cell) lead to production of less hemoglobin than normal. There are other acquired and congenital reasons, too, why microcytosis can develop. Although microcytosis is asymptomatic in itself, it often is found in association with other conditions (such as anemia) which can be mildly to severely symptomatic.

Microvascular thrombosis

"Mī´-croh-vask´-yoo-lar throm-bōs´-is." Simply put, since "thrombosis" is the $400 medical word for a blood clot and "microvascular" means small ("micro-") vessel ("-vascular"), a microvascular thrombosis simply is a blood clot in a small blood vessel.

Midodrine

"Mi´-doh-drin." Midodrine is a drug used to treat postural orthostatic tachycardia syndrome (POTS), a syndrome (of unknown cause) of a fast heartbeat (tachycardia) and low blood pressure (hypotension) (and resulting lightheadedness) upon assuming a more erect posture that is diagnosed in many mast cell disease patients prior to recognition (if ever) of their underlying mast cell disease. It is thought that midodrine helps POTS by constricting blood vessels and thus raising blood pressure, but it actually has never been clearly proven to do that in any large, well-controlled studies. All I can say is that in all of the many MCAS patients I've seen who have tried midodrine for the POTS that was diagnosed before their MCAS was found, I've never seen one who benefited from midodrine to what I would consider a significant degree.

Midostaurin

"Mi´-doh-stawr´-in." Midostaurin is an experimental drug, in the same class of tyrosine kinase inhibitors (TKIs) as imatinib, being tested for its ability to treat mastocytosis. At the time of this writing, its testing in advanced systemic mastocytosis (ASM) is at a fairly late stage and the drug has been performing well (making it the very first drug to perform well in this difficult-to-treat form of mast cell disease), so regulatory approval likely will come relatively soon, and the manufacturer (Novartis) has now begun testing of the drug in the more common form of systemic mastocytosis, namely, indolent systemic mastocytosis. As of the time of this writing, there has been no sign yet that the company is moving to test this drug (or any other drug) in MCAS.

Monoclonal gammopathy of undetermined significance

"Mon-oh-clohn-al gam-op-uh-thee" of undetermined significance, often abbreviated as MGUS. A common condition that is almost impossible to avoid as one ages ever further, MGUS is generally regarded as a precursor state to multiple myeloma, a malignancy of the body's plasma cells which serve as part of the body's immune system by being the sole producer of the body's antibodies. In multiple myeloma, there is gross excessive proliferation of one particular, turned-malignant typed of plasma cell, in turn producing a gross excess of whatever type of antibody that plasma cell had been programmed to produce. As the precursor state, though, MGUS features so little excess proliferation of a turned-malignant plasma cell, and so little excess production of antibody from those (few) malignant plasma cells, that it isn't clear in any individual patient whether the disease will ever become clinically significant, which is why it's called monoclonal gammopathy (i.e., malignant production of one particular type of antibody) of undetermined, or unclear, significance. The oft-quoted rate of progression of MGUS to the more advanced form of the disease (myeloma) is that 1% of MGUS patients per year will so progress, the implication being that if you're diagnosed with MGUS this year, then if you live another 10 years you'll have a 10% chance of your MGUS turning into myeloma, and if you live another 10 years beyond that you'll then have a 20% chance of your MGUS turning into myeloma, and if you manage to live altogether for 100 years past the point of diagnosis of your MGUS, then you are essentially guaranteed (a 100% chance, corresponding with the 100 years and the 1% annual rate of transformation) that by that 100-year post-diagnosis point your MGUS will have transformed into myeloma. Obviously, this risk is so low that most MGUS patients need to do little more than get a check-up with their doctor once every few years, and the reality of the matter is that many patients with MGUS actually don't bother with regular check-ups at all without suffering any adverse consequences. As malignancies of a component of the immune system (the plasma cell), both MGUS and myeloma are potential consequences of mast cell disease, but it is completely unknown at this point what fraction of the MGUS and myeloma populations actually harbor detectable mast cell disease as a "co-morbidity" (let alone as the underlying, causative condition), and likewise it is unknown at this point what fraction of the mast cell disease population actually harbors MGUS or myeloma. On rare occasions, for unknown reasons, MGUS will spontaneously disappear; it is thought that in most such instances, the MGUS came on as an erroneous part of the immune system's response to some infection, and once the infection was cleared, the MGUS went away, too, but fundamentally it's just not possible at present – we just don't have the scientific understanding available, let alone the testing – to ever truly prove what triggered onset of any given patient's MGUS, much less what made it spontaneously resolve.

Monocyte

"Mon´-oh-sīt." The largest of all types of white blood cells (leukocytes), the monocyte serves many purposes in the immune system including contributing to the inflammatory response to various bodily assaults and insults (e.g., trauma, infection). Unsurprisingly (given that mast cell disease in most patients induces a state of chronic inflammation), I have noticed that the number of monocytes is often increased (relatively or absolutely), at least some of the time, in patients with mast cell disease. (I have observed a similar phenomenon, though in somewhat smaller fractions of the mast cell disease population and somewhat less frequently, for certain other types of leukocytes such as eosinophils, basophils, and reactive lymphocytes.)

Monocytosis

"Mon´-oh-sī-tōs´-is." Simply put, either a relative or absolute increase in the monocytes in the blood. (A relative increase would be an increase in the percentage of monocytes relative to the percentages of other types of white blood cells, whereas an absolute increase in monocytes is defined as more than 1,000 monocytes per cubic millimeter of blood, regardless of what the total white blood cell count is and regardless of what the monocyte percentage is.) Interestingly, monocytosis is being found in an increasing number of studies to be associated with poorer outcomes in a variety of conditions including certain types of cancer such as lymphomas (both Hodgkin's and non-Hodgkin's subtypes), but that's not too surprising given that the number of monocytes increases when there is inflammation and the co-presence of inflammation with cancer seems to often result in a worse outcome from the cancer.

Montelukast

"Mon´-tee-lū´-kast." Montelukast is the prototypical leukotriene receptor blocking drug. It's an oral drug, usually taken for asthma and once daily at that, though it clearly helps some patients with mast cell disease and I've anecdotally observed that in mast cell disease patients who benefit from montelukast, more benefit seems to be gained from twice-daily dosing than once-daily dosing. See this dictionary's entry for Leukotrienes for more information.

Morphine

"Mor´-feen." Morphine, as you probably know, is a potent and commonly used narcotic, and since many mast cell disease patients suffer pain, many mast cell disease patients come to receive morphine at some point, a dicey proposition considering that in some mast cell disease patients, narcotics serve to trigger acute flares of mast cell mediator release. Morphine (and other narcotics) commonly causes an acute side effect of nausea (sometimes even vomiting), and certainly nausea can be a symptom of a flare of mast cell disease, but it's unknown what percentage of patients who experience nausea with morphine actually have an underlying mast cell disease.

Motrin

"Moh´-trin." One of the most common trade names in the U.S. for ibuprofen. See this dictionary's entry for Ibuprofen.

MPNs

See Myeloproliferative neoplasms.

MRCP

See Magnetic resonance cholangiopancreatography.

MRI

See Magnetic resonance imaging.

MRSA

Sometimes pronounced simply as the four initials "M-R-S-A" and sometimes verbally shortened further to "Mer´-suh." See Methicillin-resistant Staphylococcus aureus.

MTHFR

See Methyltetrahydrofolate reductase.

Multisystem

Standard English word, pronounced as you'd expect. Simply an adjective meaning affecting more than one system (in the body).

Mycobacterium avium intracellulare (MAC)

"Mī´-coh-bac-teer´-ee-um ā´-vee-um in´-trah-sel´-yoo-lar´-ee." MAC is a bacterium that usually only causes infection in immunosuppressed individuals. It is a common bacterium in the environment. MAC infection typically starts with a cough and can progress to include fever, fatigue, diarrhea, abdominal pain, and weight loss. It's most common in AIDS patients with poorly controlled HIV (fortunately only a small fraction of the HIV-infected population these days, at least in the first world), but it can affect other immunosuppressed individuals, too – including, yes, mast cell disease patients. MAC is just one more reason why every pulmonary or GI symptom in a patient with known mast cell disease should not be reflexively attributed directly to aberrant mast cell mediator release.

Myelodysplastic syndrome

"Mī´-eh-loh-dis-plast´-ik" syndrome. Often abbreviated as MDS, myelodysplastic syndrome is a large array of marrow-rooted diseases in which blood cells do not mature properly, usually resulting in low counts of one or more of the cell lines (red cells, white cells, and platelets). In roughly half of the cases of MDS, cytogenetics or more sensitive mutation testing (such as FISH or PCR) is able to find specific mutations known to be associated with MDS, but in the other half, no mutations via any presently commercially available testing can be found, leaving us to wonder whether such cases are due to mutations that can't be found or are due to suppressive external forces (such as inflammatory mediators) being visited upon the marrow. At present, marrow examination (i.e., marrow aspiration/biopsy) is required to diagnose MDS.

Myelofibrosis

"Mī'-el-oh-fī-brohs'-is." A type of MPN (see "Myeloproliferative neoplasms") whose dominant clinical manifestation is development of extensive scarring in the bone marrow such that normal blood cell production can no longer take place there, instead moving to the spleen and liver, which can increase enormously (and painfully) in size as a result. The severity of myelofibrosis (MF) ranges from "low grade," in which the scarring process and other consequences of the disease can take place quite slowly (over more than a decade), to "high grade," in which problems develop fairly quickly (over several months to a few years). MF can transform into acute leukemia, but most MF patients meet their demise due to consequences of the enlarged spleen or the low blood counts (red blood cells, white blood cells, and/or platelets) that often develop. MF usually is incurable, and instead doctors ask patients to try any of several medications available to help control it (probably ruxolitinib and hydroxyurea are the two most commonly used such medications). The JAK2-V617F mutation (see JAK2-V617F mutation) is found in about half of patients with myelofibrosis.

Myeloma

"Mī'-eh-lohm'-uh." Myeloma (often referred to as multiple myeloma) is a hematologic malignancy in which a malignant precursor cell leads to malignant reproduction of plasma cells, and since plasma cells are what produce the body's antibodies, most cases of myeloma wind up with excessive levels of antibody (usually IgG, less commonly IgA, and even less commonly the other isotypes of immunoglobulin) which, if high enough, can cause the blood to start sludging (instead of flowing smoothly), with all sorts of bad downstream effects. That said, the worst part of myeloma tends to be how badly it eats away at the bones, causing "lytic lesions" throughout the bones. Treatment of myeloma has advanced greatly in the last decade or so, and though it remains the case that only the rare patient can truly be cured (and only by an allogeneic stem cell transplant at that), the duration of survival of the average myeloma patient, as measured from the time of diagnosis, has roughly doubled in the last decade from roughly 3.5 years to roughly 7 years. In some cases of myeloma, a precursor condition (essentially, very early stage myeloma) called "monoclonal gammopathy of undetermined significance" (MGUS) is found many years, even decades, before overt myeloma (according to current diagnostic criteria) emerges.

Roughly 1% of all MGUS patients (in whom the only identifiable abnormality usually is a mildly elevated level of "monoclonal" antibody, also known as an M-spike on the standard test for this that's known as a serum protein electrophoresis, or SPEP) transform into myeloma in any given year, so if you can live to 100 years past the age at which you were diagnosed with MGUS, you can be guaranteed of getting myeloma. Then again, if you can live to 100 years past the age at which you were diagnosed with MGUS (which usually doesn't get diagnosed until the 50s or later), then you've had a (record-setting) long life and hopefully a good life and probably aren't interested in getting treated for myeloma. Since myeloma is a hematologic malignancy, it is one of the cancers for which one's risk is increased if one develops a mast cell disease, but there's not much point in fretting about it since there's nothing – other than recognizing and controlling the mast cell disease – that one can do (that we know of today, anyway) to reduce that risk. This is not to say, of course, that mast cell disease necessarily underlies every case (or even many cases) of MGUS and myeloma (or any other hematologic malignancy or any other cancer, for that matter), but it just says that there's not a whole lot one can do to reduce one's risk for developing MGUS and myeloma.

Myeloproliferative neoplasms

"Mī´-el-oh-proh-lif´-er-uh-tiv nee´-oh-plasms." Abbreviated as MPNs and also sometimes referred to as chronic myeloproliferative neoplasms or myeloproliferative disorders (MPDs), the myeloproliferative neoplasms are a class of cancers, originating in blood stem cells in the bone marrow, which tend to lead to excessive production of one or more types of blood cells but tend to progress less quickly than many other blood cell cancers such as acute leukemias. Chronic myelogenous leukemia (CML, the disease for which imatinib was initially developed) is considered the prototypical MPN, though others in this class include polycythemia vera, myelofibrosis, and essential thrombocytosis – and mastocytosis. The question you, the astute reader, is probably now asking, of course, is whether MCAS is an MPN or a cancer of any sort, and this is where the semantics of what "cancer" means get tricky. In general, "cancer" is taken to refer to an uncontrolled increase (whether through excessive reproduction and/or insufficient apoptosis (programmed death)) in the number of a certain type of cell due to one or more mutations acquired after conception (i.e, non-inherited/non-congenital mutations), and it matters not (with regard to considering the process as "cancer") whether the uncontrolled increase occurs quickly or slowly. So, given that MCAS is a disease of "relatively little" to "no" aberrant proliferation of mast cells, is it a cancer or not? Clearly, if the patient has a form of MCAS in which there is no identifiable aberrant proliferation of mast cells, then that patient's MCAS is not a cancer. But even if the patient has a form of MCAS in which there are mutations that drive a "little" aberrant mast cell proliferation, can that technically be called a cancer? Yes, I suppose it can, but does such labeling *matter*? In other words, just because you call it a cancer, does it need to be regarded as a life-shortening cancer and treated as a life-shortening cancer? Absolutely not. If it's a cancer that doesn't subtract any days from your life and doesn't require any cancer treatment, there's simply no point in thinking about it as a cancer. There's no surgery or radiation therapy or chemotherapy or any other kind of therapy that we presently have that will remove or kill all of these (widely, sparsely distributed!) aberrant mast cells (at least, not without killing the patient in the process), and although there are no formal studies yet that have proven this, I can say from my clinical experience, observing hundreds of MCAS patients for several years now and never having seen a single case transform into any form of mastocytosis, that it must be a very rare event for MCAS to undergo such a transformation, and even if that should happen, it is far more likely that it would transform to the most common form of mastocytosis (namely, indolent mastocytosis) rather than more advanced, aggressive forms of mastocytosis. And, like MCAS, indolent mastocytosis doesn't require any therapy other than to try to control the aberrant mast cell activity and the downstream consequences of such. So it's my opinion, which I freely offer to all patients definitively diagnosed with MCAS, that I don't consider you to have cancer. To be sure, and as discussed elsewhere in this book, *any* mast cell disease can predispose the patient to developing any type of cancer, so it's always *possible* that some other sort of cancer might develop in an MCAS or mastocytosis patient (just as is possible in a healthy person, too), but my key message on this point is that MCAS doesn't *behave* like cancers typically behave and thus doesn't warrant treatment as a cancer and doesn't warrant even *worrying* as if it's a cancer.

N

N-acetylcysteine

"en uh-seet´-il-sis´-teen." N-acetylcysteine is a drug, available by prescription or over-the-counter, and in both IV and oral forms, that is used to help combat acetaminophen (Tylenol) overdoses. It also has been used to try to protect the kidneys from damage by some of the contrast agents used in CT scanning, though a large study in 2012 seemed to suggest it really didn't have any such benefit. N-acetylcysteine also is used to help break up thick, potentially obstructing mucus that is produced in some respiratory tract diseases such as COPD and cystic fibrosis. And, finally – yes, you guessed it – it seems to have the ability to help a small minority of mast cell disease patients, though the actual molecular mechanism(s) by which it brings about such help in such cases are completely unclear.

Naprosyn

"Nah´-pro-sin." One of the most common trade names in the U.S. for naproxen. (See entry for "Naproxen" in this dictionary.)

Naproxen

"Nuh´-prox-en." Perhaps known more widely by its most popular U.S. trade names Naprosyn and Aleve, naproxen is a commonly used non-steroidal anti-inflammatory drug (NSAID) and thus can be helpful in some patients with inflammation, including some mast cell disease patients – though some degree of caution is needed since (1) NSAIDs can trigger flares of mast cell mediator release in some mast cell disease patients, and (2) taken at high-enough doses for a long-enough time, NSAIDs can cause a wide variety of adverse effects including stomach and duodenal ulcers and kidney failure. NSAIDs also impair platelet function even with just a single dose, so taking high-enough doses can lead to bleeding.

Nebivolol

"Neh-biv´-oh-lol." Nebivolol is in the class of "beta-blocker" drugs that help treat high blood pressure, or hypertension, but it has an advantage. Most beta-blocker drugs block both the β_1 and β_2 receptors, and though blocking the β_1 receptors helps a lot in relaxing blood vessel walls (particularly arterial walls) and reducing blood pressure, blockade of the β_2 receptor is what leads to most of the side effects from beta-blockers. Nebivolol, then, has an advantage in that it blocks only β_1 receptors, not β_2 receptors. In other words, it is a β_1-selective beta-blocker. Since many mast cell disease patients have hypertension, beta blockers are sometimes given to such patients (almost always without any recognition of their mast cell disease). In general, it's probably a good idea to avoid using beta-blockers to treat a patient with mast cell disease because if the patient suffers anaphylaxis and emergently needs to be given epinephrine, the effect of the epinephrine will be at least partly blocked by the presence of the beta blocker, and precious time can be lost in wondering why the epinephrine is not working better to reverse the anaphylaxis before the problem is recognized and the "work-around" drug, glucagon, is finally given.

Neoral

"Nee-or-al." Trade name for a formulation of cyclosporine commonly used in the U.S. See Cyclosporine.

Nephrology

"Neh-frol´-oh-jee." Nephrology is the study of, or the specialty in medicine that tends to problems of, the kidney.

Neuroendocrine tumor

"Nyur´-oh-en´-doh-krin too´-mer." Also called a neuroendocrine cancer or neuroendocrine malignancy. These terms refer not to a specific type of cancer but rather a specific class of cancers. As a class, neuroendocrine cancers are pretty rare relative to most other classes of cancer. Within the class of neuroendocrine cancers, carcinoid is the most common specific cancer, but there also is a wide variety of other, much less common neuroendocrine cancers such as gastrinomas, somatostatinomas, VIPomas, etc. All of the neuroendocrine cancers have symptoms which can partially mimic mast cell disease. However, in the vast majority of cases of these rare tumors, the total range and duration of symptoms, and the pattern of progression/worsening, don't come anywhere close to what's typically seen in mast cell disease. Nevertheless, in part because of the partial symptom mimicry, patients who are ultimately found to have mast cell disease often have been previously suspected of having – and thus have been intensively tested for, and sometimes even treated for – a neuroendocrine malignancy for which definitive diagnostic evidence cannot be found.

Neuroleptic malignant syndrome

"Nyur-oh-lept-ik" malignant syndrome. Sometimes abbreviated as NMS, neuroleptic malignant syndrome is a rare, life-threatening, acute illness of unknown cause in which certain drugs (mostly in the "neuroleptic" class) cause severe muscle rigidity and "autonomic instability" (high fever and possibly high heart rate and blood pressure and respiratory rate) and agitation, delirium, and even coma. Various theories have been developed as to what might cause NMS, but no such theory accounts fully for all that has been clinically observed in NMS cases. Some patients with mast cell disease occasionally present with an NMS-like emergency, but that's a long way from saying that mast cell disease is a cause of NMS. One wonders if NMS results from acute catastrophic release of certain mast cell mediators that affect brain function, perhaps akin to how Kounis syndrome and takotsubo syndrome increasingly seem to be the results of acute catastrophic release of various mast cell mediators that affect coronary artery or heart muscle function. Oh, well – another research project for the pile…

Neurology

"Nyur-ol-oh-jee." Neurology is the study of, or the specialty in medicine focusing on diseases of, nerve cells including both those in the central nervous system (brain and spinal cord) and the peripheral nervous system (out in the tissues beyond the brain and spinal cord).

Neuropathy

"Nyur-op´-uh-thee." Any condition of abnormality in one or more nerves. Central neuropathy more specifically identifies neuropathy within the central nervous system (consisting of the brain and spinal cord), potentially causing both "neurologic" effects (e.g., tremor, dystonia) and "psychiatric" effects (e.g., depression, anxiety, panic), while peripheral neuropathy more specifically identifies neuropathy within the peripheral nervous system (the nerves out beyond the central nervous system). Mast cell disease can cause a wide variety of problems throughout the central and peripheral nervous systems. The most common peripheral nervous system effect seems to be tingling/numbness paresthesias that migrate about the "distal extremities" (i.e., the hands and feet). Mast cell disease has been associated with every major psychiatric disease, but otherwise we don't yet know what the most common central nervous system effect of mast cell disease actually is.

Neutropenia

"Nū´-troh-peen´-ee-uh." Simply, a low number of neutrophils in the blood.

Neutrophil

"Nū´-troh-fil." A type of white blood cell, primarily responsible for fighting the most common types of infection, typically bacterial infections. Neutrophils are the most common type of leukocyte in the human body. Typically about 45-70% of the body's leukocytes are neutrophils.

Niacin

"Nī´-uh-sin." Also known as vitamin B_3, niacin is a vitamin that's critical in a large number of key metabolic processes in the human body including breakdown (catabolism) of fat, carbohydrate, and protein (oh, and alcohol, too), plus it also helps with development/creation (anabolism) of fatty acids and cholesterol, and it also is involved in inter-cell signaling and repair of damaged DNA. Severe deficiency of niacin leads to a disease called pellagra, endemic in more malnourished populations around the world. Mild niacin deficiency causes an insidious slowing of metabolism, causing decreased tolerance to cold, while greater levels of deficiency cause more overt symptoms and signs including nausea, skin and mouth lesions, anemia, headaches, and tiredness. Patients with pellagra suffer diarrhea, inflammatory skin lesions and skin thickening and hyperpigmentation (a blackish hyperpigmentation about the armpits is characteristic), dementia, inflammation of the mouth and tongue, digestive upset, and amnesia, irritability, poor concentration, anxiety, fatigue, restlessness, apathy, and depression. (So now you can see why a patient mast cell disease might be confused for a patient with niacin deficiency.) Sufficiently severe niacin deficiency is fatal. Absent severe alcoholism or other reason for severe malnourishment, it is quite hard in the modern world to become severely niacin-deficient. In the right clinical context, a simple niacin level blood test that finds a low level makes the diagnosis of niacin deficiency.

Nilotinib

"Nī-lot′-in-ib." Like its sister drug dasatinib, nilotinib is a so-called "second generation" tyrosine kinase inhibitor, sort of a "super-imatinib" or "super-Gleevec" that now is often used first-line to treat chronic myeloid leukemia (CML), though it originally was used only to regain control of some cases of CML that had come to resist imatinib. There also are just a few reports in the medical literature suggesting nilotinib may be able to help some patients with allergic or mast cell disease.

Nitroglycerin

"Nī′-troh-glis′-er-in." Although nitroglycerin is a key ingredient in the manufacturing of some explosives (such as dynamite), its potent ability to dilate blood vessels makes it a commonly used drug to treat certain heart diseases such as angina and congestive heart failure. Because mast cell disease can cause congestive heart failure, and because mast cell disease can cause chest pain that sometimes gets misinterpreted as angina, some mast cell disease patients come to be on nitroglycerin, whether it helps them or not.

Nizatidine

"Nī-zat′-ih-deen." Probably better known by its most popular U.S. trade name Axid, nizatadine is a pretty uncommonly used histamine H_2 receptor blocker (i.e., a drug akin to famotidine and ranitidine).

N-methylhistamine

"en meth′-il-hist′-uh-meen." *N*-methylhistamine is the principal breakdown product of histamine, and it has a longer half-life in the urine than histamine, so when one is looking in the urine for evidence of increased mast cell histamine production/release, there is a greater chance of finding an elevated *N*-methylhistamine level than an elevated histamine level, and therefore many doctors evaluating a patient for mast cell disease will (quite reasonably) only order a urinary *N*-methylhistamine level. However, doctors who are unfamiliar with the differences between histamine and *N*-methylhistamine may order just a histamine level, yielding misleadingly normal results, and laboratory staff who are unfamiliar with the differences between histamine and *N*-methylhistamine may mistakenly test a sample for histamine instead of the *N*-methylhistamine ordered by the doctor.

Non-steroidal anti-inflammatory drugs

"Non-ster-oid´-ul an´-tī (or an-tee) in-flam´-uh-tor´-ee" drugs, often abbreviated NSAIDs. The NSAIDs are a large class of drugs which, by and large, inhibit the enzymes cyclo-oxygenase 1 and cyclo-oxygenase 2 (COX1 and COX2), thereby inhibiting the formation (in quite a variety of cells) of prostaglandins, which are important inflammation-inducing molecules. Most NSAIDs (such as ibuprofen and naproxen) have reversible effects on the COX enzymes and relatively short durations of effect, but some – such as aspirin – have irreversible, longer-duration effects. Given that mast cells induce some of their inflammatory effects via production of prostaglandins, NSAIDs can be helpful in controlling some of the inflammation that arises in some mast cell disease patients, but one needs to be careful because in some mast cell disease patients, NSAIDs trigger acute flares of mast cell mediator release, and we don't yet have any way (other than going by the effects of past NSAID exposure) to predict how any given mast cell disease patient will tolerate any given NSAID.

Norepinephrine

"Nor´-ep-ih-nef´-rin." Norepinephrine is in the class of "catecholamine" molecules that have the ability to constrict blood vessels (thus driving up blood pressure) and speed up the heart rate. Elevated levels of norepinephrine are a normal part of the fear/scare/alarm/stress (or "fight-or-flight") mechanism in the human body, but elevated levels of norepinephrine are also produced abnormally in certain diseases such as the rare neuroendocrine malignancy called pheochromocytoma – and in some patients with mast cell disease, which I guess is not surprising considering that mast cells are both capable of directly making norepinephrine and are capable of influencing other cells to make norepinephrine.

Norfloxacin

"Nor-flox´-uh-sin." Like levofloxacin and ciprofloxacin, norfloxacin is in the class of "fluoroquinolone" antibacterial antibiotics to which resistance has rapidly been rising in the last decade, largely due to overuse of these antibiotics.

O

Obsession-compulsion

Standard English there, no trickiness to the pronunciation. O-C (sometimes also referred to as obsessive-compulsive disorder, or OCD) is a psychiatric illness in which the patient either is excessively interested (i.e., obsessed) in a given subject and/or feels compelled to repeatedly engage in a certain behavior. It can be a very serious illness and utterly destroy any ability to pursue a productive life. Although certain behavioral therapies sometimes can achieve improvement and even cure, most OCD is incurable and more severe cases may benefit from drug therapy. Interestingly, benzodiazepines seem to be the best treatment found thus far for controlling OCD

Occam's Razor

"Ŏk´-umz" Razor. This is the short-and-sweet phrase encapsulating a basic, universal-truth notion that among multiple possible explanations for a given set of observations, the explanation that accounts for the largest subset of the observations (ideally the entire set of observations) is the explanation that is most likely to be the true explanation, regardless of how "common" or "uncommon" that explanation might be. Occam's Razor is particularly relevant to mast cell disease because mast cell disease often presents with a very large set of symptoms, leading doctors to suspect diagnoses that account for one subset of those symptoms or another, but rarely suspecting mast cell disease either because they do not know that mast cell disease can cause many of those symptoms and/or because they think that mast cell disease is very rare and therefore is highly unlikely to be causing all of the symptoms. Importantly, though, the truth of Occam's Razor is completely independent of how prevalent/rare, or how common/uncommon, a given explanation is, and if mast cell disease can better account for a larger portion of the full range and chronicity of the patient's symptoms than any other diagnosis, then mast cell disease (far more likely MCAS than the known-to-be-quite-rare mastocytosis) is the most likely diagnosis.

Octreotide

"Ŏk´-tree-oh-tīd." A synthetic molecule very chemically similar to a natural hormone called somatostatin which can help control diarrhea, particularly when the disease called carcinoid is underlying the diarrhea. Octreotide is usually administered as a subcutaneous (under-the-skin) injection, much like an insulin injection. Like somatostatin, the normal octreotide molecule has a short half-life in the human body, so it needs to be injected typically three times a day to have a sustained effect in controlling diarrhea, but the manufacturer has also developed a long-lasting form that usually has to be injected only once every few weeks. Octreotide is sometimes referred to as the brand name Somatostatin, and the long-lasting form is sometimes referred to as the brand name Somatostatin LAR.

Octreotide scan

"Ŏk´-tree-oh-tīd scan." A special procedure in a radiology department's nuclear medicine section used for detecting the location of a rare type of cancer called carcinoid. In this test, a slightly radioactive form of a drug called octreotide (very chemically similar to a natural hormone called somatostatin) is injected into the bloodstream and the patient then reclines under a very sensitive radioactivity scanner. The radioactive octreotide binds to somatostatin receptors on the surface of carcinoid cells, allowing the scanner to thus detect the location of the radioactivity and thus the location(s) of the carcinoid cells. The radioactivity in the "tracer dose" is then soon naturally excreted out of the body, and it appears this amount of radioactivity is so low as to be harmless (to the limits of our ability to detect, anyway).

Olopatadine

"Oh´-loh-pat´-uh-deen." Olopatadine is a histamine H_1 receptor blocker marketed as an eyedrop for the treatment of irritated eyes – a symptom commonly seen in mast cell disease.

Omalizumab

"Oh´-muh-liz´-oo-mab." Known more widely by its U.S. trade name Xolair, omalizumab is a "monoclonal antibody" type of drug targeted very specifically against the type of antibody known as IgE which has the ability, upon binding with the mast cell, to activate the mast cell. At present, it is primarily used to treat certain difficult cases of asthma, and it is not presently approved to treat any form of mast cell disease (ignoring, of course, the likelihood that asthma is a form of mast cell disease). Curiously, an increasing amount of medical literature is demonstrating that the degree to which omalizumab seems to be able to benefit a patient appears to be independent of the amount of IgE in the patient's blood. Like other authors who have reported similarly in the literature, in my experience I have found omalizumab helpful for some patients with MCAS, especially those who manifest a large number of "allergies."

Omeprazole

"Oh-mep´-ruh-zōl." Known more commonly by its most popular U.S. trade name Prilosec, omeprazole is the prototypical proton pump inhibitor (PPI), and since PPIs are used to inhibit gastric acid production and since excess gastric acid production is usually suspected to be the culprit (and may actually be a culprit) in patients with symptomatic "gastroesophageal reflux" (or heartburn), it is not surprising that PPI drugs come to be applied in many mast cell disease patients long before any mast cell disease that's actually causing reflux and heartburn is discovered.

Onychodystrophy

"On´-ih-koh-dis´-troh-fee." Abnormal growth of nails. Various forms of onychodystrophy (weak/brittle nails, thin nails, ridged nails, spotted nails) are common in mast cell disease – and other diseases, too, to be sure.

Oromaxillofacial surgery

"Or-oh-max-il-oh-fā-shul" surgery. Often abbreviated as OMFS, oromaxillofacial surgery is the surgical specialty focusing on surgical treatment of diseases of the mouth, jaw, and face (as opposed to operations intended more to address cosmetic aspects of the face, which are handled primarily by plastic surgeons and dermatologists).

Osteoarthritis

"Os´-tee-oh-ar-thrīt´-is." A type of arthritis (inflammation of the joints) in which there is inflammation of both bone and joints. Unsurprisingly, many patients with mast cell disease come to be diagnosed with osteoarthritis long before their mast cell disease is recognized/diagnosed.

Osteogenesis imperfecta

"Os´-tee-oh-jen´-eh-sis im´-per-fect´-uh." Often abbreviated as OI, osteogenesis imperfecta is a rare congenital disease causing the bones to become so brittle that they often spontaneously fracture. Although there is no cure yet, it is possible to test for the presence of the underlying mutations that cause OI. Given that mast cell disease can drive weakening of the bones, sometimes to such a point as to cause spontaneous fractures, it is not surprising that some such patients come to be suspected of having OI long before their mast cell disease is suspected and diagnosed.

Osteonecrosis

"Os´-tee-oh-neh-krohs´-is." A severe bone condition in which the bone literally dies. Severe infection and other disease processes can do this, but medications in the bisphosphonates class can do it, too.

Osteonecrosis of the jaw

"Os´-tee-oh-neh-krohs´-is" of the jaw. Often abbreviated ONJ, osteonecrosis of the jaw is a deterioration of the jawbone (more commonly mandible than maxilla), a rare but potentially life-threatening condition most commonly seen in the wake of treatment with a bisphosphonate drug (such as pamidronate or zoledronate or risedronate) or anti-RANKL drug (such as denosumab) ironically given with intent to strengthen bone that is weakening due to one disease or another. ONJ appears to be even more likely to develop in patients who have significant dental or periodontal disease or who have undergone invasive dental procedures during, or in the several weeks prior to, treatment with bisphosphonate or anti-RANKL therapy. ONJ can be so devastating a consequence of ordinarily quite innocuous bisphosphonate or anti-RANKL therapy that obtaining "clearance" by a dentist prior to initiation of such therapy is now the standard of care.

Osteopathy

"Os´-tee-op´-uh-thee." By adding "-opathy" (something wrong) to "osteo-" (bone), you get the medical word for describing a state of there being something wrong with one or more of the patient's bones. Examples include osteopenia, osteoporosis, and osteosclerosis.

Osteopenia

"Os´-tee-oh-peen´-ee-uh." A bone condition in which the bone gets moderately thinned and thus weak, potentially causing some pain and some risk for fracture either spontaneously or with less stress than it would normally take to fracture a bone. As with osteoporosis, there can be a lot of reasons why this thinning might happen, but mast cell disease is one of the possible causes. Although vitamin D and calcium supplements can help to strengthen osteopenic bone, sometimes bisphosphonate therapy is used, too.

Osteoporosis

"Os´-tee-oh-por-ohs´-is." A bone condition in which the bone gets severely thinned and thus very weak, causing pain and quite a risk for fracture either spontaneously or with just slight stress. As with osteopenia, there can be a lot of reasons why this thinning might happen, but mast cell disease is one of the possible causes. Although vitamin D and calcium supplements can help to strengthen osteoporotic bone, bisphosphonate therapy is often used, too, when the bones get this thin.

Osteosclerosis

"Os´-tee-oh-scler-ohs´-is." A bone condition in which the bone gets abnormally thickened, which actually (because of the way bone is structured at the microscopic level) can make it weaker than usual and more prone to pain and fracture. As with osteopenia/osteoporosis, there can be a lot of reasons why this thickening might happen, but mast cell disease is one of the possible causes. Actually, it's even possible for mast cell disease to cause osteopenia/osteoporosis in some areas of the bones while simultaneously causing – in the very same patient, at the very same time – osteosclerosis in other areas of the bones. Although vitamin D and calcium supplements and bisphosphonate medication can help with osteopenia and osteoporosis, treating osteosclerosis is trickier and usually involves going after the root problem, be it mast cell disease or whatever else is driving it in the individual patient.

Otic

"Oh´-tik." An adjective referring to the ear.

Otitis

"Oh-tīt´-is." Otitis is simply inflammation of the ear. Otitis externa refers to inflammation of the outer (visible) part of the ear, while otitis media refers to inflammation in the middle part of the ear. Like any other type of inflammation, otitis can be of infectious or sterile origin, but most doctors reflexively assume it to be of infectious origin when they see it, and thus many patients whose mast cell disease causes episodic otitis wind up getting many courses of antibiotics that they probably don't need.

Otolaryngologist

"Oh´-toh-lar´-in-gol´-oh-jist." A doctor who specializes in otolaryngology.

Otolaryngology

"Oh´-toh-lar´-in-gol´-oh-jee." Otolaryngology is the study of, or the specialty in medicine focusing on diseases of, the ears, nose, and throat. (Technically, it would have to be "otorhinolaryngology" to refer to the ears, nose, and throat, but on a practical basis, "everybody just knows" that the shorter term "otolaryngology" also includes the nose.)

Ovarian torsion

"Oh-vār-ee-un" torsion. Simply put, a twisting of the ovary about the stalk of tissue (containing the ovarian artery and ovarian vein) from which the ovary dangles. And yes, to you male readers, it causes women as much pain as men experience from impact to the scrotum, the difference being that for men the pain from scrotal impact usually fades within a few minutes, while for women it often takes surgery to fix the torsion.

Oxcarbazepine

"Ox´-car-baz´-eh-peen." Known more widely by its most popular U.S. trade name Trileptal, oxcarbazepine is primarily used as an anti-seizure drug but also is used to treat bipolar (manic-depressive) disorder, anxiety disorders, and significantly bothersome tics. Small wonder, then, that some mast cell disease patients come to be tried on oxcarbazepine long before their mast cell disease is recognized/diagnosed.

Oxycodone

"Ox´-ee-coh´-dōn." Oxycodone is a commonly used narcotic, and since many mast cell disease patients suffer pain, many mast cell disease patients come to receive oxycodone at some point, which is a dicey proposition considering that in some mast cell disease patients, narcotics serve to trigger acute flares of mast cell mediator release.

P

Palpitations

"Pal´-pih-tā´-shuns." A sensation of the heart beating either faster than expected or irregularly. Palpitations are a common sensation among MCAD patients, even though objective testing for cardiac rhythm irregularities (dysrhythmias) in such patients usually find no dysrhythmias at all, let alone in correlation with the periods when the patients are sensing palpitations. That said, a borderline to mild increase in heart rate, at baseline, is very common among MCAD patients, and many such patients who have not yet come to be diagnosed with MCAD will consult a cardiologist for their borderline tachycardia (among consultations with many other specialists for many other problems caused by MCAD), and it is almost a given that the cardiologist will not find any cardiac-rooted explanation for the problem no matter how much cardiac testing is pursued, which isn't surprising since the tachycardia almost certainly is not rooted in the heart itself and instead the heart is merely responding (normally) to the stressed/inflamed milieu that MCAD creates. For example, I often see mild elevations in plasma free norepinephrine levels in MCAD patients, and increased norepinephrine can influence the heart to speed up, but it's highly likely that it's a far more complex assortment of direct and indirect effects from dysfunctional mast cells that drives the borderline tachycardia seen so commonly in MCAD patients.

Pamidronate

"Pah-mih´-drōn-āt." Pamidronate is one of the (older, IV) bisphosphonates sometimes used to treat the bone-weakening states called osteopenia or osteoporosis often seen in MCAD patients.

Pancreatic insufficiency

"Pan´-kree-at´-ik in´-suh-fish´-in-see." This term refers to inadequate production by the pancreas of (1) the enzymes needed to digest food that's coming down from the stomach through the duodenum, and/or (2) various hormones (e.g., insulin) needed to maintain proper metabolic balance of many systems in the body. Pancreatic insufficiency can develop due to lots of reasons including chronic inflammation, scarring (i.e., fibrosis), or autoimmune attack.

Pancreatitis

"Pan'-kree-uh-tīt'-is." Simply put, inflammation ("-itis") of the pancreas. This can be acute or chronic. When severe enough, it causes pain (acute or chronic), though often in MCAS there's only a subclinical pancreatitis that can be seen in merely modest elevations in key pancreatic enzymes such as lipase and/or amylase.

Pantoprazole

"Pan-toh'-prah-zōl." More commonly known by its most popular U.S. trade name Protonix, pantoprazole is one of many drugs in the proton pump inhibitor (PPI) class that dramatically reduces acid production in the stomach.

Paraneoplastic

"Par'-uh-nee'-oh-plast'-ik." This adjective technically describes any phenomenon that develops as a consequence of a malignancy, but it's most commonly applied to unusual autoimmune or hormonal/metabolic illnesses that are caused by a malignancy and thereafter operate largely independently of the malignancy but sometimes can improve if the malignancy goes into remission. A classic example is when a type of lung cancer called small cell lung cancer causes a rare autoimmune disorder targeting the Purkinje cells in the cerebellum (a part of the brain at the back of the head), causing the patient to lose balance, which might be the first clinical symptom. If the lung cancer isn't found and put into remission quickly, the autoimmune disorder can get so bad so fast that the resulting problem with maintaining balance can become permanent.

Paranoia

"Par'-uh-noi'-uh." A psychiatric state of irrational perception of threat.

Paresthesia

"Pahr'-us-theez'-ya." Abnormal sensation. Most commonly used to describe an abnormal tingling and/or numbness, which happens to be a very common intermittent neurologic abnormality in MCAD patients, mostly felt in the hands/fingers and/or feet/toes.

Paroxetine

"Pahr-ox´-eh-teen." More commonly known by its popular U.S. trade name Paxil, paroxetine is one of many drugs in the class of anti-depressant drugs called selective serotonin reuptake inhibitors, or SSRIs. Many MCAD patients are diagnosed as suffering from depression (either because they truly are suffering from a real "major depressive disorder" as defined in psychiatrists' diagnostic manuals or because their doctors interpret their fatigue as depression since they can't imagine what else might be causing it) and therefore wind up getting chronically prescribed, or at least trying, various SSRIs including paroxetine.

Paroxysmal nocturnal hemoglobinuria

"Par´-ox-is´-mal noc-turn´-ul heem´-oh-glōb´-in-yur´-ee-uh." That's quite a mouthful, so it's usually referred to by the initials PNH. PNH is a rare, odd, potentially life-threatening disease in which a mutation develops in the gene for a key blood cell membrane protein called PIG-A, with the end result being that red blood cells start spontaneously breaking down ("hemolyzing") and sometimes abnormal blood clots form, too. It's been my experience that many PNH patients also suffer many symptoms that can't possibly be explained by red blood cell hemolysis or blood clots but which instead are well explained by MCAS, and I have found laboratory evidence of MCAS in almost every PNH patient I've tested for such. Although the mutations that drive PNH are quite distinct from the mutations that drive MCAS, I wonder if the same genetic fragility state (driven by epigenetic mutations) that we're beginning to think underlies MCAS might also "permit" the emergence of PNH.

Partial thromboplastin time

Partial "throm´-boh-plast´-in" time. More commonly referred to by its initials ("PTT"), this is a common blood test that tells the doctor in part how well the "intrinsic" pathway in the coagulation system is working. A similar sounding test, the prothrombin time (PT), is commonly ordered along with the PTT and tells the doctor in part how well the "extrinsic" pathway in the coagulation system is working. Some MCAD patients present modest abnormalities (high or low) in the PT and/or PTT, and such abnormalities sometimes are clues to the presence of an uncommon autoimmune disorder called an anti-phospholipid antibody, which in some such patients becomes clinically significant because sometimes that sort of an antibody can cause enough dysfunction in the clotting system to result in abnormal clotting (or, much less commonly, abnormal bleeding).

Parvovirus B-19

"Par´-vo-vī´-rus" B-19. This is a virus that causes the common childhood "fifth disease" ("slapped cheek syndrome"), but it sometimes causes a wide range of problems beyond rash, and where it most intersects with a hematologist's life is when it causes "red cell aplasia," a state where the bone marrow has given up making red blood cells.

Paxil

"Pax´-il." The most common trade name in the U.S. for paroxetine.

Pegylated

"Peg´-il-āt´-ed." This adjective describes a particular chemical modification of a molecule (usually a protein) that renders the molecule more resistant to metabolism in the body. Pegylated drugs such as interferon or filgrastim can last for a week or longer compared to only a day or so for the non-pegylated form.

Pelger-Huet

"Pel´-ger-Hyoo´-et." The Pelger-Huet anomaly is a congenital condition in which the nucleus in each of the body's neutrophils divides (abnormally) into only two lobes instead of the usual three or four lobes. As best as we can tell, it's a harmless anomaly. On the other hand, there is the pseudo-Pelger-Huet anomaly that features the same bi-lobed abnormality in some of the body's neutrophils, often a hint that a myelodysplastic syndrome (see Myelodysplastic syndrome) may be present.

Penicillin

"Pen´-ih-sil´-in." This drug is considered by many to be the first antibiotic ever discovered. Many MCAD patients are allergic to penicillin and related drugs.

Pentosan

"Pen´-toh-san." Also known by its most common U.S. trade name Elmiron, the drug pentosan is most commonly used to inhibit activation of urinary tract mast cells which leads to release of inflammatory mediators creating a sterile, non-infectious "interstitial cystitis" which often is mistaken for a urinary tract infection since the symptoms of IC and a UTI are so similar and most doctors are taught that such symptoms (e.g., painful urination) are caused by UTIs and are never taught that such a thing as IC even exists, much less what causes it.

Periactin

"Per´-ee-act´-in." See Cyproheptadine.

Periodontal

"Per´-ee-oh-dont´-ul." For all practical purposes, this adjective refers to the gums. In a fashion similar to how many MCAD patients suffer deterioration of the teeth for mysterious reasons despite good attention to dental hygiene (and usually without any recognition by patient or dentist that MCAD is afoot), some MCAD patients also suffer gum deterioration.

Peripheral neuropathy

See Neuropathy.

PET scan

"Pet" scan. See Positron emission tomography.

PET/CT scan

"Pet see tee" scan." See Positron emission tomography.

Petechiae

"Peh-teek´-ee-ī." Plural of "petechia" (pronounced "peh-teek´-ee-uh"). Tiny red dot in the skin as a result of a tiny amount of bleeding into the skin. Usually seen only when the patient has severe thrombocytopenia (a very low platelet count).

Pharyngitis

"Fār´-in-jīt´-is." Simply put, pharyngitis is inflammation ("-itis") of the pharynx, or throat. Bottom line: sore throat (of any cause). Many MCAD patients complain of at least intermittent (and sometimes constant) pharyngitis.

Phenazopyridine

"Fen-az´-oh-pir´-ih-deen." More commonly called by its most popular U.S. trade name Pyridium, this drug essentially anesthetizes the urinary tract, so it should be no surprise that in a disease like MCAD that can cause chronic inflammation of any part of the body, including the urinary tract, phenazopyridine is sometimes used to help provide symptomatic relief when antibiotic therapy (given for a presumed urinary tract infection) doesn't help. If the patient isn't forewarned, though, she may become quite alarmed when she sees her urine turning orange shortly after starting to take this drug.

Phenylalanine

"Fen´-el-al´-uh-neen." One of the 20 "amino acid" building blocks used to build human proteins. In the disease polycythemia vera, a mutation of the DNA making up the JAK2 gene (which guides a cell's protein-assembling machinery to make the JAK2 protein) usually causes the mistaken use of the amino acid phenylalanine in place of the correct amino acid valine at position 617 in the unique sequence of amino acids that defines the JAK2 protein.

Pheochromocytoma

"Fee´-oh-krōm´-oh-sī-tohm´-uh." This is a rare type of cancer – one of the so-called "neuroendocrine cancers" – that causes episodic flushing and severe hypertension, so you can see why MCAD patients very often have undergone evaluation for pheochromocytoma before mast cell disease is suspected.

Phlebotomy

"Fleh-bot´-uh-mee." Drawing of blood from a patient. Medical professionals distinguish between diagnostic phlebotomy (the commonly performed drawing of a small blood sample for the purpose of running one or more tests on the sample) and therapeutic phlebotomy (the rarely performed drawing of a large amount of blood, typically done as part of the treatment for the relatively rare diseases of polycythemia vera and hemochromatosis).

Piebaldism

"Pī´-bald-ism." Piebaldism is a congenital abnormality, due to mutations in KIT, that causes improper development of the pigment-bearing "melanocyte" cells in the skin that give skin its color. As a result, white patches develop about various parts of the skin and hair, most characteristically a forelock of hair and a triangular patch on the forehead.

Pituitary

"Pih-too´-ih-tār´-ee." The pituitary is a key gland, located at the base of the brain (roughly smack dab in the middle of the head), that's responsible for production of a number of key hormones which in turn regulate a wide array of critical processes in the body.

Plasma cell

"Plas´-muh" cell. Plasma cells, derived from the type of lymphocyte called a B lymphocyte (or simply "B cell"), are the part of the immune system responsible for manufacturing antibodies (specialized proteins that can bind to specific things and summon other parts of the immune system to the site to break down the thing (such as a bacteria) to which the antibody has bound). Ordinarily, each plasma cell is subtly different from every other plasma cell and thus makes a different antibody, but sometimes the B cell from which a plasma cell is derived becomes malignant, leading to lots of copies of the same plasma cell and thus way more of one very specific type of antibody than there should be. When at an advanced stage, this sort of plasma cell malignancy is called multiple myeloma, though other types of plasma cell malignancies are also seen sometimes. MCAD patients seem to be at increased risk for development of malignancy, especially hematologic malignancy, which includes plasma cell malignancies.

Platelet

"Plāt´-let." A type of small blood cell (well, not really a cell, but it's best here to just think of it as a small blood cell) that's chiefly responsible for ganging up ("aggregating") with others of its own kind, whenever there's a break in a blood vessel and bleeding starts, to plug the hole and stop the bleeding. Other processes then help stabilize and strengthen the platelet plug and eventually heal the vessel, but proper formation of a platelet plug is a critical first step toward stopping any bleeding.

Polycythemia vera

"Pol'-ee-sī-theem'-ee-uh vehr'-uh." A type of blood cell cancer, rooted in the bone marrow (where all of the body's blood cells are made), in which the primary issue is the uncontrolled excessive manufacturing of red blood cells, though sometimes excessive numbers of white blood cells (leukocytes) and/or platelets can be seen, too. Usually shortened to "P. vera" ("pee vehr'-uh") or just the initials "PV" in conversation amongst medical professionals, it's a low-grade cancer in most of the patients who have it, with the average patient living a decade or more with it. Some PV patients don't even need treatment and can just be watched, though those who need treatment usually do fine with relatively mild treatment such as phlebotomy (occasional draining of excess blood) or a mild chemotherapy drug called hydroxyurea. Issues from PV can include general plethora (redness, or a flushed appearance) in the face and other aspects of the skin, abnormal blood clots (e.g., a deep venous thrombus, a pulmonary embolus, or a stroke), and headache and vision problems. Occasionally, PV transforms into acute leukemia. In 2006 it was discovered that virtually all PV patients bear mutations in a gene called JAK2 ("jack-2") which contributes to the development of the disease. Usually the mutation in the JAK2 gene in PV results in the cell's protein-assembling machinery, when assembling the long sequence of amino acids that uniquely defines the JAK2 protein, making use of the wrong amino acid at position #617 in the sequence, and thus medical professionals talk about the common "JAK2-V617F" (or JAK2^{V617F}) ("jack-2-vee-6-17-eff") mutation in PV (see JAK2-V617F mutation). ("V," or valine, is the amino acid that *should* be in position 617 in the JAK2 protein, but due to the mutation in the JAK2 gene that's usually found in PV, "F," or phenylalanine, is the amino acid that actually gets used at position 617, and this one simple change results in a JAK2 protein that's always "turned on" (or, medically speaking, "constitutively activated") rather than the normal JAK2 protein that waits for appropriate signals before turning on to exert its normal activities in the cell.) New medications called JAK2 inhibitors are in development as potential new treatments for controlling PV.

Polycythemic

"Pol'-ee-sī-theem'-ik." Generally refers to a state of having too much hemoglobin and too many red blood cells in the bloodstream, though if there are too many white blood cells and/or platelets, too, then the term is taken to refer to all of the blood cell increases that are present.

Polymorbidity

"Pol´-ee-mor-bid´-ih-tee." Since morbidity means illness, polymorbidity means multiple illnesses. I commonly describe the overall clinical picture of MCAD as a chronic multisystem polymorbidity of a generally, but not necessarily, inflammatory theme.

Polyp

"Pol´-ip." A growth of excess tissue (most commonly found in the large intestine, also known as the colon) which, given enough time, may turn frankly malignant/cancerous. Since mast cells are integrally involved in regulating normal growth and development of all tissues, and since mast cell disease leads to all sorts of abnormal tissue growth in various patients, it shouldn't be surprising that polyps are sometimes found in some MCAD patients – though since polyps are a very common finding in the general population, it's impossible (at least at present) to say whether any given polyp emerged because of underlying mast cell disease.

Porcine

"Por´-seen." This adjective refers to things that are related to a pig. For example, heparin used for pharmaceutical, blood-thinning purposes is commonly obtained from the intestinal tissues of pigs, so it's sometimes referred to as porcine heparin.

Porphyria

"Por-fir´-ee-uh." Not really a single disease so much as a class of (rare) diseases, porphyria of one sort or another develops when one or another of the multiple enzymes needed by the body to manufacture hemoglobin aren't working properly, a situation which virtually always is due to a mutation producing either a quantitative deficiency or a qualitative defect in the enzyme in question. Although each form of porphyria has certain distinguishing clinical and laboratory characteristics making for a unique – and typically quite mysterious and odd – presentation, the different forms also share many features including abdominal pain whose pattern can easily mimic what's seen in MCAD. And thus it's not uncommon to find that patients who are ultimately shown to have MCAD have been previously tested for, and sometimes even diagnosed as having, porphyria. So how can somebody be mistakenly diagnosed as having porphyria? Easy. The "porphyrin metabolites" that are strongly elevated in the blood and urine (and, in some forms of porphyria, also the stool) are commonly mildly elevated in MCAD because it's a normal phenomenon for porphyrin metabolites to mildly elevate whenever the body is suffering any stress, and if you don't think that pain and other discomforts that go on for years and years without definitive diagnosis doesn't cause stress, then you're not terribly familiar with the human condition. So it's quite common that after a patient has been suffering intermittent abdominal pain of unclear origin for many years, some bright physician finally remembers from his days in medical school that there's a rare disease called porphyria that can cause mysterious abdominal pain, so he runs the blood and/or urine screening test for porphyria, he finds mildly elevated porphyrin metabolites, and he triumphantly tells the patient, "I think we've got it. I think you have porphyria, and you need to go see a porphyria specialist," of which there are precious few in any country, even the U.S., and in most cases the patient winds up seeing either a hematologist (or perhaps a gastroenterologist) who has virtually no experience with such a rare disease. But repeat testing soon shows that the porphyrin metabolite levels in most such patients never get anywhere close to the marked elevations that hallmark true porphyria, and thus the patient's hopes of finally getting a definitive diagnosis are dashed once again. And of course MCAD is virtually never then considered in such patients because the vast majority of doctors were and are trained to know only about mastocytosis, not MCAS, and they know that mastocytosis is a rare disease the presents with otherwise inexplicable anaphylaxis and flushing, which porphyria patients usually don't show.

Positron emission tomography

"Poz´-ih-tron ee-mish´-un toh-moh´-grah-fee." This is an imaging technique, useful especially in the diagnosis and management of cancer, in which a very slightly radioactive sugar solution is introduced into the patient's bloodstream via an IV and then the patient is placed under a radioactivity detector (the "PET scanner") to try to detect where the radioactivity is concentrating in the body. Because cancers, through their abnormally rapid cell/tissue growth, are consuming more energy than normal cells/tissues, and because sugar is a key source of energy for cell/tissue growth, the infused sugar tends to concentrate in malignant areas, and thus a picture of where the radioactivity is concentrating belies the places in the body where malignancies are present. It's a good, if expensive, test – but it's certainly not a perfect test, as other processes that drive cells to consume more energy – such as inflammation, which often is seen in various tissues as a result of MCAD – can also cause "hot spots" to appear on a PET scan.

Postural orthostatic tachycardia syndrome

Postural "or´-thoh-stat´-ik tak´-ih-card´-ee-uh" syndrome, often abbreviated POTS. Like chronic fatigue syndrome, fibromyalgia, and dozens, if not hundreds, of other "syndromes" of unknown cause, POTS is a (strangely increasingly common) syndrome in which the patient suffers acute onset of an unusual (and typically symptomatic) degree of speeding of the heart rate, and lowering of the blood pressure, upon assuming a more vertical position (i.e., going from lying down (supine) to sitting, or going from sitting to standing). It's normal, of course, for heart rate to increase and blood pressure to fall when going through such a maneuver, but the issue is the degree of the change. Normally, only small changes in blood pressure and heart rate are seen with such maneuvers and the heart and blood vessels rapidly adjust to compensate for the inevitable interaction between gravity and the change in position, leaving the patient completely asymptomatic. In POTS, though, the changes are to a larger degree and the compensation mechanisms don't work well, creating acute onset, for some period, of symptoms of a fast heartbeat and low blood pressure. The symptom of a fast heartbeat – the thumping in the chest of a heart beating rapidly – can be mildly annoying, but by itself it's usually harmless. Rather, it's the low blood pressure – causing dizziness, weakness, lightheadedness, and perhaps even frank loss of consciousness – that's obviously the truly troublesome symptom. POTS is typically diagnosed by a "tilt table test" in which the patient is secured to a rotating table that's initially in the horizontal position, and after the patient is connected to blood pressure and heartrate monitors and baseline vital signs are obtained, the table is swung to a more vertical position, and if the heartrate rises by a certain amount and/or the blood pressure falls by a certain amount, then POTS is "diagnosed." The problem with this diagnosis in some patients, though, is that there often is spontaneous onset of symptoms at times *other* than when moving from a more horizontal position to a more vertical position, i.e., non-postural, non-orthostatic tachycardia and hypotension. And such symptoms do often lead doctors to test patients for various cardiac and neurologic abnormalities, but when such tests prove unrevealing, focus returns to the posturally related episodes, leading to a diagnosis of POTS. Of course, as you now know, mast cells can release – quite acutely – various mediators that can cause precisely the clinical events seen in POTS, so it's quite common for patients who are ultimately shown to have MCAD to have been previously diagnosed with POTS. Also in the "of course" category, it's not at all uncommon for such patients to have failed to significantly improve with any of the various medications used to treat POTS, which typically target blood vessel tension and salt/water balance in the body. All of that said, in my experience some POTS specialists are increasingly recognizing the possibility of MCAD in some of their patients, particularly those with symptoms beyond POTS which are best explained by MCAD.

Potassium

"Poh-tas´-ee-um." This natural element is critically involved in a vast array of metabolic processes in the body, and it's important for the body to keep potassium levels in various tissues, including the blood, within pretty narrow limits. As mast cell disease can affect so many different processes in the body in so many different ways, it's never surprising to me when I see abnormal potassium levels – either high or low – in an MCAD patient, though fortunately such abnormalities tend to be mild, perhaps reflecting just how hard the body strives to maintain proper balances of potassium.

Pramipexole

"Pram´-ih-pex-ol." Better known by its most common U.S. trade name of Mirapex, pramipexole is a medication that mimics dopamine and fits into cell-surface dopamine receptors (typically on nerve cells) to help treat Parkinson's disease and restless leg syndrome – and since the range of neurologic symptoms and problems in some MCAD patients certainly includes "restless leg syndrome," it's not surprising that some MCAD patients come to be on, or at least have tried, pramipexole long before diagnosis of their MCAD.

Prasugrel

"Pras´-oo-grel." More commonly known by its one U.S. trade name at present of Effient, prasugrel is a medication that inhibits platelet function, and since platelets are intimately involved in formation of blood clots including the clots that obstruct coronary arteries to cause myocardial infarctions (i.e., heart attacks), prasugrel is commonly prescribed to patients who have suffered heart attacks. And since the cholesterol-based plaque that builds up, through inflammatory processes, in arteries as a precursor to such clots can develop as a consequence of mast cell disease, it's not surprising that some heart attack survivors who are found to have MCAD have long been on prasugrel (or at least have been tried on prasugrel at some point in the past).

Prednisone

"Pred´-nih-sōn." This immune-system-suppressing medication is probably the most widely prescribed oral glucocorticoid, or steroid, drug. It is useful for suppressing inflammation and an overactive immune system (and thus is certainly a reasonable drug to consider using in some flares of mast cell disease) and is usually tolerated fairly well in the short run, but it has many harmful side effects in the long run. Some inflammatory and autoimmune conditions, though, just can't be adequately managed without prednisone (or another steroid), and it becomes quite a challenge for patient and physician to manage those long-term side effects.

Pregabalin

"Pre-gab´-uh-lin." Known more widely by its most common U.S. trade name Lyrica, pregabalin is a medication used to treat various neurologic conditions including certain types of seizures and certain pain syndromes which seem to be of primary neurologic origin (so-called "neuropathic pain"). It also is used in fibromyalgia and diabetic peripheral neuropathy. In some countries it even is used for treatment of certain anxiety disorders. Since MCAD can cause seizures and mysterious pain syndromes, it's not surprising that some MCAD patients come to be on (or at least have been tried on) pregabalin prior to diagnosis of MCAD.

Presenile dementia

"Pre´-seen´-īl dee-men´-shuh." Also known as Alzheimer's disease, presenile dementia is a chronic loss of general cognitive abilities ("dementia") occurring at an earlier age than usual ("presenile"). Accumulation in the brain of a certain type of abnormal protein seems to be a hallmark, consistent feature of Alzheimer's disease and seems to play some role in causing the impairment of neuron functioning that manifests as dementia, but the root cause of the process remains unknown. Interestingly, some drugs that inhibit misbehaving mast cells (e.g., masitinib) are also appearing, in early clinical trials, to have some positive effects on Alzheimer's disease patients, but that's a long, *long* way from saying that Alzheimer's disease is an MCAD-driven process.

Presyncope

"Pre´-sin´-koh-pee." Presyncope is a sensation, usually of acute/episodic onset, of feeling lightheaded, as if one is near fainting, and is commonly reported by patients who are diagnosed with dysautonomia or postural orthostatic tachycardia syndrome (POTS). It is almost always due to an acute drop in blood pressure, a phenomenon which can be caused by mast cell disease (usually by release of blood-vessel-dilating mediators from mast cells located in or near blood vessel walls), so it's not surprising that presyncope is a common symptom reported by MCAD patients. Sometimes presyncope becomes so severe as to result in frank syncope, or full fainting/loss-of-consciousness.

Prevacid

"Prev´-uh-sid." The most common trade name in the U.S. for lansoprazole.

Prilosec

"Pril´-oh-sek." The most common trade name in the U.S. for omeprazole.

Primidone

"Prim´-ih-dōn." Perhaps known better by its most common U.S. trade name Mysoline, primidone is an old medication initially used primarily to help control some seizure disorders (i.e., epilepsy), though it also has come over time to be used for a variety of other problems including essential (or benign or idiopathic) tremor, depression, bipolar disorder, psychosis, and even the cardiac rhythm disturbance known as long QT syndrome (LQTS).

Prolapse

"Proh´-laps." A condition in which part or all of an organ is pushed out of its normal place. The term is most commonly applied to the uterus ("uterine prolapse" in which the uterus descends into, or even protrudes out of, the vagina) or the rectum ("rectal prolapse" in which the rectum descends into, or even protrudes out of, the anus).

Prolia

"Proh´-lee-uh." Along with Xgeva, Prolia is one of the two trade names for denosumab in the U.S. See Denosumab.

Promethazine

"Proh-meth´-uh-zeen." Known much more widely by its common U.S. trade name Phenergan ("fen´-er-gen"), promethazine is an anti-nausea drug with a fairly short half-life and some mild abilities to block the histamine H_1 receptor.

Pronormoblast

"Pro-norm´-oh-blast." The pronormoblast, also known as a proerythroblast, is one of the stages of blood cell development on the way from the stem cell to the red blood cell. When red blood cell development fails in the rare disease called pure red cell aplasia, it's commonly due to infection in pronormoblasts by a virus called parvovirus B-19 which causes "giant pronormoblasts" to be seen in the bone marrow sample which almost inevitably will be obtained by the hematologist who's trying to figure out why red blood cell production has failed. Pure red cell aplasia is occasionally seen in MCAD, but it's due to mast cell release of red-blood-cell-production-suppressing inflammatory mediators rather than infection.

Propranolol

"Pro-pran´-oh-lol." More commonly known by its most popular U.S. trade name Inderal, propranolol is a classic "beta blocker" medication used to treat high blood pressure (hypertension), fast heart rates (tachycardia), and other conditions. Since hypertension and tachycardia are often seen in MCAD patients, it's not unusual for such patients to have been tried on propranolol at some point before diagnosis of their MCAD.

Prostaglandin D_2

"Pros´-tuh-glan´-din" D2. An inflammatory mediator produced by mast cells (and, in lesser amounts, by a few other types of cells), prostaglandin D_2 has a very short half-life and quickly breaks down upon exposure to heat, so getting an accurate measurement of the prostaglandin D_2 level in blood or urine is challenging, requiring careful chilling of the specimen. Neverthless, if an elevated prostaglandin D_2 level can be found, it's a pretty reliable sign that a heightened state of mast cell activation is present.

Prothrombin time

"Pro-throm´-bin" time. More commonly referred to by its "PT" initials, the prothrombin time is a common, simple test of the part of the coagulation system known as the "extrinsic pathway." Many patients with an excessive tendency for blood clotting require chronic blood thinning, or anticoagulation, therapy, and one of the most commonly used such drugs is warfarin (also widely known by its most popular U.S. trade name Coumadin), whose effectiveness is carefully monitoring in such patients by regular measurement of the PT. When no PT-affecting medications are present, modest abnormalities (high or low) in the PT can reflect various clotting system abnormalities including, sometimes, the erroneous generation by the immune system of so-called "anti-phospholipid antibodies" which can target various proteins in the coagulation system to cause excessive clotting (or, much less commonly, excessive bleeding). MCAD can cause excessive clotting and excessive bleeding by various mechanisms, including anti-phospholipid antibodies, so when an abnormal PT (or its sister test, the partial thromboplastin time, or PTT) is found in an MCAD patient, it's reasonable to perform additional testing for the presence of anti-phospholipid antibodies.

Proton pump inhibitor

"Pro´-ton" pump inhibitor, often referred to by its initials, PPI. The PPIs are a class of medications (such as omeprazole, pantoprazole, and lansoprazole) which impede production of acid in the stomach even more potently than the histamine H_2 receptor blockers (such as famotidine and ranitidine). Many MCAD patients overproduce stomach acid (a consequence of excessive histamine production and release by dysfunctional mast cells), and many other MCAD patients feel as if they overproduce stomach acid even though they're proven not to (a feeling that's probably consequential to release of other, inflammatory mediators from dysfunctional mast cells), and such patients often come to be chronic PPI users even though many such patients don't appear to be helped much by these drugs.

Pruritus

"Prur-īt´-us." This is the medical word for the sensation of itchiness.

Pseudoxanthoma elasticum

"Sū´-doh-zan-thohm´-uh ee-last´-ih-cum." Sometimes known as PXE, this rare genetic disease, usually stemming from a mutation in a gene called ABCC6, causes abnormal hardening and breakdown of elastic fibers in various tissues resulting in various problems in the skin, the eyes, and premature atherosclerosis in blood vessels. A PXE-like problem with premature atherosclerosis is also occasionally seen in patients with various hereditary abnormal hemoglobin conditions such as sickle cell anemia and thalassemia, though since mast cell disease can cause premature atherosclerosis and mast cell disease can co-exist with sickle cell anemia and thalassemia, one has to wonder whether the premature atherosclerosis seen in sickle cell anemia and thalassemia might in fact be due to mast cell disease rather than an odd case of PXE not featuring any of the mutations known to cause PXE.

Psoriatic arthritis

"Sor´-ee-at´-ik" arthritis. This is a type of joint pain (arthritis) syndrome that also features psoriasis-type skin lesions. It's yet another one of the hundreds of known chronic idiopathic inflammatory conditions for which no cause has yet been identified, raising the possibility that at least some cases might be due to MCAD.

Psychosomatic

"Sī´-koh-soh-mat´-ik." This adjective describes a state in which a patient's symptoms are thought (usually by people other than the patient) to be imaginary or not "real." Because clear abnormalities in the physical exam or lab tests often cannot be found (by physicians unfamiliar with MCAD) to correlate with the complaints put forth by an MCAD patient, such symptoms are often erroneously presumed by such physicians (and, often, the patient's acquaintances and even family) to be psychosomatic. Of course, feeling a symptom but not being able to find any correlating objective abnormality, and then being accused of "making it up," leads to great stress since such patients can't imagine what they're doing that might lead their brains to fabricate such "false" symptoms, and thus they can't see any path forward toward easing such symptoms. Psychosomatism is a real psychiatric disorder, but it is rare; MCAD is a real disorder, but it (especially MCAS) is common. As such, patients who have assortments of symptoms that cannot be explained by most routine testing – especially when they are symptoms of a generally inflammatory and/or allergic nature – should be carefully evaluated for MCAD before anyone begins suspecting the symptoms are psychosomatic.

Pulmonary embolus

"Pul´-moh-nār´-ee em´-bōl-us." More commonly referred to by its "PE" initials, a pulmonary embolus (plural: pulmonary emboli, "pul´-moh-nār´-ee em´-bōl-ī") is a blood clot in the pulmonary artery (leading from the heart's right ventricle to the lungs) or one of its branches. If it's a big enough clot that blocks enough blood flow to the lungs, a PE of course can be (rapidly!) fatal. As abnormal blood clotting is a common complication of inflammation, some mast cell disease patients have a tendency toward excessive blood clotting and thus suffer, or at least are at risk for suffering, a PE. Doctors are well trained to consider the possibility of a PE when a patient complains of shortness of breath, particularly when it's of acute onset and accompanied by chest pain.

Pulmonic valve

"Pul-mon´-ik" valve. The pulmonic valve sits at the base of the pulmonary artery which provides the conduit for blood being pumped out of the heart's right ventricle to travel to the lungs in order to off-load waste carbon dioxide and pick up a fresh supply of oxygen. Without the presence and proper operation of the (one-way) pulmonic valve, a lot of the blood pumped forward into the pulmonary artery with each beat of the heart (i.e., with each contaction of the right ventricle) would simply fall back into the right ventricle, dramatically reducing blood flow to the lungs and causing substantial impairment in delivery of oxygen to tissues throughout the body. This causes fast breathing (tachypnea) and a bluish discoloration of the skin.

Pulmonology

"Pul´-mon-ol´-oh-jee." This is the study of the lungs, or the specialty focusing in lung disease.

Pure red cell aplasia

Pure red cell "ā′-plā′-zha." Sometimes known by its "PRCA" initials, pure red cell aplasia is a disease in which the bone marrow at least temporarily (and sometimes, more seriously, permanently) stops making red blood cells, while production of other types of blood cells remains essentially unimpaired. PRCA is usually caused by an infection of red blood cell precursor cells in the bone marrow called pronormoblasts, and it's usually a virus called parvovirus B-19 that's the culprit in such infections. Sometimes, though, PRCA can be caused by other mechanisms, including autoimmune disorders (typically seen in conjunction with a rare type of cancer of the thymus gland in the center of the chest (i.e., in the mediastinum) called a thymoma) as well as severe inflammatory conditions. Rarely, mast cell disease can produce such strong inflammation as to cause the appearance of PRCA.

Pyridostigmine

"Pir′-ih-doh-stig′-meen." Known more commonly by its most popular U.S. trade name Mestinon, pyridostigmine is an inhibitor of a key enzyme for proper nerve cell functioning called cholinesterase. It's used to treat the rare autoimmune neurologic condition called myasthenia gravis, to treat postural orthostatic tachycardia syndrome (POTS), and to reverse the effects of exposure to certain "nerve gas"-type chemical warfare agents.

Q

Quercetin

"Kwer′-seh-tin." Quercetin is a natural component of many foods, especially certain vegetables such as broccoli. It is a type of molecule classified as a "flavonoid" that has anti-inflammatory properties. It is available as an inexpensive over-the-counter "supplement" and can help some patients with mast cell disease. The precise mechanisms by which it inhibits mast cell activity (at least in some patients) are unclear.

R

Radiotherapy

"Rā′-dee-oh-ther′-uh-pee." Simply put, radiotherapy is treatment of a disease (usually cancer) by radiation of one type or another.

Ranitidine

"Ruh-ni´-ti-deen." Also known by its most popular trade name Zantac, the drug ranitidine is a histamine H_2 receptor blocker (see the entry for "histamine" for more information). Ranitidine has more drug-drug interactions than the other most popular H_2 blocker, famotidine.

Red cell distribution width

Standard English words there, no tricky pronunciation, but it is a bit tricky to explain what the "RDW" actually is. The RDW is one of the numbers usually reported on a complete blood count (CBC), and simply put, it's a measure of how monotonously sized the red blood cells in the blood sample are. If most of the red blood cells in the sample are about the same size (regardless of whether that size is normal (normocytic), larger than normal (macrocytic), or smaller than normal (microcytic)), then the RDW will be normal. As the number of red blood cells of sizes different from the average size increases in the sample, the RDW increases. Putting together the hemoglobin, hematocrit, the red blood cell count, the average red blood cell size (otherwise known as the mean corpuscular volume, or MCV), and the RDW – especially when *trends* of these numbers are available – can often give the doctor a pretty good idea of how well red blood cell production in the bone marrow is working, including some ideas of specific underlying causes if there are abnormalities seen in any of these parameters.

Relapsing polychondritis

Relapsing "pol´-ee-kon-drīt´-is." Sometimes known by its "RP" initials, relapsing polychondritis is a rare multisystem condition, usually diagnosed and managed by rheumatologists, most prominently featuring chronic inflammation of unknown cause affecting a type of connective tissue present widely throughout the body called cartilage. Many of the symptoms of RP mimic what can be seen in MCAD, and since nobody knows the cause of RP, it's possible that some variant of MCAD is the underlying issue in some portion of the RP population. (Another project for the research pile, eh?)

Retinitis

"Ret´-in-īt´-is." Simply put, retinitis is inflammation ("-itis") of the retina, the thin tissue at the back of the eye that transforms light into electrical impulses that travel down the optic nerve to the brain, which interprets those impulses as the images we see. As such, retinitis usually causes visual impairment. If not identified and corrected soon enough, it can cause permanent blindness.

Rheumatoid arthritis

"Room´-uh-toid" arthritis. Often referred to by its "RA" initials, rheumatoid arthritis is a particular (and common) type of inflammatory condition most commonly affecting the joints but sometimes also other tissues such as the lungs.

Rheumatology

"Room´-uh-tol´-oh-jee." Rheumatology is the study of joints and connective tissues, or the medical specialty focusing in diseases of the joints (such as arthritis) and connective tissues including the "collagen vascular disorders" (such as lupus). Given the generally inflammatory theme with which mast cell disease commonly presents, it's not surprising that many MCAD patients have been previously evaluated by a rheumatologist before their MCAD is diagnosed.

Rhinosinusitis

"Rī´-noh-sīn´-yoo-sīt´-is." Simply put, this is inflammation ("-itis") of the nose ("rhino-") and sinuses. Especially given that mast cells tend to site themselves at the environmental interfaces and then abnormally produce and release inflammatory mediators, rhinosinusitis is a common complication of mast cell disease.

Rhizotomy

"Rī-zot´-oh-mee." A rhizotomy is a surgical procedure in which selected nerve roots emerging from the spinal cord are destroyed (typically by simply severing them) in an effort to relieve symptoms of dysfunction in such nerves such as various spastic and pain conditions.

Ribonucleic acid

"Rī´-boh-noo-clā´-ik" acid. Far more commonly referred to by its abbreviation RNA, ribonucleic acid is the critical intermediate between a specific strand of DNA (i.e., a specific gene) and the specific protein coded for by that specific strand of DNA. The string of DNA that defines a gene is transcribed into a corresponding string of RNA, and that string of RNA is then translated into a corresponding string of amino acids which define a given protein and which can actually accomplish things inside a cell. The discovery (by the team at the University of Bonn led by Dr. Gerhard Molderings) that virtually every MCAS patient bears mutations in the KIT protein in the patient's mast cells was made by analyzing sequences of KIT RNA extracted from such patients' mast cells.

Right upper quadrant

Standard English words there, no tricky pronunciation. Often abbreviated as RUQ, this simply refers to the right upper part of the abdomen, where such parts of the anatomy as the liver and gallbladder are usually found. Thus, RUQ pain or swelling can be sign of a problem in the liver and/or gallbladder, but it also can be a sign of a problem in other structures in the area such as the small or large intestinal tract.

Risedronate

"Ris-eh´-drōn-āt." Known more widely by its most popular U.S. trade name Actonel, risedronate is yet another bisphosphonate for protecting bones against weakening. It's taken orally, typically once a week or even once a month.

RNA

See Ribonucleic acid.

Rohypnol

"Roh-hip´-nol." The most commonly recognized trade name in the U.S. for flunitrazepam. See Flunitrazepam.

Rosette

"Roh-zet´." In its most basic meaning, a rosette simply is a pattern in which a given sub-pattern is replicated and arrayed around a central feature. In medicine, the word is usually applied to a cellular pattern in which a certain type of cell (typically a red blood cell) is arrayed around a cell (which may be the same type, or a different type, of cell (such as another red blood cell, or a white blood cell). Red blood cell rosetting can be a sign of certain conditions or diseases such as a difference in the Rh blood type between mother and fetus, or the presence of malaria.

S

Salmonella

"Sal´-moh-nel´-uh." *Salmonella* is a class of common bacteria. Some of the specific bacteria in this class can cause food poisoning. Because a flare of MCAD can sometimes mimic an incident of food poisoning, some MCAD patients – usually before they're actually diagnosed with MCAD – come to be suspected of suffering *Salmonella*-based food poisoning. Of course, since MCAD can interfere with proper functioning of the immune system and thus render the patient more susceptible to infection, true *Salmonella* infections are possible in an MCAD patient (just like in somebody who doesn't have MCAD), but in my experience such infections are no more common in MCAD patients than in people who don't have MCAD.

Sandimmune

"Sand´-im-yoon." Trade name for a formulation of cyclosporine commonly used in the U.S. See Cyclosporine.

Sarcoid

"Sar´-coid." Also known as sarcoidosis, sarcoid is yet another interesting inflammatory disease of unknown origin despite decades of study. It's usually just an acute issue that resolves on its own, but sometimes it becomes a chronic disease which can progress to a fatal point. Sarcoid features abnormal collections of inflammatory cells, known as granulomas, that accumulate in various organs such as the lungs and lymph nodes. As is the case regarding many chronic idiopathic inflammatory diseases, I have my suspicions that, at least in some sarcoid patients, MCAD is the root issue. (Yes, add this one, too, to the list of research projects to be done.)

Satiety

"Suh-tī´-eh-tee." Satiety is a sense of fullness. "Early satiety" is when you get a sense of fullness during eating sooner than you'd expect to based on how much you ate, and it can be a sign of any of a number of problems including a stomach cancer or an enlarged spleen or liver.

Sclerae

"Skler´-ī." The whites of the eyes, surrounding the colored iris. These areas can assume other colors in various states of illness, such as a yellow-brown color when an excess of bilirubin accumulates in the blood, or a bloody red when there is bleeding into the sclerae (a condition called a hyphema). Sometimes a pattern of engorged tiny blood vessels comes to stand out against the white fields; this is an inflammation of the sclerae called scleritis, or scleral conjunctivitis. MCAD occasionally causes various problems that lead to abnormal coloring of the sclerae.

Scopolamine

"Scoh-pol´-uh-meen." Also known by its popular trade name Dramamine, this drug is a sedating histamine H_1 receptor blocker (see "histamine" for more information). Its most widely known use is to prevent the nausea of seasickness.

Secretin stimulation test

"See´-kreh-tin" stimulation test. This is a test, usually administered by gastroenterologists, that helps detect whether a rare type of neuroendocrine cancer called a gastrinoma is present. Gastrinomas, usually located in the stomach, produce the hormone gastrin in an unregulated fashion. Gastrin drives the acid-producing cells of the stomach – the parietal cells – to produce acid. As you might imagine, ordinarily the production of acid is a highly regulated process, but the production of gastrin by a gastrinoma is an unregulated process, and thus the stomach makes far more acid than it should, and this leads to problems of ulcers (which sometimes bleed) and abdominal pain even apart from the basic problem that a gastrinoma is a cancer that can spread (metastasize) and eventually kill the patient. Ordinarily, the stomach's parietal cells turn down their production of gastrin when they sense an increased level in the blood of another hormone, secretin. (Secretin, as you might expect, is produced by certain specialized cells in the duodenum (just a little ways down the intestinal tract from the stomach), where they are perfectly positioned to sense stomach acid production and increase secretin production if the juices coming down the intestinal tract from the stomach are getting too acidic.) Of course, since production of gastrin by gastrinoma tumor cells – as opposed to parietal cells – is unregulated, there is no suppression of acid production by gastrinoma tumor cells when the secretin level increases. Therefore, you can now imagine how the secretin stimulation test works. After a catheter that can measure acidity is threaded through the patient's nose or mouth, down through the throat, esophagus, and stomach and finally into the duodenum, the baseline acidity level is measured and then secretin is infused into the patient's bloodstream while the acidity level continues to be monitored. If there is no gastrinoma present, the acidity should ease up as the secretin infusion continues, but if the juices persist in being just as acidic as they were at baseline in spite of the secretin infusion, then it's a pretty good bet that a gastrinoma is present. Because MCAD often leads to excessive levels of acid production that can lead to ulcer disease, sometimes a gastrinoma is suspected before MCAD is suspected, and thus an occasional MCAD patient comes to have a secretin stimulation test done as part of the thousand (or two) tests they undergo, over years and years, to try to figure out why they're so sick in so many different ways.

Septicemia

"Sep´-ti-seem´-ee-uh." Septicemia is the general term for infection (usually by bacteria, though sometimes by a fungus or another unusual microorganism) that's present in the blood. Without effective treatment, septicemia is often fatal. There are many different paths by which MCAD can (fortunately only occasionally) lead to septicemia.

Serotonin reuptake inhibitors

"Seer´-oh-tōn´-in re-up´-tāk" inhibitors. Also known as selective serotonin reuptake inhibitors, or SSRIs, these very commonly prescribed medications were developed to treat depression and generally have been pretty successful at doing so. It was originally thought that the SSRIs treat depression by blocking "serotonin reuptake elements" (SREs) on the surfaces of presynaptic nerve cells, thereby increasing the amount of the signaling molecule serotonin in the neural synapse available for binding to, and thus activating of, post-synaptic nerve cells, and by stimulating such post-synaptic neural activity, depression can be lifted. In more recent times we've been discovering the presence of SREs on the surfaces of other cells, too, including – you guessed it – the mast cell. Therefore, whether it's through stimulating nerve cells which then help settle down hyperactive mast cells, or by directly binding with and inhibiting hyperactive mast cells, it's not surprising that SSRIs help settle down at least some mast-cell-related symptoms in some MCAD patients. Commonly prescribed SSRIs include fluoxetine (Prozac) and paroxetine (Paxil), but there are lots of other SSRIs that have been developed and approved for marketing.

Serotonin

"Seer´-oh-tōn´-in." This is a key signaling molecule in regulating activity of nerve cells, and we've been learning more recently that it also binds to, and thus participates in the regulation of, many other types of cells, too, including mast cells.

Sickle cell anemia

Standard English words there, no tricky pronunciation. This is an inherited disease in which a single mutation in the gene for making beta globin (one of the components of hemoglobin) leads to the formation of an abnormal hemoglobin molecule that's unusually sticky when it doesn't have a molecule of oxygen that's bound to it. As a result, in a poor-oxygen environment (such as the blood that's found in veins as opposed to arteries), these abnormal hemoglobin molecules stick to one another, causing hemoglobin to clump up instead of floating apart from one another in the fluid environment inside the red blood cell, and such clumping, or polymerizing, causes the red blood cell to deform in a way that, when visualized through a microscope, resembles a sickle. When red blood cells deform in this way, they don't flow through the tiniest blood vessels, called capillaries, in normal fashion. In fact, they get stuck in, and plug up, the capillaries, which obvious impairs blood flow through those capillaries and thus impairs delivery of oxygen and other nutrients that blood brings to the various tissues throughout the body. Unsurprisingly, as tissues starve for oxygen and nutrients, they start dying, and it hurts. This is the sickle cell pain crisis that you may have heard about, and it is pure misery. The curious thing about sickle cell anemia, though, is that even though every sickle cell anemia patient has exactly the same beta globin mutation, roughly 15% of such patients have a really rough course (a "poor phenotype") of the disease, while the other 85% or so have a much easier time (though certainly no picnic), implying that there must be *something else* going on in the 15% that makes their course so much worse. A few years ago I began realizing that most poor-phenotype sickle cell anemia patients have symptoms that are much easier for MCAS to explain than sickle cell anemia, and when I tested them for MCAS, I found it in most of them, and I also began finding that treating such MCAS would sometimes enable a poor-phenotype sickle cell anemia patient to "transform" into a good-phenotype sickle cell anemia patient. (Yes, I did eventually publish these findings, in the *American Journal of the Medical Sciences* in late 2014.) Of course, there remains a great amount of further research to be done in this area.

Sideroblastic anemia

"Sid´-er-oh-blast´-ik uh-neem´-ee-uh." Sideroblastic anemia is a disease in which one or more of various proteins needed to facilitate the incorporation of iron into hemoglobin (in the process of manufacturing hemoglobin and thus the process of manufacturing a red blood cell) are not working properly, whether by quantitative deficiency or qualitative defect. Sideroblastic anemia can be a congenital disease, but it also can be an acquired disease, and in the latter case, it's considered to be a type of myelodysplastic syndrome (MDS). I have seen the acquired form of sideroblastic anemia develop as a consequence of MCAD in a few patients, though it's not yet at all clear how mast cell disease is actually causing this. Yet another research project…

Silodosin

"Si-lōd´-uh-sin." Perhaps known better in the U.S. by its trade name Rapaflo, silodosin is a medication that treats poor urine flow in men caused by a non-cancerous enlargement of the prostate gland called benign prostatic hyperplasia (BPH). Because MCAD can reduce urine flow through a number of mechanisms, including BPH, it's not surprising that some MCAD patients come to be on (or at least come to have been tried on) silodosin (usually before their MCAD is diagnosed).

Simvastatin

"Sim´-vuh-stat´-in." Better known by its most popular U.S. trade name Zocor, simvastatin is a widely prescribed cholesterol-lowering medication. Because many MCAD patients suffer from progressive (and likely MCAD-driven) build-up of cholesterol-laden plaque in the arteries called atherosclerosis, it's not surprising that many such patients come to be on simvastatin or one of its sister drugs (e.g., lovastatin or atorvastatin). Interestingly, more recently it has been discovered that these "statin" drugs cause a mild general reduction in inflammation in the body, though how they do so remains a mystery.

Singulair

 "Sing´-yoo-lār." The most common trade name for montelukast in the U.S.

Sinus histiocyte

 Sinus "his´-tee-oh-sīt." This is a type of inflammatory cell found in lymph nodes. Mast cell disease sometimes causes reactive inflammation in lymph nodes leading to an increased number of sinus histiocytes that sometimes can mislead a pathologist, looking at a lymph node biopsy under a microscope, to think that the patient has a rare type of cancer called histiocytosis.

Sinusitis

 "Sīn´-us-īt´-is." Simply put, this is inflammation ("-itis") of the sinuses, and since mast cells tend to site themselves at the environmental interfaces (which certainly includes the sinuses), it's no surprise that sinusitis is a common consequence of misbehaving mast cells.

Sjögren's syndrome

 "Syoh-grenz" syndrome. This is a relatively rare autoimmune disease, usually managed by rheumatologists, in which the autoantibody that's erroneously generated by the immune system attacks, among other targets, key cells in the tear ducts and salivary glands that produce fluid and mucus. This leads to dry eyes, a dry mouth, and many other consequences as well. Since MCAD can lead to the development of potentially any autoimmune disease, and since MCAD can also cause "burning mouth syndrome" which can lead to suspicion of Sjögren's syndrome (even though Sjögren's syndrome is only rarely found to be the cause of burning mouth syndrome), it's not surprising to see the possibility of Sjögren's disease being contemplated and investigated at some point along the course in some patients with MCAD.

Sodium

 "Soh´-dee-um." Sodium, of course, is an element that's essential to human life (indeed, essential to most forms of life), and the concentration of sodium must be maintained within a narrow range in various tissues (such as blood). Sodium levels can increase above normal or decrease below normal in a huge range of disease processes, and thus it's not surprising that many of the illnesses driven by MCAD also lead to abnormalities in sodium levels. Of course, just as with potassium, an abnormal sodium level by now means implies that a mast cell disease is necessarily present. Careful evaluation is required to identify why a sodium level is abnormal – and identification of the reason why a sodium level is abnormal is of course crucial to selecting the right therapy that will help restore the level o normal.

Solifenacin

"Sohl'-ih-fen'-uh-sin." Known more widely by its U.S. trade name Vesicare, solifenacin is a medication that reduces the tension of bladder muscle, allowing the bladder to retain larger volumes of urine and reducing urinary problems resulting from excess bladder muscle tension such as frequency, urgency, and incontinence. Because these are urinary problems seen in many patients with mast cell disease, it's not surprising that some such patients come to be tried on solifenacin (usually before their MCAD is diagnosed).

Soluble interleukin-2 receptor

"Sol'-yoo-bul in'-ter-lūk'-in 2" receptor, often abbreviated sIL2r. Although the protein that serves as a receptor for the mediator called interleukin-2 is usually integrated into the surface of various cells (especially lymphocytes), a certain amount of this protein also circulates freely in the blood, detached from any cells. It has been discovered that the sIL2r level in blood escalates substantially in an acute, severely inflammatory disease of unknown origin called hemophagocytic lymphohistiocytosis (HLH). Because some MCAD patients also manifest acute episodes of severe inflammation, it is not surprising that on occasion (usually before their MCAD is diagnosed) they are suspected of suffering HLH, and thus an sIL2r level is obtained as part of the diagnostic evaluation for HLH.

Solu-Medrol

"Sol'-yoo-meh'-drol." One of the most commonly recognized trade names in the U.S. for methylprednisolone. See Methylprednisolone.

Somatiform

"Soh-mat'-ih-form." Somatiform essentially is a synonym for psychosomatic (see Psychosomatic).

Somatostatin

"Soh-mat´-oh-stat-in." Produced in the stomach, intestines, and pancreas, somatostatin is a natural human body hormone which has a very wide range of "braking" effects in the body including (and trust me, this is just a small subset of the total set of effects caused by somatostatin) inhibiting pituitary gland secretion of growth hormone (GH) and thyroid-stimulating hormone (TSH), inhibiting the stomach's release of gastrin, and inhibiting the release of insulin from the pancreas. In view of these effects, there obviously are receptors for somatostatin on the surfaces of cells in the pituitary gland, the stomach, and the pancreas – and there also are receptors for somatostatin on the surface of the mast cell which can inhibit mast cell activation and thus inhibit the production and release of the mast cells' vast repertoire of mediators, including histamine. Thus, the drug octreotide (see the entry for such in this dictionary), which is chemically similar to somatostatin, can help control mast cell activation in mast cell disease, though it's typically used only for mast cell disease that is producing symptoms similar to what the neuroendocrine malignancy called carcinoid typically produces (otherwise uncontrollable diarrhea, flushing, and/or wheezing) since carcinoid is a type of cancer that typically responds fairly well to octreotide.

Spindle cell

Standard English words there, no tricky pronunciation. Simply put, spindle cells are cells that assume a spindle-like shape. Different cells can do this, including – you guessed it – the mast cell. Unless special testing is used, the pathologist who is seeing spindle cells in a tissue sample under the microscope may be very hard pressed to figure out when they're actually mast cells – and he has no reason to do that special testing unless the doctor who sent him the tissue sample has told him that mast cell disease is suspected – except that most doctors have no reason to suspect such unless the patient presents with the classic mastocytosis symptoms of otherwise unexplained anaphylaxis and flushing.

Splenomegaly

"Splen´-oh-meg´-uh-lee." Enlargement of the spleen. Sometimes seen in MCAD, but usually not to any remarkable, or symptomatic, extent.

Sprycel

"Sprī´-sel." The trade name in the U.S. for dasatinib. See Dasatinib.

Statin

"Stat´-in." The statin drugs help lower cholesterol levels, reduce formation of the cholesterol-laden plaque in arteries known as atherosclerosis (thus reducing the chance of arterial obstruction and resulting heart attack or other catastrophic blood-vessel-occluding events), and reduce inflammation.

Subclavian vein

"Sub-clāv´-ee-un" vein. This is a major vein in the body, located in the upper part of the chest, one on each side.

Subcutaneous

"Sub´-kyoo-tān´-ee-us." This is the $400 medical word for "under the skin."

Sublingual

"Sub-lin´-gwul." And this is the $400 medical word for "under the tongue."

Sucralfate

"Sū´-cral-fāt." Probably better known by its most common U.S. trade name Carafate, sucralfate is a medication commonly used to treat increased stomach acid, and since MCAD patients commonly suffer increased stomach acid (or at least commonly suffer pain in the area of the stomach that's thought to be due to increased stomach acid even though sometimes it's actually a result of inflammation), it's not surprising that some MCAD patients come to be tried on sucralfate at some point before their MCAD is diagnosed.

Suicidality

"Sū´-ih-sī-dal´-ih-tee." As you probably guessed, this is the inclination of a (severely depressed) patient to commit suicide.

Sunitinib

"Sū-nit′-in-ib." More widely known by its U.S. trade name Sutent, sunitinib is a tyrosine kinase inhibitor (a somewhat distant cousin of dasatinib) that's approved for treatment of kidney cancer and imatinib-resistant gastrointestinal stromal tumor (GIST), which is relevant to mast cell disease because the key gene that's mutated in GIST – KIT – is also the key gene that we think is mutated in most cases of MCAD. Thus, while there haven't been any published reports yet of sunitinib being tried (much less proving helpful) in mast cell disease, there is a theoretical basis for suspecting it might indeed be helpful in MCAD. And, in fact, as of the time of this writing, I am aware of one MCAD patient who has tried sunitinib and found it very helpful (furthermore, just as is usually the case with imatinib, sunitinib was helpful in this patient at a dose much lower than is typically used to treat cancer).

Supine

"Su′-pīn." The horizontal position. The patient is in the supine position when the patient is lying down.

Supraventricular tachycardia

"Sū′-prah-ven-trik′-yoo-lar tak′-ee-card′-ee-uh." Commonly referred to by its "SVT" initials, this is a cardiac rhythm abnormality in which the heart beats at an abnormally fast rate due to a disturbance in electrical conduction in the atrial chambers in the heart that are responsible for pumping blood into the ventricular chambers before the blood is then pumped further forward into the pulmonary artery (from the right ventricle) or the aorta (from the left ventricle). There are many different specific types of SVT that can be distinguished on electrocardiogram (ECG, or EKG), and different types of SVT require different treatment. Symptoms can include palpitations, chest pain, shortness of breath, dizziness, and loss of consciousness, so you can see how some patients with MCAD can be suspected instead of having SVT.

Syncope

"Sin′-koh-pee." Transient loss of consciousness that usually comes about from acute major dilation of blood vessels leading to a substantial drop in blood pressure. Flares of MCAD can occasionally cause syncope, but more common is a milder drop in blood pressure (causing just dizziness or lightheadedness rather than actual loss of consciousness). Such milder episodes are called presyncope.

Synthroid

"Sin´-throid." The most commonly recognized trade name in the U.S. for levothyroxine. See Levothyroxine.

Systolic

"Sis-tol´-ik." This is the peak blood pressure (i.e., the first of the two numbers always reported in a blood pressure reading) stemming from the part of the cardiac cycle in which the ventricles contract and eject blood into the pulmonary artery (carrying blood away from the right ventricle toward the lungs) or the aorta (carrying blood away from the left ventricle toward all the other tissues of the body).

T

T-cell lymphoma

T-cell "lim-fohm´-uh." A less common subtype of lymphoma (a cancer of the "lymphocyte" type of white blood cell) in which the "T-cell" type of lymphocyte is at the heart of the malignancy. Among lymphomas, B-cell lymphomas are far more common and tend to present in more predictable ways and respond better to treatment. T-cell lymphomas are much less common, present in more variable and odd ways, and do not respond as well to the treatments we have available today.

T-cell-receptor gene-rearrangement studies

Standard English words there, no tricky pronunciation. Often abbreviated TCRGR. TCRGR is a laboratory test that can tell whether the T cells in a blood or tissue sample are "clonal" or not. Ordinarily, lymphocytes are supposed to be different from one another with regard to the foreign invaders that they've been bred to recognize and react against. A malignant lymphocyte (of any type, whether B-cell or T-cell or other, less common types), though, is, like any cancer, a precise copy of another malignancy lymphocyte, and there is various testing that can be done to see if the lymphocytes in a sample contains bunches of lymphocytes that all recognize the same foreign invader in the same way. If so, we label such identical bunches of cells to be "clonal" lymphocytes, and though many situations of clonality drive

434

malignancy, not all do, and one needs to be careful about making a diagnosis of malignancy based on a positive test for clonality. Different tests are used to discover clonality in B-lymphocytes as opposed to T-lymphocytes. TCRGR is one of the tests used to discover T-lymphocyte clonality, and when the test is positive *in the right clinical context*, it can help support a diagnosis of T-cell lymphoma or T-cell lymphocytic leukemia – but it can be tricky because in about 20% of the times when the TCRGR test is positive, it's actually a false positive.

Tachycardia

"Tak´-ee-card´-ee-uh." The medical word for a heart rate faster than normal. Doctors are trained that the "normal" range for the heart rate is about 60-100 for an adult (faster for children), but the truly healthy adult is going to have a heart rate more in the 60-80 range. This becomes relevant to MCAS because many MCAS patients have heart rates in the 80s and 90s, sometimes even the low 100s, and they often undergo extensive evaluation for such tachycardia in which usually no other cause is ever found – and of course mast cell disease is never suspected because doctors aren't trained about MCAS and they're not even trained that mastocytosis can cause tachycardia. Most doctors are trained (for about 30-60 seconds out of their decade of medical schooling/training) that mastocytosis is rare and is the only mast cell disease and causes anaphylaxis and flushing and a high tryptase level, and that's it. So it's no wonder that no general doctor or cardiologist ever thinks about mast cell disease as a potential cause of tachycardia or any of the many other cardiovascular abnormalities that mast cell disease can cause.

Takotusbo syndrome

"Tak´-oh-sū´-boh" syndrome. This is an uncommon – and unusual form of – heart failure which tends to come on acutely (as opposed to the far more common chronic pattern of heart failure) and literally causes a ballooning of heart's ventricles, forming quite a distinctive picture on the echocardiogram that's almost always done when a patient presents with symptoms and signs of heart failure. Takotsubo heart failure is increasingly coming to be understood to be a consequence of acute flaring of mast cell activation, but the specific mediators that are being released to cause the heart to do all of the odd things seen in the syndrome remain to be identified. In keeping with the general observation that mast cell activation tends to flare shortly after one major (physical or psychological/emotional) stressor or another, so, too, does takotsubo syndrome tend to be seen only after a major stressor.

Tambicor

"Tamb´-ih-kor." The most recognized trade name in the U.S. for flecainide. See Flecainide.

Tasigna

"Tah-sig´-nuh." The trade name in the U.S. for nilotinib. See Nilotinib.

Telangiectasia macularis eruptiva perstans

"Teel-anj´-ee-ek-tā´-zha mak´-yoo-lar´-is ee-rup´-tiv-uh per´-stanz." Typically abbreviated as TMEP, this is a form of cutaneous mastocytosis producing a pattern of skin lesions somewhat different from urticaria pigmentosa (UP).

Tendinitis

"Ten´-din-īt´-is." Take any part of the body, tack "-itis" to the end, and you get a medical word for inflammation of that part of the body. Thus, tendinitis refers to inflammation of one or more tendons. While mast cell disease can cause tendinitis, various rheumatologic diseases can do this, too, and it can even be seen as an unusual side effect of certain medications (most notoriously, the fluoroquinolones such as ciprofloxacin (Cipro)).

Tetrahydrocannabinol

"Teh´-trah-hī´-droh-kan-ab´-in-ol," often abbreviated as THC. This is the primary active ingredient in marijuana. It binds with cannabinoid receptors on human cells to cause a wide variety of effects. The mast cell surface features (inhibitory) cannabinoid receptors, making me wonder whether at least some of the chronically ill patients out there who claim that the only thing that makes them feel better is marijuana might be unrecognized MCAS patients in whom THC's binding with the cannabinoid receptors on their dysfunctional mast cells leads to a quieting of the activity of those cells and thus a lessening of symptoms.

Therapeutic Phlebotomy

See Phlebotomy.

Thrombocytopenia

"Throm´-bo-sīt´-oh-peen´-ee-uh." This is the medical word for a low platelet count.

Thymoma

"Thy-mohm´-uh." This is the medical word for a tumor of the thymus gland, a small organ in the middle of the chest which is responsible for certain functions in the immune system.

Thyroid

"Thy´-roid." This is the gland, located in the front of the neck, responsible for producing thyroid hormone, which drives a lot of processes in the body. When thyroid hormone production is diminished (which can happen due to one or more of a multitude of processes), many things can go awry, starting with a sense of fatigue, generalized weakness, and feeling cold much of the time – all symptoms that can be seen in mast cell disease, too. No wonder, then, since most physicians receive a decent amount of training about thyroid disease and almost no training about mast cell disease that when they see a patient with these symptoms, they often suspect thyroid disease, and set about testing for such, but never suspect mast cell disease.

Tics

"Tiks" Abnormal brief isolated neurologic motor activities such as contractions of one muscle or another (for example, a tic in an eyelid muscle might make it appear as if the patient is winking at times for no reason). Tics are sometimes seen in patients with neurological effects from mast cell disease, but they can be effects of a vast array of other neurological abnormalities, too. I'm not aware of any tic behaviors which are specific for mast cell disease.

Tinnitus

"Tin´-ih-tus." A state of true abnormal hearing (i.e., not a hallucination) in which a particular sound is constantly heard for either a period of time (often recurrent) or indefinitely. The tinnitus sufferer – who can be hearing, hearing-impaired, or even deaf – often "hears" a high-pitched tone, but sometimes it is a "shushing white noise" or even a "jet engine roar." Tinnitus can be present in either or both ears, and the intensity of tinnitus can range from trivial to insanity-inducing. Tinnitus is a common complaint in those with mast cell activation disease, though the mechanism by which the symptom is produced, and the mechanism by which the disease causes the symptom, remain quite mysterious.

Tizanidine

"Tih-zan´-ih-deen." Known better by its most popular U.S. trade name Zanaflex, tizanidine is a muscle relaxant, and since many patients with mast cell disease complain of widespread soft tissue pain, and since excessive muscle tension can be painful, it's not surprising that many patients with mast cell disease get empirically tried on tizanidine (and/or other muscle relaxants) at some point in their typically very long course before they finally get accurately diagnosed with mast cell disease.

TNF-alpha

"T-N-F alf´-uh." TNF-alpha is one of the body's major inflammatory mediators. It is produced by mast cells and many other types of inflammatory cells. Levels of TNF-alpha in the blood can sometimes be found to be elevated above normal in patients with MCAD as well as patients with many other inflammatory diseases.

Tonsillectomy

"Ton´-sil-ect´-uh-mee." Another group of lymph nodes at the back of the throat. See Adenoidectomy for more information.

Tramadol

"Tram´-ah-dol." Perhaps known more commonly by its U.S. trade name Ultram, tramadol (usually taken orally) helps to treat pain not only by binding to one of the body's opioid (narcotic) receptors but also by inhibiting reuptake of key signaling molecules serotonin and norepinephrine. It seems to be a relatively safe pain-reliever for MCAD patients to try, and especially in a disease in which both non-steroidal anti-inflammatory drugs and narcotics can often trigger symptomatic flares, it's a good drug for the mast-cell-treating physician to keep in his back pocket, so to speak.

Tranexamic acid

"Tran´-ex-am´-ik as´-id." A fibrinolytic inhibitor medication. See Fibrinolysis and Aminocaproic acid.

Transaminitis

> "Trans-am´-in-īt´-is." This is a bit of a slang term, referring to elevation(s) in the enzyme aspartate aminotransferase (AST) and/or the enzyme alanine aminotransferase (ALT). Most doctors reflexively think that elevations in AST and/or ALT necessarily stem from inflammation in the liver (hepatitis), but AST and ALT are present in a many other tissues besides the liver. For example, elevations in AST and/or ALT can be seen in inflammation of muscle tissue and in the abnormal breakdown of red blood cells known as hemolysis.

Transfusion

> "Trans-fyoo´-zhun." Transfusion is the transfer of blood, or a component of blood (such as red blood cells, platelets, or plasma) from one person to another. Transfusions often are lifesaving treatments, but on occasion they can cause various, and sometimes very severe or even fatal, illnesses.

Transient ischemic accident

> Transient "is-keem´-ik" accident. More commonly referred to by its "TIA" initials, this is a medical event in which there is transient blockage of a blood vessel. Even though the term technically applies to transient blockage of *any* blood vessel, in practice it is applied only to transient blockage of large or small blood vessels in the head supplying blood to the brain. A TIA thus clinically appears similar to a stroke except that because the blockage is only transient in a TIA, most or all of the symptoms from a TIA usually resolve pretty quickly and without specific treatment, whereas the symptoms from a stroke often resolve little or even not at all.

Triamterene/hydrochlorothiazide

> "Trī-am-ter-een hī-droh-klor-oh-thī-uh-zīd." A combination of two different, relatively weak diuretic (urination-inducing) medications. In some patients it is helpful in controlling hypertension. Its most common trade name in the U.S. is Maxzide.

Tricyclic antidepressant

> "Trī-sik´-lik an´-tī-dee-pres´-ent," sometimes referred to simply as a "tricyclic." The tricyclic antidepressants are a class of medications (one commonly used example being amitriptyline)

that have been used for decades to treat depression and other ailments (such as insomnia). One of the reasons why they can bring the benefits they do is that they chemically function as sedating histamine H_1 receptor blockers, among other effects.

Triglyceride

"Trī-glis´-er-īd." Triglyceride is a type of lipid, or fat carrier, that helps transport fat and sugar from liver to fat tissue and vice versa. Elevated lipids in the blood (i.e., hyperlipidemia) are an extremely common problem whose most widely recognized adverse consequence is build-up of potentially obstructing atherosclerotic plaque in arteries. Now, I'm certainly not saying that all, or even most, cases of hyperlipidemia are due to mast cell disease, but for reasons I don't yet understand, I have seen some mast cell disease patients who present with elevated levels (sometimes extremely so) of one type of lipid or another, and then once the patient's mast cell disease was diagnosed and effective therapy was found (therapy other than traditional lipid-lowering therapy, to be sure), the hyperlipidemia mostly or completely resolved. Clearly, then, in at least some mast cell disease patients, either the disease has the ability to directly or indirectly drive hyperlipidemia and/or some other process which is independent of the mast cell disease and which is driving the hyperlipidemia coincidentally turns out to be responsive to the same drug that's able to control the mast cell disease. And since I have learned well that it is always unwise to bet against Occam, I will bet that it is the mast cell disease in those patients that is driving their lipid elevations. It will be an interesting research project for the future to clearly define what percentage of hyperlipidemia patients bear mast cell disease and how much better those hyperlipidemias can get when such mast cell disease is treated. It also is interesting to note that the most commonly used class of lipid-lowering medications, the "statins," seem to fairly consistently reduce total body inflammation, raising many questions vis-à-vis mast cells such as, "As part of their inflammation-reducing effect, do statins inhibit mast cell activation? If so, is such inhibition accomplished by direct interaction of the drug with the cell, or by indirect interaction, or both? How much of a statin's ability to lower blood lipid levels is due to the drug's interaction with fat cells (adipocytes) vs. interaction with mast cells?" etc. etc. etc.

Tryptase

"Trip´-tās." Among all of the many mast cell mediators
discovered thus far, tryptase is pretty unique in that, as far as
anybody has found thus far, it seems to be produced only by the
mast cell and no other types of cells. Although initially (i.e.,
when discovered in the 1980s, by Dr. Lawrence Schwartz at
Virginia Commonwealth University) the level of tryptase in the
bloodstream (i.e., the "serum tryptase") was thought to primarily
reflect the total (summative) state of activation of the body's mast
cells, in the last decade a new perspective has resulted from
ongoing research and now it is thought that the serum tryptase
level far dominantly reflects simply the total number of mast cells
in the body and far less the summative activation state of the
body's mast cells. Curiously, despite a few decades of research
now, the primary purpose of tryptase in the biological functioning
of the human body remains unclear.

Tylenol

"Tī´-len-ol." The most popular brand name in the U.S. for
acetaminophen (see Acetaminophen).

Tyrosine kinase inhibitors

"Tī-roh-seen kī-nās" inhibitors. The tyrosine kinase inhibitors
(TKIs) are a class of generally extremely expensive medications
(more than $100,000 per year, at least in the U.S.) that inhibit
proteins, called tyrosine kinases, which control a wide range of
functions in various cells including cell growth (i.e.,
reproduction) and activation. TKIs typically are oral drugs. The
prototypical TKI is imatinib (see Imatinib), originally developed
to control chronic myeloid leukemia (and wildly successful at
doing so, the rare "grand slam home run" in cancer therapy) but
soon found to also be helpful in certain (but clearly not all)
patients with mast cell diseases of various types as well as some
other diseases, too. Imatinib is considered the primary example
of "first-generation" TKIs. The "second-generation" TKIs,
helpful in some patients whose disease has escaped control of
first-generation TKIs, include dasatinib, nilotinib, sunitinib, and
others. Now there are "third-generation" TKIs such as bosutinib
and ponatinib, and fourth-generation TKIs are in development as
well. Generic versions of imatinib are expected to begin hitting
the market in 2015, and they likely will be less expensive than the
original manufacturer's imatinib, but how much less expensive is
anyone's guess at this point. (The manufacturers of the TKIs

have certainly been pilloried in the academic and popular press for what they charge for these drugs, and some countries (e.g., India) have actually forced severe price controls on these manufacturers.)

U

Upper respiratory infection

Standard English words there, no tricky pronunciation, but a mouthful nonetheless and thus often abbreviated in writing and speaking as URI. Obviously, this is an infection in the upper respiratory tract, i.e., the mouth, nose, sinuses, and/or throat, but not the lungs, which constitute the lower respiratory tract. A history of frequent upper respiratory "infections" is common in patients with mast cell disease, but the real question is how many of those alleged "infections" actually were just flares of sterile inflammation driven by mast cell disease. A true infection almost always generates fever. If a "URI" isn't accompanied by fever and is attributed to a "virus" (and with no positive viral testing to prove such a guess), one has to wonder – especially in a patient shown to have MCAS – whether such an "infection" might actually have just been a flare of MCAS in the upper respiratory tract.

Urethra

"Yur-eeth-rah," adjective form "urethral." This is a part of human anatomy, the tube through which urine flows from the bladder to the outside world. The urethra, just like any other part of the body, can get inflamed due to a wide variety of infections, but it also can get inflamed for non-infectious reasons, and I'll bet you're already thinking of one possible such non-infectious reason (yes, MCAS). Either way, infection or not, inflammation is inflammation and an inflamed urethra is going to make for painful urination. Of course, doctors are trained to almost reflexively associate painful urination with infection (since they receive virtually no training about non-infectious causes of urethral inflammation and they of course almost certainly receive no training about MCAS), so it is very common for patients who are ultimately shown to have MCAS to report a history of frequent urinary tract "infections" in which, quite oddly, the urinalysis and urine culture failed to show any signs of the infection that was expected based on the symptom of painful urination (a.k.a. dysuria). Also of course, such patients go through many courses of antibiotics for such "UTIs," and because such non-infectious inflammation of the urethra is not going to respond particularly well to an antibiotic, these are the patient who puzzle their primary care doctors and urologists with regard to how curiously resistant their "infections" are, and how long the courses of antibiotics need to be to get rid of such "infections," and how many different courses of antibiotics are needed to get rid of such "infections," and how quickly such "infections" are to relapse. Be careful, though: mast cell disease does often create an increased susceptibility to infection, so anytime a patient – even a proven MCAS patient – presents with dysuria, infection needs to be ruled out, because if the patient actually does have an infection and an appropriate antibiotic is not provided, the infection can become a much more serious (even life-threatening) problem.

URI

See Upper respiratory tract infection.

Urinalysis

"Yur´-in-al´-ih-sis," plural urinalyses (pronounced "yur´-in-al´-ih-seez"). A very common lab test in which the patient's urine is analyzed for a wide range of parameters including its degree of acidity and the presence of red and white blood cells, glucose, protein, bacteria, bilirubin, etc. Many diseases affect the urine, and thus results from the urinalysis can be instructive in the diagnostic process. There is no one specific way in which mast cell disease affects the urine; many different alterations in the urine are possible in different variants of mast cell disease, and actually it's not the mast cell disease itself that directly causes such changes in the urine but rather other disease processes induced by the mast cell disease that lead to changes in the urine. As such, a routine urinalysis per se is not a routine process for diagnosing mast cell disease – though, to be sure, analyzing the urine for various mast cell mediators (e.g., histamine, N-methylhistamine, prostaglandin D_2, and 9,11-β-prostaglandin-$F_{2\alpha}$) is a routine part of diagnostically assessing a patient for mast cell disease.

Urinary tract infection

Standard English words there, no tricky pronunciation. Although a "UTI" technically refers to an infection anywhere along the urinary tract, in practice an infection of the ureter, bladder, and/or urethra is called a UTI, while infection of the kidney itself is called pyelonephritis ("pī´-el-oh-nef-rīt´-is"). UTIs are commonly seen in mast cell disease because mast cell disease, through its effects on the immune system, increase the risk for infection of all types. See the entry for Urethra above for further comments on aspects of UTIs vis-à-vis mast cell disease.

Uroporphyrin

"Yur´-oh-por´-fir-in." Uroporphyrin is a molecule that basically is one of the intermediate stages on the path toward building a hemoglobin molecule. In some of the "porphyria" diseases (see the entry in this dictionary for Porphyria), there is a build-up of uroporphyrin that can be detected in laboratory testing.

Urosepsis

"Yur´-oh-seps´-is." This medical word refers to severe, life-threatening infection of the urinary tract.

Urticaria

"Ur´-tih-kār´-ee-uh." This is the medical word for hives, a skin rash of pale red, raised, itchy bumps.

Urticaria pigmentosa

"Ur´-tih-kār´-ee-uh pig´-men-tōs´-uh." This is a form of cutaneous mastocytosis in which there is darker (typically brownish) coloring of hives, or urticaria.

Uterine prolapse

"Yoo´-ter-in pro´-laps." See Prolapse.

UTI

See Urinary tract infection.

V

Valine

"Vāl´-een." One of the 20 "amino acid" building blocks used to build human proteins. Among its many, many other uses in human proteins, valine is the amino acid that should be normally found at position 617 in the normal human JAK2 protein. In the disease polycythemia vera, a mutation of the DNA making up the JAK2 gene (which guides a cell's protein-assembling machinery to make the JAK2 protein) usually causes the mistaken use of the amino acid phenylalanine in place of the correct amino acid valine at position 617 in the unique sequence of amino acids that defines the JAK2 protein.

Vanillylmandelic acid

"Vah'-nil-il-man-del'-ik" acid. A real mouthful that's usually abbreviated as VMA, vanillylmandelic acid is an end-stage metabolite of the catecholamines epinephrine and norepinephrine. The level of VMA is typically tested when pheochromocytoma (whose flares can often make the patient look as he might look with mast cell disease) is suspected. Therefore, it is not all that uncommon to find that VMA has been tested (and, of course, usually found to be normal or only minimally abnormal) in a patient who ultimately is found to have a mast cell activation disease of one form or another.

Vasoactive intestinal peptide

"Vā'-soh-act'-iv in-test'-in-al pep'-tīd," often abbreviated VIP. This interesting mediator is released by various intestinal cells that can become cancerous (a "VIPoma"), sometimes leading to overproduction of VIP that can produce abdominal pain and chronic diarrhea, and thus you can see how a patient who is ultimately found to have mast cell disease might at some point in his work-up come to be suspected of possibly having a VIPoma (one of the rare "neuroendocrine" cancers that may overproduce chromogranin A, too) and thus might have a VIP level checked.

Vaso-occlusion

"Vā'-soh-oh-kloo'-zhun." Simply put, blockage of a blood vessel from potentially any cause. Vaso-occlusion most common occurs because of (abnormal) blood clots, because of atherosclerotic plaque build-up in arteries, and because of sickle red blood cells in sickle cell anemia.

Venlafaxine

"Ven'-lah-faks'-een." More commonly known by its most popular U.S. trade name Effexor, venlafaxine is an "atypical anti-depressant" that is used for a wide variety of purposes beyond just depression. For example, it's often used to help suppress menopausal hot flashes, and since patients with mast cell disease often suffer spontaneous sweats, it's not all that unusual to find the venlafaxine has been empirically tried at some point in the mast cell disease patient's history (before the mast cell disease was diagnosed and effectively controlled with mast-cell-directed therapy, which usually then takes care of the sweats).

Ventricular ectopy

"Ven-trik´-yoo-lar ek´-toh-pee." This is the medical word referring to extra, but typically benign, beats of the heart's left and/or right ventricle. Ventricular ectopy sometimes is what underlies the sense of palpitations which mast cell disease patients often report intermittently experiencing.

Ventolin

"Ven´-toh-lin." The most common trade name in the U.S. for albuterol. See Albuterol.

Ventricular tachycardia

"Ven-trik´-yoo-lar tak´-ee-card´-ee-uh." This is an acutely life-threatening type of abnormal heart rhythm. If ventricular tachycardia is not promptly recognized and corrected, the patient suffering this abnormal rhythm likely will die within minutes.

VIP

See Vasoactive intestinal peptide.

VIPoma

Sometimes pronounced "vip-ohm-uh," and sometimes pronounced "V-I-P-ohm-uh." This is a tumor of intestinal cells that produce vasoactive intestinal peptide. Again, see Vasoactive intestinal peptide.

Vistaril

"Vist´-er-il." One of the most common trade names for hydroxyzine in the U.S. See Hydroxyzine.

VKORC1

Usually pronounced "vee-kork-1." This is a drug-processing enzyme which, together with CYP2C9 (see this dictionary's entry

446

for CYP2C9), is responsible for the majority of the metabolism of the very commonly used anticoagulant drug warfarin. Mutations in VKORC1 can increase or decrease (more commonly decrease) the metabolism of warfarin, and of course a decrease in warfarin metabolism would lead to a build-up of the drug and thus more anticoagulant effect than desired/expected for a given dose, and that could lead to serious bleeding complications. Anytime the blood gets thinner (as measured by a rise in the prothrombin time (PT) and related international normalized ratio (INR) tests) than expected for a given dose of warfarin, the possibility that there might be mutations in CYP2C9 and VKORC1 needs to be considered. There is blood testing routinely available now which can detect such mutations.

VMA

See Vanillylmandelic acid.

W

Waldenstrom's macroglobulinemia

"Wal´-den-stromz mak´-roh-glob´-yoo-lin-eem´-ee-uh." This is a relatively unusual type of blood cell cancer in which malignant plasma cells are substantially overproducing an IgM type of antibody, and since IgM is a pretty big protein, you get a build-up of so much protein in the blood that the blood starts becoming more viscous (i.e., "sludging"), and when the blood doesn't flow normally like a fluid, a whole variety of troubles can develop pretty fast. Waldenstrom's patients sometimes also see some enlargement of their spleens.

Warfarin

"War´-fer-in." Often called by its most popular U.S. trade name Coumadin ("Koo´-muh-din") even when the brand the patient is taking isn't really Coumadin, warfarin is one of the oldest blood thinners, or anticoagulants, there is. Although it's pretty cheap and, when properly managed, can be very helpful in treating and preventing abnormal blood clotting, it is a challenging drug to manage properly, with a tendency to lead to major changes in the degree of blood clotting it's causing depending on many different factors including interactions with a very large number of other drugs, so the amount of blood thinning one is getting from it has to be monitored by checking a particular blood test (the "INR," or international normalized ratio, a number that gets calculated from the actual "prothrombin time" (PT) blood test) relatively frequently.

Wegener's granulomatosis

"Weg´-eh-nerz gran´-yoo-lohm´-uh-tōs´-is." Wegener's is an autoimmune disease in which the immune system erroneously generates a particular antibody (called an anti-neutrophil-cytoplasmic antibody, or ANCA ("ank´-uh")) targeting certain elements of the lungs and kidneys, principally, and sometimes also the joints, skin, and nervous system. It can be fatal, but most patients who get this these days manage to survive because of relatively good treatment consisting of suppression of an immune system gone berserk.

X

Xanax

"Zan-ax." The most common trade name in the U.S. for alprazolam. See Alprazolam.

Xgeva

"Eks-jee´-vuh." Along with Prolia, Xgeva is one of the two trade names for denosumab in the U.S. See Denosumab.

Y

Yes…

…we have no bananas. No, that makes no sense and has nothing to do with mast cell disease, but it sure seemed like we needed *something* in the Y's. But, oh, wait a second, I think I just thought of what might actually be a legitimate Y entry (see the next entry).

You…

…likely know somebody who has MCAS. Yes (hey, there's a legitimate use of a Y word relevant to mast cell disease), MCAS is suspected (at least by some specialists) to really be so prevalent that the average person likely knows somebody else who has it, regardless of whether either of them realizes it. In fact, after reading this book, I'll bet you can recognize the diagnostic possibility in your acquaintances better than their own doctors can. And, You can do something about MCAS. You can do something about it if you have it (or at least suspect you have it) (see the chapters on diagnosing and treating MCAS), and You can do something about it if somebody You care about has it or is likely to have it (see the final chapter, "What's Next?").

Z

Zafirlukast

"Zaf´-ir-lū´-kast." Probably known more widely by its U.S. trade name Accolate ("Ak-oh-lāt"), this is a "second generation" version of montelukast and thus is a leukotriene receptor blocker.

Zetia

"Zet´-ee-uh." The most common trade name in the U.S. for ezetimibe. See Ezetimibe.

Zithromax

"Zith´-roh-max." The most common trade name in the U.S. for azithromycin. See Azithromycin.

Zocor

"Zoh´-kor." The most common trade name in the U.S. for simvastatin. See Simvastatin.

Zoledronate

"Zōl-eh´-drōn-āt." Known more widely by its predominant U.S. trade name Zometa, zoledronate is probably the most popular injectable bisphosphonate ("bis-fos´-foh-nāt") medication because it can be given in just a few minutes compared to 2-4 hours for its older sister drug pamidronate (trade name Aredia). Since the bisphosphonate drugs help retard progression of the bone weakening called osteopenia or osteoporosis, and since osteopenia and osteoporosis are common consequences of mast cell disease, use of bisphosphonate drugs is common in managing mast cell disease. Some mast cell disease patients have trouble tolerating the bisphosphonates, though, and a new class of bone-strengthening drugs called the anti-RANKL antibodies that accomplishes the same end effect through a different mechanism is now starting to show up, beginning with denosumab (trade names Prolia and Xgeva). I haven't seen any mast cell disease patients prove intolerant to denosumab yet, but that's just my anecdotal experience.

Zolpidem

"Zol-pih´-dem." Far better known by its most popular U.S. trade name Ambien, zolpidem is a sleep inducer in the class of imidazopyridine drugs, and even though the general chemical structure of this class of drugs is different from the benzodiazepines, the imidazopyridines nevertheless bind to benzodiazepine receptors, which means part of the effectiveness of zolpidem might be due to a calming effect on mast cells as much its calming effect on neurons.

Zometa

"Zō-meh´-tuh." The most common trade name for zoledronate. See Zoledronate.

Appendix 2: Diagnostic Criteria for Mastocytosis and Mast Cell Activation Syndrome

---

WHO 2008 Diagnostic Criteria for Systemic Mastocytosis

Major Criterion:
1. Multifocal, dense aggregates of MCs (15 or more) in sections of bone marrow or other extracutaneous tissues and confirmed by tryptase immunohistochemistry or other special stains

Minor Criteria:
1. Atypical or spindled appearance of at least 25% of the MCs in the diagnostic biopsy
2. Expression of CD2 and/or CD25 by MCs in marrow, blood, or extracutaneous organs
3. KIT codon 816 mutation in marrow, blood, or extracutaneous organs
4. Persistent elevation of serum total tryptase > 20 ng/ml

Diagnosis of SM made by either (1) major criterion + any one or more minor criteria, or (2) any three minor criteria.

Proposed Diagnostic Criteria for Mast Cell Activation Syndrome

Valent et al. Criteria
(per *International Archives of Allergy and Immunology* 2012)

1. Chronic/recurrent symptoms (specifically: flushing, pruritus, urticaria, angioedema, nasal congestion or pruritus, wheezing, throat swelling, headache, hypotension, and/or diarrhea) consistent with aberrant MC mediator release
2. Absence of any other known disorder that can better account for these symptoms
3. Increase in serum total tryptase of [20% above baseline, plus another 2 ng/ml] during, or within 4 hours after, a symptomatic period
4. Response of symptoms to histamine H_1 and/or H_2 receptor antagonists or other "MC-targeting" agents such as cromolyn.

Molderings et al. Criteria
(per *Journal of Hematology and Oncology* 2011)

Major Criteria:
1. Multifocal MC aggregates as per WHO major criterion for SM
2. Clinical history consistent with chronic/recurrent aberrant MC mediator release (symptoms per Table 3, Molderings et al., *Journal of Hematology and Oncology* 2011)

Minor Criteria:
1. Abnormal MC morphology as per WHO SM minor criterion #1
2. CD2 and/or CD25 expression as per WHO SM minor criterion #2
3. Detection of known constitutively activating mutations in MCs in blood, marrow, or extracutaneous organs
4. Elevation in serum tryptase or chromogranin A, plasma heparin or histamine, urinary N-methylhistamine, and/or other MC-specific mediators such as (but not limited to) relevant leukotrienes (B4, C4, D4, E4) or PGD_2 or its metabolite 11-β-$PGF_{2\alpha}$.

Diagnosis of MCAS made by either (1) both major criteria, or (2) the second major criterion plus any one of the minor criteria, or (3) any three minor criteria.

Appendix 3: Idiopathic Diseases, Syndromes, and Symptoms Which Since 2009 I've Come to Wonder Might Be (In At Least Some Cases) Assorted Variants of, or At Least Indirectly Due To, Mast Cell Activation Syndrome

Given how mast cell disease has the potential to impact every system in the body in a myriad different ways, and given its common clinical presentation with multisystem inflammation and odd reactivities, I think I can be excused for wondering whether the following diseases *might* be assorted variants of MCAS. Ultimately, though, it of course will require a formal research project with a group of patients with each of these disease, testing them very carefully to see if they do indeed have MCAS and then trying to establish some connection as to *how* MCAS seems to cause these diseases, before we will be able to say confidently that MCAS indeed is the root cause of these diseases.

Acute lymphoid leukemia
Acute myeloid leukemia
Adenomyosis
Allergic rhinitis
Anemia of chronic inflammation
Anti-phospholipid antibody syndrome
Aplastic anemia
Asthma
Attention-deficit and attention-deficit/hyperactivity disorders
Atypical angina
Atypical nephrolithiasis
Autism spectrum disorders
Benign ethnic leukopenia
Bipolar affective disorder
Blurry vision (episodic)
Budd-Chiari syndrome
Burning mouth syndrome
Burning scalp syndrome
Cataplexy
Chronic constipation (idiopathic)
Chronic cough (idiopathic)
Chronic diarrhea (idiopathic)
Chronic dyspepsia (idiopathic)
Chronic fatigue syndrome
Chronic inflammatory demyelinating polyneuropathy
Chronic low back pain (idiopathic)
Chronic lymphoid leukemia
Chronic myeloid leukemia
Chronic nausea (idiopathic)
Chronic rhabdomyolysis

Colon cancer
Combined variable immunodeficiency
Complex regional pain syndrome (CRPS)
Congestive heart failure
Conversion disorder
Coronary and peripheral artery disease
Cronkhite Canada syndrome
Delayed-type hypersensitivity drug reaction
Depression
Dercum's disease
Diabetes insipidus and mellitus (types 1 and 2)
Difficult/complicated sickle cell anemia
Diverticulitis
Dysautonomia
Dystonia
Ehlers-Danlos syndrome Type III
Endometriosis
Epilepsy/pseudoepilepsy
Erectile dysfunction
Essential hypertension
Essential tremor
Fibromyalgia
Fibrous histiocytoma
Focal segmental glomerular sclerosis
Functional abdominal pain
GastroEsophageal Reflux Disease (GERD)
Gastroparesis
Gilbert's syndrome
Gout (some forms)
Granuloma annulare
Hemophagocytic syndrome/hemophagocytic lymphohistiocytosis
Heparin-induced thrombocytopenia
Hidradenitis suppurativa
Histiocytosis X and Erdheim-Chester syndrome
Hodgkin's lymphoma
Human seminal protein allergy (HSPA)
Hyperemesis gravidarum
Hypersensitivity vasculitis
Hypertriglyceridemia (some cases)
Idiopathic adenopathy
Idiopathic bradycardia
Idiopathic conjunctivitis
Idiopathic delayed puberty
Idiopathic edema
Idiopathic elevated erythrocyte sedimentation rate or C-reactive protein
Idiopathic glomerulonephritis

Idiopathic hemochromatosis

Idiopathic hemorrhagic or embolic stroke or transient ischemic accident

Idiopathic hypercoagulability

Idiopathic hypereosinophilic syndrome

Idiopathic hypokalemia

Idiopathic hypomagnesemia

Idiopathic hypotension

Idiopathic hypothyroidism

Idiopathic immunodeficiency

Idiopathic nonspecific autoimmunity

Idiopathic/"neurogenic"/"pathogenic" pain

Idiopathic pancreatitis

Idiopathic paresthesias

Idiopathic pruritus

Idiopathic pulmonary fibrosis

Idiopathic splenomegaly

Idiopathic tachycardia

Idiopathic transaminitis

Idiopathic weight gain

Idiopathic weight loss

Inflammatory bowel disease

Interstitial cystitis

Irritable bowel syndrome

Kidney failure

Lactose intolerance

Leukocytosis (idiopathic)

Leukopenia (idiopathic and "benign ethnic")

Lobular carcinoma in situ

Lupus

Macrophage activation syndrome

Medullary thyroid cancer

Merkel cell carcinoma

Micronutrient malabsorption

Migraine headaches

Miscarriage

Mixed connective tissue disease

Monoclonal gammopathy of undetermined significance

Morgellons disease

Multiple chemical sensitivity syndrome

Multiple sclerosis

Myasthenia gravis

Myelodysplastic syndrome (especially cases of normal-cytogenetics MDS)

Myelofibrosis

Myeloma

Narcolepsy (idiopathic)

Night chills (idiopathic)

Night sweats (idiopathic)
Nocturnal leg cramps (idiopathic)
Non-Hodgkin's lymphoma
Nonspecific arthritis
Nonspecific myalgias
Nonspecific vasculitis
Obesity
Obstructive sleep apnea (especially in non-morbidly-obese patients)
Panic disorder
Periodic hypokalemia
Periodic paralysis
Polycystic kidney disease
Polycythemia (without JAK2 mutation)
Polymyalgia rheumatica
Post-traumatic stress disorder
Postural orthostatic tachycardia syndrome (POTS)
Pre-eclampsia/eclampsia
Prostate cancer
Pseudoxanthoma elasticum
Pure red cell aplasia not due to parvovirus B-19 infection
Refractory dizziness
Relapsing polychondritis
Reflex sympathetic dystrophy (RSD)
Restless leg syndrome
Rheumatoid arthritis
Sarcoidosis
Schizophrenia
Scleroderma
Senile purpura
Sensory processing disorder (e.g., hyperacusis)
Severe postprandial fatigue
Sickle cell anemia patients (and, especially, patients with variants of sickle cell anemia) which behave much worse than expected and/or in ways difficult to attribute to sickling
Sickle nephropathy
Sickle pulmonary hypertension
Sjögren's disease
Somatism/psychosomatism
Stromal tumor of uncertain malignant potential
Substance abuse (IMPORTANT: Note I said in the title to this section, "Some Cases")
Tachy-brady syndrome and perhaps some cases of other cardiac dysrhythmias
Temporomandibular joint (TMJ) syndrome
Thrombocytopenia (idiopathic/immune)
Thrombocytosis (idiopathic and essential)
Tics (idiopathic)

Tn polyagglutination syndrome
Unchelatable sickle transfusional hemosiderosis
Unspecified connective tissue disease
Unspecified porphyria
Unspecified sideroblastic anemia
Uveitis
Waldenstrom's macroglobulinemia

Author Bio

Dr. Afrin earned a B.S. in computer science at Clemson University in 1984 and then an M.D. at the Medical University of South Carolina (MUSC) in 1988, where he also pursued internal medicine residency and hematology/oncology clinical and research fellowships. While on faculty at MUSC from 1995-2014, he was active in undergraduate and graduate medical education, educational and information technology administration, and practice and research in hematology/oncology and medical informatics. Since the mid-'00s, his clinical work has increasingly focused in hematology, especially mast cell disease.

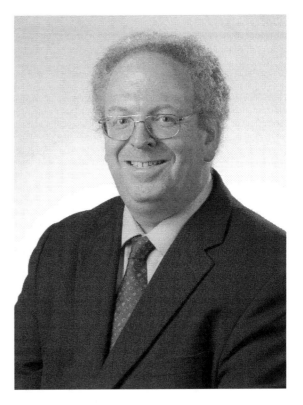

In 2008 Dr. Afrin started coming to understand that a newly recognized type of mast cell disease, now called mast cell activation syndrome (MCAS), was the underlying diagnosis in many patients he was seeing who were each suffering large assortments — quite different from one patient to the next — of chronic multisystem inflammatory illnesses of unclear cause. Dr. Afrin soon gained experience that MCAS is far more prevalent than the only mast cell disease previously known to medicine (the rare disease of mastocytosis) and that most MCAS patients, once accurately diagnosed, can eventually find significantly helpful medications targeted at the disease. The frequency and magnitude of the improvements Dr. Afrin has seen — even the relief that comes from finally having a unifying diagnosis other than "psychosomatism" — have spurred him to focus in this area, not only tending to the needs of his patients but also pursuing research to advance our understanding of the disease and helping to educate other professionals who in turn can help even more of the many people who have long been suffering not only the symptoms of the disease but also the natural concern of not understanding why one would be so "unlucky" to have acquired so many medical problems. As it turns out, such patients are not so unlucky and truly have just one root issue (and a very common one at that) which has the biological capability to develop, directly or indirectly, into most or all their previously diagnosed problems.

There is a great deal yet to learn about this, but even with just the present very limited understanding, the opportunity to diagnose and help patients with MCAS seems to be enormous and Dr. Afrin felt a description of the disease, written for the general public, might help lead some MCAS patients on a journey to diagnosis and improvement sooner rather than later. He joined the University of Minnesota in 2014 to further his interests in this area. He has an extensive record of peer-reviewed publications and has spoken widely in his areas of interest.

Dr. Afrin hopes this book will help people who might have, or do have, MCAS. A portion of the proceeds of purchases of this book will go to support research and education in this area.

If you have questions pertaining to Dr. Afrin's book, or would like more information, please email info@mastcellresearch.com.

You can also visit www.mastcellresearch.com.

Or, find us on Facebook @facebook.com/mastcellresearch/, and Twitter @MastCellHelp.

Made in the USA
Middletown, DE
06 November 2020